Human Reproduction and Society

by the same author

FUNDAMENTALS OF OBSTETRICS AND GYNAECOLOGY
Volume I Obstetrics
Volume II Gynaecology

EVERYWOMAN
A Gynaecological Guide for Life

PEOPLE POPULATING

Human Reproduction and Society

DEREK LLEWELLYN-JONES

OBE MD MAO FRCOG

Associate Professor of Obstetrics & Gynaecology
University of Sydney, New South Wales
Australia

Honorary Obstetrician & Gynaecologist at
the Women's Hospital (Crown Street)
Sydney

Lately, Senior Obstetrician & Gynaecologist
Maternity Hospital, Kuala Lumpur
Malaysia

FABER AND FABER
3 Queen Square
London

First published in 1974
by Faber and Faber Limited
3 Queen Square London WC1
Printed in Great Britain by
Butler and Tanner Ltd, Frome

ISBN 0 571 10358 8

Preface

The exponential growth rate of human population, together with ecologically faulty productive technology, poses a major threat to mankind's survival in the next half century. The rapidly increasing population growth rate has resulted from the technological advances in sanitary engineering and medicine which have occurred since 1940. These have had the effect of prolonging the life of adults, but more important, of enabling an increasing number of infants and children to escape the dangers of infectious disease. The consequence has been that an increasing number of children reach puberty, and being human, marry and reproduce. The changes in human population, usually its growth, are termed population dynamics.

In the past six years I have been fortunate enough to be asked to join World Health Organization teams which have been charged with investigating the teaching of human reproduction, population dynamics and family planning in medical schools, so that the help needed could be assessed. In 1969 I visited India, in 1970 Thailand and in 1971 Indonesia. The courtesy with which we were received, and the hospitality given to us was heart-warming, as was the dedication of the majority of medical educators.

But the visits did disclose that, by and large, efforts to interest students of medicine in these important matters were making a slow impact. In part, this was because of a lack of suitable written material; in part, it was because the introduction of a new subject meant that it had to compete for time, in an overcrowded curriculum, with other subjects, some of which were more suitable for the curriculum of a European medical school, four decades ago.

The enthusiasm of many medical educators, and the needs of the community, made me increasingly aware that attitudes towards the delivery of health care required drastic revision. The 'god-doctor' of the past must be replaced by the health team, in which the doctor is only one—if a most important—member.

With this experience, on my return to Australia from Indonesia in April, 1971, I determined to write a book on the demographic and social problems of human reproduction. The readers I had in mind were students of medicine and the other members of the health team, the nurses, social workers, physiotherapists, health visitors and occupational therapists; but I also believe that the book should be of interest, and I hope value, to the intelligent general reader. The more people there are today who are informed on the vital matters of population growth, its causes and its control, the greater is our chance of overcoming the challenge posed by exponential population growth.

The preparation of the manuscript involved me in a considerable amount of travel, and in discussions with a variety of people. I must give particular gratitude to Professor J. C. Caldwell, and Dr. L. Ruzicka of the Department of Demography at the Australian National University who gave me help and encouragement in the section of the book dealing with demography. I must also acknowledge the courtesy with which I was received at the Bureau of Census and Statistics, Commonwealth of Australia, and especially the help given me by Mr. R. Watson who showed me how the 1971 census was organized. Mr. Michael Giles, and other officials in the Bureau, kindly read the manuscript and made helpful comments. I am grateful to them. My visit to Mauritius would not have been as valuable as it was had it not been for Mr. R. K. Nair and his colleagues in the Mauritius Family Planning Association.

Miss Pamela Roberts and her colleagues in the Social Work Department of The Women's Hospital were, as usual, most helpful, and our discussions on the social problems associated with abortion and with unwanted pregnancy did much to clarify my thoughts.

The dull, but necessary, work of obtaining books and journals for me was done by Miss Patricia Neill, Miss Sue Willis and Mrs. Robyn Matson of the Department of Obstetrics and Gynaecology, The University of Sydney. The typing, and retyping, was done by my secretaries, Miss Irene Kowalski initially, and latterly Mrs. Shirley Pitfield. Mrs. Pitfield typed the final draft and helped me in many ways. I am most grateful to her. Jenny Robinson prepared the index.

PREFACE

The book has an extensive bibliography, but the references in the text are rather unusual. I believe that lists of names with dates in the text, or keyed numbers, tend to distract the reader from the flow of the narrative, and hinder clear reading. I have therefore placed only the senior author's name in parentheses, and have tried to select the most useful reference when they were multiple.

Finally, I must acknowledge the forbearance of my wife, for during much of the eighteen months it took to write *Human Reproduction and Society*, she has had to put up with journals, books, notes and papers scattered around the house, with strict instructions that none was to be moved.

In many nations, health workers are key people in promoting social change. In no area of society is change more urgently needed than in our attitudes to natality. In *Human Reproduction and Society* I have tried to set out the facts, to show how population is measured, how its growth may be controlled, and what social problems are found in human reproduction.

DEREK LLEWELLYN-JONES

Sydney,
Australia,
1973

Contents

PART ONE

Population Dynamics

Figures

Tables

TABLES

TABLES

PART 1
Population Dynamics

A French riddle for children illustrates another aspect of exponential growth—the apparent suddenness with which it approaches a fixed limit. Suppose you own a pond on which a water lily is growing. The lily plant doubles in size each day. If the lily were allowed to grow unchecked, it would completely cover the pond in 30 days, choking off the other forms of life in the water. For a long time the lily plant seems small, and so you decide not to worry about cutting it back until it covers half the pond. On what day will that be? On the twenty-ninth day, of course. You have one day to save your pond.

The Limits to Growth
MEADOWS, D. H., Potomac, 1972

The growth of world population during the next twenty-five years, therefore, has an importance which transcends economic and social considerations. It is at the very heart of the problem of our existence.

The Future Growth of World Population
United Nations Publication, 1958
(Population Studies Series No. 28)

ONE

The Problem of Growth

In this last quarter of the twentieth century, man, more than ever before, is experiencing an accelerating growth phenomenon in population and in the production of manufactured goods. Population is growing exponentially, so is production, so is consumption, so is waste and so is land occupancy. In no finite system—and planet Earth is finite—can this unlimited growth continue. Eventually the limits to growth are reached.

The limits to growth have been analysed recently by a team of scientists from the Massachusetts Institute of Technology, with the help of models and computers. These models were constructed to investigate 'the five major trends of global concern —accelerating industrialization, rapid population growth, widespread malnutrition, depletion of non-renewable resources, and a deteriorating environment' (Meadows). The scientists point out the trends are interconnected in many ways, and their exponential increase threatens our future. Population cannot grow without food. Food production is increased by growth of capital, which provides the needed inputs of water, fertilizer and new strains of seeds. Capital is produced by increasing industrialization, but this requires that more of the finite mineral resources of the world are used. These resources are converted into consumer goods and the profits provide the capital to replace outmoded equipment, to finance research and to provide capital for food production. The discarded resources, the waste of the products of manufacture and the residues of food production produce increasing pollution. Pollution interferes with the quality of life, with health, with the growth of population and the production of food. All have finite growth limits.

The M.I.T. scientists in their simulated computer analysis say, with some confidence, that 'under the assumption of no major change in the present system, population and industrial growth will certainly stop within the next century at the latest'. The transition from unlimited growth to rapid decline will lead to increasing crises, disasters and final collapse. They show that technological discoveries can delay the date of the collapse, but cannot prevent it. Some of the strategies available are discussed in Chapter 9 of this book, and in greater detail in Meadows' *The Limits to Growth*, which should be read.

The consensus is that to survive we must change our attitudes to reach a state of global population equilibrium, in which births and deaths are equal, and in which simultaneously industrial growth is reduced so that capital investment equals capital depreciation. This does not mean a dull, uniform society. Only population and capital need to be kept in equilibrium. Any human activity which does not use large quantities of non-renewable resources, or produce severe environmental pollution, can continue to grow. It means that technological advances to conserve, rather than to exploit, will be needed. It means that the stimulation of the spirit will largely replace the greed for goods. But it also means that there must be a more equal distribution of the available goods. This, in turn, implies that the gap between the rich and poor nations must be drastically reduced. The rich nations must get poorer so that the poor nations can become richer. The rich nations must eat less and consume fewer goods, so that the poor nations may have more.

The greatest hindrance to this is the rapid rate of population growth. Dedicated economists are currently concerned to procure, in the shortest possible time, a state of capital equilibrium. Human biologists seek to achieve a state of population equilibrium. That is what this book is about.

Exponential Population Growth

Demographers and human biologists have known for some years that the rate of growth of human population has speeded up, so that the time interval for population doubling has diminished progressively. This is exponential growth. The population is increasing by a constant percentage of the whole in a constant time period, like the water lily in the French riddle quoted earlier. We have reached the penultimate day.

In the year 1650, the population of the world was about 500

million. By 1850, 200 years later, it had doubled to 1,000 million. In the 75 years between 1850 and 1925, it had doubled again to 2,000 million. In the next 35 years, up to 1960, it had risen to 3,000 million, and in the next 15 years, by 1975, it is expected to reach 4,000 million. This means that it will have doubled in the 50 years between 1925 and 1975. By the year 2001 it is likely to be 6,000–7,000 million and by the year 2010 it could have doubled in only 35 years to reach 8,000 million (Figure **1/1**). This unprecedented growth rate, which the United Nations estimates to be about 2 per cent per annum, is unique in human history (Table **1/1**).

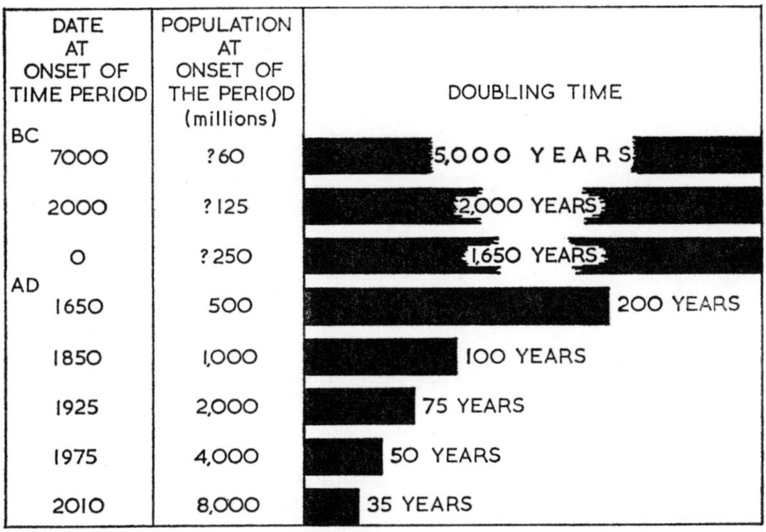

Figure **1/1** The progressive reduction of the time taken to double the population of the world since 7000 BC.

A growth rate of 2 per cent per annum may not appear to be serious until it is realized it is *exponential* and until the *scale* of the growth rate is considered. The population of the world in 1970 was 3,634 million. If the 2 per cent annual growth rate is applied, by mid-1971 the population had increased by 0·02 times 3,634 million, or 73 million people. This 73 million is added to the 3,634 million to give 3,707 million as a base, in calculating the mid-year population for 1972 and so on. Thus at later dates, the increase will be even larger, even if the rate of

Table 1/1

Estimates of world population to 2000 AD (in millions)

Year (Christian Era)	*World Total*	*Hungry developing nations*				*Affluent developed nations*				
		Total	*Asia*	*Latin America*	*Africa*	*Total*	*Europe & U.S.S.R.*	*North America*	*Oceaina*	*Japan*
2000E	6,494	5,115	3,645	652	818	1,372	871	333	35	133
1990E	5,438	4,168	3,052	500	616	1,289	835	299	30	125
1980E	4,457	3,299	2,465	377	457	1,169	768	261	24	116
1970	3,634	2,582	1,955	283	344	1,055	705	228	19	103
1960	2,986	2,040	1,557	213	270	947	639	199	16	93
1950	2,518	1,766	1,381	163	222	752	572	166	13	*
1900	1,650	1,145	930	65	150	506	423	81	2	*
1850	1,240	945	810	35	100	293	265	26	2	*
1800	960	750	630	20	100	208	200	6	2	*
1750E	750	592	480	12	100	153	150	1	2	*
1650E	545	439	327	12	100	106	103	1	2	*
1000E	360	290	230	6	50	70	70	—	—	*
0E	250	200	170	3	30	50	50	—	—	*

Source: *World Population Situation 1970* Table 15, U.N., 1971.
* = included in 'Asia'
E = Estimated

growth is held to 2 per cent; for example, in 1975, the world population is expected to be 4,000 million. The annual addition in that year will be 0·02 times 4,000 million, or 80 million people, so that in mid-1976, there will be 4,080 million people in the world. The consequences of a population increase of this magnitude threaten us all.

The current rate of population growth, which has resulted from the reduction of the death rate of infants, children and adolescents, without an equivalent reduction in the birth rate,

Table 1/2

Population doubling time for various annual rates of increase

Annual increase (per cent)	*Years needed to double a population*
0·1	600
0·2	300
0·5	140
1·0	70
1·5	47
2·0	35
2·5	29
3·0	24
3·5	21
4·0	17

The doubling time approximately equals 70 divided by the growth rate.

is the highest the world has known. One way of demonstrating the effects of this is to estimate the time it takes the population of a nation to double given a known annual population growth rate. An annual growth rate of 2 per cent means that the population of any nation will double in about 35 years, but that if this can be reduced to 0·8 per cent, it will take 100 years to double the population and give more time to solve the problems of population growth (Table **1/2**). Currently, mankind needs all the time we can obtain.

To the economist, the current rate of population growth poses a unique situation. This was succinctly summarized in 1972, in a

World Bank Sector Working Paper *Population Planning*. The report stated that 'There is no reason to believe that current rates of growth will fall fast enough to relieve the pressures on developing countries, arising from the need to use significant and rising proportions of their resources simply to maintain the average standard of living of growing numbers, leaving less for further improvement. . . . The decline of mortality in most developing countries has resulted in the survival of more adults, who would otherwise have had a shorter life span, and an increase in the number of surviving infants. The respective contributions of these two groups to the postwar population increase cannot be accurately calculated, but probably they are about equally significant. The economic impact of their survival is quite different, however, more adults living longer increase the potential labor force and create an immediate demand for jobs and supporting services. They also add to the numbers in the reproductive age group, with a potential impact upon fertility. More children surviving mean a rise in the dependency burden and, at a later stage, a further relative increase in the reproductive age groups. Thus while any fall in the infant mortality rate is to be welcomed on humanitarian grounds, it adds burdens to weak economies which can be lessened only by reducing fertility. To do so, and thus lessen the dependency burden, leads to large economic benefits. This is the heart of the economic case in favor of programs to limit fertility.' To the ecologist the needs of the 'growth' economists will mean increasing environmental pollution, increasing aggregation in urban areas, increasing congestion of roads, houses and lungs; and increasing threats of an ecological doomsday. To the demographer the consequences of this growth rate are that the children born today will themselves start having children in the next 15–25 years, and a multiplier effect on population will result. To the physician, the population growth imposes strains on the provision of preventive health care and of medical care. To the politician, population growth gives promise of dissent and turbulence as undernutrition, malnutrition, unemployment and underemployment increase, with potential revolutionary situations in many countries. To the affluent nations, the rate of population growth in the world offers a further threat. As will be seen, the rate of growth is not uniform throughout the nations. The developed countries have already reduced their growth rate considerably, but in the developing countries the growth rate is disproportionately high, so that the great burden of population growth falls on those nations least able, economically, to cope with the problem.

Two-thirds of the world's people live in the developing nations, and as their population increases exponentially, more and more do they threaten the current values of the developed nations. Possessions become threatened by people. Even the aid given by the affluent nations (as much to aid their exports and to damp down dissent in the developing regions, as to increase employment and productivity), is swallowed up in the quicksands of expanding populations, with little real effect on improving the lot of the majority of the people (Hayter). Food scientists, at huge expense, have developed new strains of wheat and rice—two of the three cereal staples of the world—which offer hope of avoiding increasing undernutrition. But the populations are increasing as rapidly as, or more rapidly than, harvest yields, so that little progress is being made to increase the calorie intake of the people. And more than calories are needed. The intake of the most important constituent of diet, protein, has also failed to increase. The situation is such that 'continued malnutrition mocks the basic aim of development and hinders its effective realisation. . . .', to quote the Director of the Food and Agriculture Organization, speaking in 1971.

At this time, environmental pollution is mainly a problem of the developed nations. In the industrial nations of the Atlantic seaboard and in Japan, the skies over the cities are becoming increasingly contaminated with industrial smog. Open land is being swallowed up to be covered with concrete to make highways on which cars can travel, discharging pollutants as they speed between new raw suburbs of brick and concrete. Rivers, and the ocean, are being increasingly polluted with the industrial effluent resulting from the manufacture of products which custom and advertising induce an acquisitive society to believe it needs. The need to possess more material goods dominates the need to live in harmony with the environment. Forests are cut down and minerals dug up to satisfy the insatiable demand for paper and packaging which add considerably to the cost of the goods and are discarded haphazardly over the land. The disposal of this garbage is becoming an increasing problem. The need for water is outstripping the water resources so that recycling is now becoming a necessary concept. 'What I drank and urinated today, my brother will drink tomorrow' is becoming the norm.

The congestion of people in the decaying cities places stresses on them resulting in an increased consumption of tobacco and alcohol and an increase in psychosomatic disorders, the symptoms of which are treated by sedatives, stimulants and tranquillizers, whilst the causes remain largely unprobed. These three social problems appear to be increasing. Population density is

Table 1/3

The population of the world, by regions, in 1970, with other vital data

Region	*Population (in millions)*	*Percent of world's population*	*Estimated*		*Implied annual growth rate*	*Years to double population*
			Birth rate	*Death rate*		
World	3,634	100·0	34	14	2·0	35
Africa	344	9·7	46	20	2·6	28
North America	228	6·3	18	9	1·2	65
Latin America	283	7·8	39	10	2·9	25
Asia	2,056	55·9	38	15	2·3	30
U.S.S.R.	242	6·8	18	8	1·0	70
Europe	462	13·0	18	10	0·8	100
Oceania	19	0·5	24	10	2·0	35

damaging human dignity. At present the self-destructive urge of unlimited production and unbridled consumption is confined to the countries of North America, Europe and Japan, but there is evidence that many developing countries are taking them as a model for their own development. If such models are applied to countries whose growth rate is high, the disastrous effect will be infinitely greater.

As has been mentioned, there are striking regional differences in the rate of population growth (Table 1/3). In 1970, Africa had a population of 344 million. Between 1961 and 1970 the growth rate was calculated to be an average of 2·5 per cent, but because of the unreliable statistics from many African nations it is likely that both the population and the growth rate are higher. This supposition has been confirmed by those nations which have made a census recently. These have shown that previous population estimates were too low. For the continent, as a whole, in the period 1961–70, the birth rate was over 45 per 1,000 and the death rate about 20 per 1,000.

Emerging from a period of colonial rule, the African nations south of the Sahara are anxious to implement health measures to reduce the high death rates of infants and children, but in general show little enthusiasm for reducing the birth rate. Despite the world's highest infant and childhood mortality rates, with tribal societies, large families are a source of pride, and high fertility a cultural norm. As the continent has one quarter of the earth's surface, but only one-tenth of its population, many African leaders find difficulty in believing that population growth poses a problem. As far as density of population is concerned there is no problem; however, the urban population is growing at a rate of 5 per cent per annum, and in rural areas the available land has very limited agricultural potential. The fertile lowlands are relatively small in area and, apart from Australia, Africa is the driest of the continents. In addition, an increase in the reproductive growth rate is inevitable due to the age structure of the population and to better death control. Economic development and the expansion of social services are lagging increasingly behind the population growth rate, with potentially severe problems likely to arise, unless a massive investment programme can be mounted. In the present climate of African opinion, control of population growth is unlikely to be accepted, except as a part of a programme of maternity and child health; and the population growth rate may be expected to be about 3 per cent per annum during this decade. Caldwell, who has made a particular study of Sub-Saharan Africa, is cautiously optimistic that changes can occur. He writes 'there can be little doubt that most of the "ideological" resistance to family planning will crumble as enough African precedents are established to demonstrate that family planning is compatible with the African way of life or government'. The unanswered question is: will the change in attitude come about quickly or slowly? Major determinants of change are probably the increasing rate of urbanization and the increasing demand for education.

Africa is not the fastest growing region at this time. This dubious distinction must go to Latin America (including Central America and the Caribbean area). With the exceptions of Argentina, Cuba, Jamaica and Uruguay, every Latin American nation has a high rate of population growth. In 1970, the population of Latin America was estimated to be 283 million, an increase of 71 million over the 1960 estimate. This implies an annual growth rate of 2·9 per cent. Although the birth rate of 40 per 1,000 is lower than that found in Africa, the death rate of 11 per 1,000 is also lower, so that the annual population growth rate exceeds that of Africa. The population problems of Latin America are far greater than those of Africa, for more and more Latin Americans are migrating to the cities, seeking jobs which do not exist, and adding to the congestion of the insanitary urban slums. The social problems arising from this internal urban migration, coupled with uncontrolled fertility, are immense. Both within the cities and in the rural areas, social programmes in health, education and welfare are unable to meet the basic needs of the population, as the rate of population growth outstrips the investment in social services.

The situation in North America is different. Population growth in Canada and the U.S.A. is steady but not excessive. However, in an intensely consumer society, which survives only by importing raw materials from the developing nations, environmental pollution problems are increasing rapidly, and are causing considerable concern. It has been calculated that one American child will consume, and pollute, in his lifetime, twenty-five to fifty times the quantity consumed and polluted by one Indian child.

Asia, excluding the U.S.S.R., contains 56 per cent of the world's population. In 1971, over 2,000 million people lived in Asia, and the annual population growth rate, between 1961 and 1971, was 2·1 per cent. This means that over 40 million people are added to Asia's population each year. The birth rate has tended to remain constant since 1950, at about 36 to 38 per 1,000, but the death rate has continued to decline, so that the annual growth rate is increasing slightly. Within Asia, the reproductive growth rate varies between 1·2 and 2·8 per cent per annum. The world's most populous nation, the People's Republic of China, seems to have made considerable headway in reducing its rate of population growth to less than 1·4 per cent per annum, which is a remarkable achievement. Japan, too, must be excluded from the general statement about Asia. In fact, Japan is now classed, together with Israel, as a developed nation. Asian governments face increasing problems of land hunger, under-employment and unemployment, increasing inequalities of income and increasing urban growth.

Europe, including the U.S.S.R., with 700 million people, has the lowest birth rate of all the regions, a low death rate and the lowest annual growth rate. The problems facing Europe are those of urbanization and environmental pollution rather than population growth, but these problems are of considerable magnitude, and currently defy resolution. At a meeting held in the Netherlands in 1971, the degree of pollution of the North Sea and its effects on the ecology of the region provoked an intense argument, but no answers for urgent action.

Oceania is the least populated region with only 19 million inhabitants, and one in which land is available. But in the largest nations of the region, Australia and New Zealand, 85 per cent of the people live in towns of 25,000 inhabitants or more, and 66 per cent live in the five largest metropolitan conglomerations. In Australia, the problems of urban congestion and environmental pollution are beginning to be serious.

The problems of the non-Caucasian nations in Oceania are considerable. Papua-New Guinea, which achieved semi-independence in 1972, has an estimated 2·4 million inhabitants. The birth rate is unknown, but estimates range from 38 to 53 per 1,000 of population. The death rate is falling, so that a reproductive growth rate of over 3 per cent per annum is anticipated. The next largest nation, Fiji, has a population of 500 thousand and the next, Samoa, one of 160 thousand people. In both these nations, family planning measures have been implemented, as population growth presses on land, jobs and resources.

It can be seen that in all the continents, population growth and the distribution of the population are creating problems which threaten the well-being, perhaps the survival, of all mankind, and these are compounded by the current desire of most nations to increase economic growth.

There are, of course, solutions, which may or may not work. They are suggested in this book and if they are accepted, and if they do work, this will be known within the lifetime of most readers. If the solutions are wrong or fail to work, a disaster of unprecedented magnitude will sweep the earth, and the readers of this book or their children will not be spared.

Population dynamics is the study of population change. Currently, and generally in history, this means population growth rather than population decline. Since the rate of population growth is the major problem facing the entire world today, an understanding of the components of population growth, and an examination of current trends should enable the reader to appreciate, more readily, the possible solutions.

Mauritius—A Microcosm

A microcosm of the world problem is shown by the island of Mauritius. Until 1721, Mauritius was uninhabited by people. The animal life was large, the dodo was unique, but no humans had managed to establish a settlement. In that year the French occupied the island. They imported slaves from Madagascar and Mozambique, a few artisans from India, and some landowners from France to establish a spice industry, and later introduced sugar cane. Sugar prospered, and by 1821 the population had grown to 80,000. Meanwhile in 1810, the British had replaced the French as colonial rulers of Mauritius and in 1835 they abolished slavery. This caused considerable industrial problems as over 30,000 of the 70,000 black slaves refused to work the sugar plantations, and moving into the inland mountainous area took land for small-scale farming. To obtain labour for the cane fields, the British encouraged a large-scale migration of Indians with the result that the population quadrupled to 320,000 by 1871. At this point, reduced immigration and the inadvertent introduction of malaria, cholera and enteric diseases from India slowed the rate of population growth, which stabilized at 370,000 in 1891 and remained at that level till 1921. At this time, better sugar prices, and a more enlightened colonial government, enabled money to be allocated to sanitary control, with the consequence that the death rate fell and the population rose, reaching 450,000 in 1951. High sugar prices increased the wage rates with resulting improved childhood nutrition; malaria and cholera were eradicated; and a vigorous campaign against infectious disease was mounted with the result that the infant mortality fell from 142 per 1,000 live births in 1944 to 80 per 1,000 live births in 1954, the crude death rate falling from 27 per 1,000 to 16 per 1,000 over the same period. The health measures of the 1930s also meant that

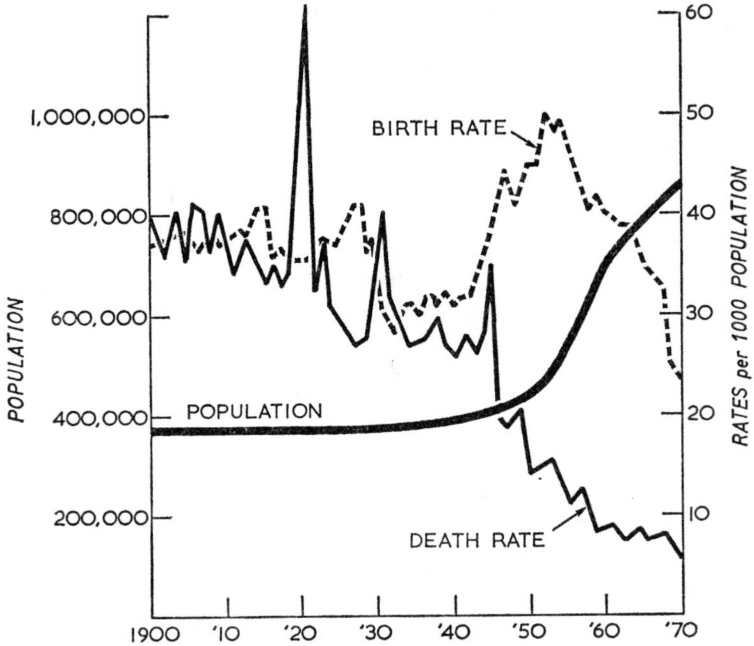

Figure **1/2** Birth rate, death rate and population growth in Mauritius, 1900–70.

many more children survived to reach puberty, and as they married the birth rate increased. As a consequence, the population growth rate rose precipitously to above 3 per cent per annum by 1958.

The alarming rate of population growth led to the appointment of a committee to consider its effects on the economic resources, the employment problems and potential production of the island. The report was sombre. The committee calculated that the island would have a population of one million by 1975 unless action was taken urgently, and noted that the growth of population was exceeding the expansion of the island's productivity. It contended that at least 15,000 more people would need to be employed each year, and that housing and the primary school population would grow to unmanageable numbers. To solve the problem the Committee rejected emigration, as they could see no possible acceptor nations, and recommended that the Government made the people aware of the problem by a propaganda campaign, and offered family planning as part of the social services.

The population of Mauritius is divided into three main groups. Twenty-eight per cent of the population are Creole or White, and are mainly Roman Catholic; 53 per cent are Hindu Indo-Mauritians; 16 per cent are Muslim Indo-Mauritians, and 3 per cent are Chinese. Because of strong action by the Roman Catholics, who dominated the Government, and by the Muslims, the recommendations were rejected.

By 1958, the population exceeded 600,000 and unemployment was rising. To investigate the twin problems, a further study was made. In this report, it was noted that in 1952, children under the age of 14 had formed 38 per cent of the population, but by 1958, they had increased to 44 per cent, a rise of 38 per cent as compared with an increase of 20 per cent for the population as a whole. Commenting on the report, the Government suggested that if economic viability was to be maintained, if unemployment was to be reduced, and if food per capita was to be increased, a major objective must be 'to slow down and if possible arrest the increase in the population'. Because of continued opposition by the Roman Catholics, again no action was taken other than to appoint two technical missions, one to investigate the social and demographic problems, the other the economic problems of Mauritius.

In 1961, the two reports were published. Both strongly recommended urgent Government action in establishing family planning as an integral part of the health and welfare programme. It was the 'most important single measure' that they had to propose.

'Had the Government started such a service in the early 1950s, the future of Mauritius might have looked less sombre than it did at that time.' The author of the socio-demographic report, Professor Titmuss, also declared that 'no alternative presents itself but action, immediate and sustained, to develop population policies on as broad a scale as possible designed to slow down the rate of population growth'. Families had to be limited in size by voluntary measures, information and assistance being provided by the Government as an integral part of the health and welfare services, and within the reach of every mother and father in the island. The economic report by Professor Meade concluded: 'The scheme would not make much sense to the people nor have much success unless the family planning measures were accompanied by vigorous economic and social planning.' Unless all these measures were initiated, Professor Titmuss saw 'economic, social and political disaster'. That disaster would occur was emphasized by Professor Meade. He foresaw the 'terrifying prospect' of a population of 3 million by the year 2000 unless action was taken urgently. He declared 'the economic future of Mauritius is dominated by its population problem. . . . Unless resolute measures are taken to solve it, Mauritius will be faced with a catastrophic situation. Even if one makes the "optimistic" assumption that the three-child family will rapidly become the general pattern in Mauritius, it will be necessary to find work for a 50 per cent increase in the population of working age over the next 15 years and to find school accommodation etc. over the same period for a 20 per cent increase in those under 15 years of age.'

The debate on the reports was long and bitter, but a change in attitudes was evident—family planning was accepted by all groups, although on a very limited scale.

The population continued to grow, the problems increased, but so did the concern of the people. In 1965, international agencies offered support, and the Government gave funds to the Mauritius Family Planning Association and the Roman Catholic Action Familiale (which taught the rhythm method of birth control). The Mauritius Family Planning Association initiated a campaign for population control by means of education, training and the establishment of family planning clinics. Film shows and talks on family planning were given in most villages. Letters were sent to all village and district councils, to social welfare centres and to doctors inviting their support. By 1970 the campaign to educate and inform had been expanded so that each marriage or birth notified to the Registrar General led to a letter, and to a visit by a field worker to the wife to explain the purpose of family planning. In 1970, 50,000 visits to women were made. In addition, talks were given on TV (each month) and radio (every alternate week) and discs were cut which were played at appropriate times, such as weddings. 'Drop-outs' were visited, and a coupon system was introduced. Field workers were given books of coupons, and if women were introduced to family planning and used an appropriate method for six months, the field worker received 6 rupees for each acceptor. Cartoon films lasting 10 minutes, made by Disney, were shown in commercial cinemas. In 1970, a total of 146 shows were made, and were seen by over 70,000 people. By 1971, 20 centres and 62 clinics had been established, mainly by using existing Maternity and Child Health facilities on a sessional basis. Over 4,200 clinic sessions were held, supervised by 5 full-time doctors. These attracted over 40,000 clients. At the clinics, oral contraceptives were made available at a nominal fee of U.S. 10c per month and a pilot scheme of injectable contraceptives was initiated. Condoms were made available at clinics, but more usefully were sold at tailor and barber shops. In 1970, 128,091 condoms were sold at a cost of 3 for U.S. 50c. IUDs were introduced but were less popular than oral contraceptives. The total new patients registered at clinics in 1970 was 8,230. Four thousand of these had come because of canvassing and 1,500 had been referred from MCH clinics. In the 1970 report of the Mauritius FPA, 20,600 women were noted to be current clients. This is 12 per cent of the 191,000 women aged 15–49 in the island. Assuming that 24 per cent of these were unmarried, widowed, divorced or separated, the proportion protected increases to 15 per cent. By mid-1971, there were 24,700 current clients; of these over 75 per cent chose to use oral contraceptives.

Action Familiale was established in 1963 to help couples understand the 'importance of sex education and self-control' and to aid in limiting the rate of population growth by teaching the rhythm method. The educators of Action Familiale aimed 'to help the couples to use the temperature method correctly, but to be able after a certain period to be on their own. When they can read out their chart without fail, when they can differentiate between the fertile and infertile periods, they become autonomous.' A survey was conducted in 1969 when the 2,649 registered 'autonomous' couples were investigated, 470 of these could not be found. Action Familiale claim that 83 per cent of those contacted still used the method. By December, 1969, a total of 6,197 couples were still in the scheme. Action Familiale methods were followed by about 15 per cent of all women currently using birth control measures.

The effect of all these measures has led to a decline in birth rate, despite the fact that increasing numbers of girls are entering the reproductive era. It has been calculated that 10,600 females enter the reproductive era and 3,500 leave it annually—a net gain of 7,100 potential mothers.

In 1971, two further matters of considerable importance occurred. The first was that the Government, at last after 20 years, decided to enter the field of family planning actively. Supported by the United Nations Agencies, it proposed to integrate family planning into Maternity and Child Health services, and to include the Family Planning Association personnel in the Ministry of Health.

Perhaps even more important in the long term is the 1971 'Four-Year Plan for Social and Economic Development'. This plan notes, in discussing the economy, that better jobs and a higher standard of living can only come about 'through curbing the rate of increase in the labour force'. To achieve this, the report recommends that 'a population policy for Mauritius must aim at reducing fertility rates to levels comparable to those in the industrialized countries over the next 10 to 15 years, in order to improve the age structure of the population and to give those born a better chance of life'. To do this, the rate of population growth must be cut to 1·6 per cent per annum, which implies a population of 980,000 by 1980 and one of 1,071,000 by 1985. So that this may be achieved, the Government promises to make family planning 'means and the know-how more widely available', and, echoing Titmuss and Meade, observes that 'a population policy cannot be independent of a strategy for the economic and social development of the island as a whole'.

The converse is also true. A strategy for economic and social survival of a nation cannot be independent of a population policy. This hard lesson is being accepted slowly, but increasingly, by leaders of the nations of the world. In microcosm, Mauritius faces the problem which confronts most other nations in this age of 'population explosion'. The history of Mauritius in the last twenty years is a model of what has happened in many nations. Firstly, there is a reluctance to believe that a problem exists. Secondly, there is a belief that increased economic growth and increased food production will solve the now identified problem of the rate of population growth. Thirdly, when it has been realized that economic policies must be related to population policies, resistance to birth control by large and influential groups on ideological grounds appears. Fourthly, public opinion begins to accept that action is needed to slow the rate of population growth. Fifthly, there is a sudden awareness that, because of the delay which has occurred, the problems have multiplied, have become more complex, and perhaps defy solution. Sixthly, the hope arises that population policies based on humane principles will succeed, before the inhuman solutions of famine, pestilence and civil or international war reduces the population, by increasing deaths rather than by decreasing births.

The peace of nations, and the dignity of man are dependent on how Mauritius and other nations, particularly the giants—China, India, Indonesia, Brazil, Bangladesh, Nigeria and Pakistan—solve the problems of acute population growth. There is no other way.

TWO

The Development of Demography

The scientific study of population is a fairly recent phenomenon, although Confucius, Aristotle and Plato had speculated about the problem indirectly. Up to the time of the devastating epidemics of plague which swept into Europe from Central Asia, births and deaths had been considered natural events occasioned by acts of God, for which man had no responsibility. The 'Black Death' reached Europe in about 1346, and raged with increasing violence throughout the next six years, the peak mortality being in 1348. It has been estimated that during this time one quarter of the population of Europe died. No treatment was available, and quarantine was started too late to be effective. Europe was in panic. Townships became deserted, fields were left untilled, flocks and herds of animals wandered at will. The wrath of God was considered the cause; Jews were accused of poisoning the wells, and many were burnt alive; religious fanatics scourged themselves for their sins. But the concept that perhaps man might have some effect on his own natality and mortality was also considered.

Over the next three centuries, epidemics recurred at frequent intervals in various countries. For example, plague broke out in England in the late sixteenth and early seventeenth century. It culminated in 'The Poores Plague' of 1665, which was the most virulent epidemic since 'The Black Death' 300 years earlier. The name was apt, for the epidemic started in the fetid wooden slums of London, which had neither water supplies nor sanitation, and spread through the city. Control measures were instituted: infected houses were locked and guarded, the inhabitants being forced to remain within; many people fled the city, spreading the plague to the villages of England. John Evelyn in his diary records under the date 7 September, 1665, 'Came home, there perishing neere 10,000 poore creatures weekly. I went all along the City and suburbs from Kente

Street to St. James's, a dismal passage, and dangerous to see so many coffines expos'd in the streets, now thin of people; the shops shut up, and all in mournful silence, as not knowing whose turn may be next.' In an effort to measure the effects of the epidemic, 'Bills of Mortality' were used. These had been initiated during the plagues of the late sixteenth century. In effect they were weekly reports of burials compiled by parish clerks. Through the sultry summer of 1665 they showed a steadily rising death rate, reaching a notified peak of 8,300 in September, although informed observers such as Dr. Nathaniel Hodge, who stayed in London throughout, thought that the real figure was nearer 12,000. From that date on, the epidemic diminished, and following the Great Fire, London was free from infection.

The Bills of Mortality, which also contained some information about christenings, formed the basis of an analysis of births and deaths by John Graunt who published the first demographic study: *Natural and Political Observations Made upon the Bills of Mortality* in 1662, three years before 'The Poores Plague' struck. He observed that in London deaths exceeded births, but in the country the reverse was true. He also noted that the causes of death varied from place to place and year to year, but that in all places there was a high mortality rate in infancy and childhood. He attempted to project the growth of London's population and identified migration in addition to births and deaths as an important factor. Progress in demographic studies was slow, and in the next 130 years, only Sussmilch's *Die Gottliche Ordnung* (The Divine Order) gave any evidence of an original mind applied to population problems. Sussmilch, a Lutheran clergyman, sought to demonstrate that a divine orderliness controlled vital events. To obtain evidence for this he studied trends in births, deaths and marriages, both in urban and rural areas. After surveying the evidence, and after enlisting the help of Euler, a distinguished mathematician, Sussmilch concluded that the population had a strong tendency to increase, and this increase was part of the Divine Order for peopling the earth. It was also God's method of countering the effects of war, famine, floods and pestilence. The Divine Order demanded that nothing would hinder the principle that men will multiply on earth. Like Graunt before him, and Malthus after him, the accuracy of Sussmilch's study was marred by inadequate, and inaccurate, recording of the essential data.

The Malthusian Controversy

The place of Thomas Malthus (1766–1834) in demographic theory remains contentious. One group of contemporary demographers give him a place of honour; their opponents claim that 'it is difficult to point to anything original, either methodological or substantive, in the writings of Malthus that can be cited as a major contribution of lasting influence in shaping either theory or research'; and again 'the main charge against him must be he was a bad observer of his fellow human beings'.

The problem of determining Malthus' place is that his original book *The Principle of Population* was in fact not a treatise on demography but a rebuttal of the theories which Godwin, a radical philosopher, had advocated in his book *Political Justice*. Godwin, who had been much influenced by the French revolutionary writers, had advocated political anarchy, social justice, the reign of reason and the abolition of private property. Once these measures had been taken, he declared the perfectibility of man would become apparent. Reason, in harness with science, would produce a delightful society. His optimism held that in this perfect society, the people themselves would find a way in which to regulate population growth, and because no man owned property, hatred and avarice would wither away. First published in 1793, *Political Justice* had had a considerable impact on intellectual thought in England, and Malthus' rebuttal was based on discussions he had had with his father about Godwin's beliefs. In fact, the full title of Malthus' book was *An Essay on The Principle of Population as it Affects Future Improvement of Society, with remarks on the Speculations of Mr. Godwin, M. Condorcet and other Writers*. His concern with the speculations is shown by the fact that over 60 per cent of the essay discusses the 'speculations', and in only 40 per cent does population receive attention.

The choice of those whom Malthus attacked is interesting. His father was a landed proprietor, an intellectual who was the friend of Jean Jacques Rousseau, of David Hume and of Condorcet. His son was brought up in a stimulating domestic atmosphere, and educated at home by two clergymen, who had a marked influence on his opinions.

Yet, in his essay, Malthus showed little sympathy for the liberal views of Godwin. By 1793, the population of England and Wales had grown to nearly 9 million—a 75 per cent increase on that of 1700. This increase had occurred over a period of time when the enclosure of common land and its use for pasture, rather than the growth of cereals, had driven many families into the new industrial towns, which had arisen with the development of steam power. The conditions in the towns were bad, the respect of the countryman for his superiors was diminishing, and prices of food were rising more rapidly than wages. These factors had led to the Gordon riots of 1780, which had struck fear into the propertied classes. The French Revolution, with its egalitarian philosophy, had increased the fear that their property might be taken from them. Godwin's book gave an English emphasis to a French philosophy, and gave intellectuals the hope that a perfect society would result.

Malthus, despite his liberal upbringing, was a member of the landowning class. His opinions were those of the landowners, his attitudes theirs. He feared the rising power of the poor, he lauded the ethic of work, he believed in a God-ordained hierarchy, and held that the poor were poor because of a defect of character and because of God's will.

In his twenties, Malthus became even more conservative, and this increased after he was ordained as an Anglican clergyman. But he continued to read widely, particularly when he determined to answer Godwin's belief in the perfectibility of man. To do this he chose as his illustration, his principle of population which stated: 'First, that food is necessary to the existence of man. Second, that the passion between the sexes is necessary and will remain nearly in its present state. Assuming then my postulata as granted, I say that the power of population is indefinitely greater than the power in the earth to produce subsistence for man. Population, when unchecked, increases in a geometrical ratio. Subsistence increases only in an arithmetical ratio. A slight acquaintance with numbers will show the immensity of the first power in comparison of the second. By that law of our nature which makes food necessary to the life of man, the effects of these two unequal powers must be kept equal. This implies a strong and constantly operating check on population from the difficulty of subsistence. This difficulty must fall somewhere; and must necessarily be severely felt by a large portion of mankind.'

In working out these ratios, Malthus contended that the population could double every 25 years (which implies an annual increase of 3 per cent) provided no factors impeded its growth, whilst food production could only double in the first 25 years, but after this would lag significantly behind population growth. Thus in 100 years, the population could have increased 16 times, but food production would only have increased four times above its original level. These ratios, which are biologically incorrect, have dazzled his defenders and critics, and have complicated discussion.

Malthus himself had noted that the postulated increase in population would not occur in real life because of two types of checks, one positive and the other preventive. He identified the positive checks as those of famine, pestilence and war, which he termed misery and vice. As a Christian, he could not accept that these checks were applicable to civilized man, and therefore recommended preventive checks, which would apply particularly to the labouring poor, for he had observed that they were the most prolific of all sections of the community. To reduce their population growth he suggested late marriage, with sexual continence prior to marriage. But he considered that both checks should operate.

The main purpose of the *Essay* was to establish that Godwin's Utopia could never be achieved, as the pressure of population would always exceed that of food. Since man could only hope to achieve a balance between population and subsistence by misery, and vice, 'the argument is conclusive against the perfectibility of mankind'. The perfect society would be wrecked by the increase of its own numbers without a corresponding increase in food. Society was divided into a class of proprietors and a class of labourers, and the latter, by increasing too rapidly, would destroy the whole fabric of civilization. Their growth must, therefore, be kept in check by restraints, or all mankind would suffer misery. There was nothing particularly original in Malthus' views. Similar views had been stated in 1677 by Matthew Hale, again in 1753 by Wallace and in 1786 by Joseph Townsend. Their books had had a small circulation and had made little impact. The effect of Malthus' book was quite different.

The Principle of Population was published at a most appropriate time. The small landowners and shopkeepers of England feared that the ideas which had led to the French Revolution would take hold amongst the labouring poor of England and their property would be endangered. In describing the principle of population, Malthus not only denied the perfectibility of man, but defended the principle of private property. God was supreme, the Divine order suggested by Sussmilch was apparent, the status quo was pre-ordained. Men were born into their appropriate station, and poverty and indigence were most men's inescapable lot, to which God had assigned them. The poor were poor because of a defect of character, and none of them should marry until able to support a family. Not only did Malthus demolish Godwin's advocacy of French revolutionary ideas, but he provided a religious basis for his alternative view, an economic basis for reducing taxation and an intellectual basis for preserving the status quo. To the conservative landowners and entrepreneurs of England, the essay on population gave comfort. What they did in self-interest was clearly approved by Divine Providence as enunciated by Thomas Malthus. At a time when repression of discussion and of association was becoming more intense, Malthus' book offered a reactionary solution, yet appeared to be progressive. It suited the time. The perfect society of the French was an intellectual mirage, and a practical failure. The ever present capacity of people to multiply more rapidly than food supplies meant the checks of vice, misery or moral restraint would always be needed. Moral restraint, by which Malthus meant postponement of marriage until a man had sufficient means to support his family, 'and a strictly moral conduct towards sex in the interval', was the most important check, and one which was under the control of 'man and the institutions of society'. 'Unnatural passions' (prior to marriage) and 'improper acts to prevent the consequences of irregular connections' were vices. Along with infanticide, war, plague and famine, they led to misery. There could be no better defence of the existing society—at least from the viewpoint of the ruling classes—and Malthus had no idea how or what the poor thought.

Yet this very book, which defended the status quo, sparked off a far-reaching controversy, and stimulated a vigorous discussion, often acrimonious, on the relationship between population dynamics and socio-economic change. Malthus wrote clearly and well, that was his strength; he communicated his ideas, and stimulated further thought, that was his importance in economic thought and in demography. He omitted data which were becoming evident, such as technological discoveries, which was his weakness.

His book was republished between 1798 and 1825 in seven editions. In each edition Malthus restated his original theme, stuck to his ratios, but then varied his attack. For example, in the second edition of 1803, he had ceased to be concerned with Godwin, but was much concerned with the payment of money to the unemployed poor, which he contended would have disastrous results, as it would lead to an increased population without any increase in production. The fear of hunger (rather than hunger itself) was a considerable spur to moral restraint. Take away that fear and man would indulge his sexual passions. For example, taxing the rich and giving the tax to the poor would have the effect of increasing the marriage rate and hence the natality of the poor, so that the numbers of the labouring poor increased. This would have the effect of a surplus of poor in the next generation and the consequent depression of wages. This in turn would lead to increased poverty and to the reduced ability of the poor to buy the increasingly scarce supply of food. The remedy for poverty lay in the hands of the poor themselves. There was no salvation in increasing the food supply as the increase in population would always surpass it. The only real remedy was to reduce the number of potential labouring poor, and the best method was to encourage moral restraint by abolishing the subsidies given to the poor under the poor laws.

The fact that many of Malthus' projections were wrong means that he is not unique amongst demographers, and the only data he could obtain were certainly inadequate. The fact that many of the ideas he supposed to be original were not, is again not unique. As an example, Bertrand Russell, writing about the English philosopher John Locke, says: 'In Locke's theory of government, there is, I repeat, little that is original. In this, Locke resembles most of the men who have won fame for their ideas. As a rule, the man who first thinks of a new idea is so much ahead of his time that everyone thinks him silly, so that he remains obscure and is soon forgotten. Then gradually the world becomes ready for the idea, and the man who proclaims it at the fortunate moment gets all the credit.' This applied to Malthus, but at least he had the honesty to acknowledge his debt to others. In the preface to the second (1803) edition of his *Essay on the Principle of Population*, he wrote: 'In the course of this inquiry I found that much more has been done than I had been aware of, when I first published the Essay. . . . The poverty and misery arising from a too rapid increase of population had been distinctly seen, and the most violent remedies proposed so long ago as the times of Plato and Aristotle. And of late years the subject has been treated in such a manner by some of the French Economists, occasionally Montesquieu, and among our own writers by Dr. Franklin, Sir James Stewart, Mr. Arthur Young and Mr. Townsend, as to create a natural surprise that it had not excited more of the public curiosity.'

'A SUMMARY VIEW'

In the final version of his essay which he entitled *A Summary View of the Principle of Population*, and which he wrote in 1830, four years before his death, Malthus had modified his initial views to some extent. The intellectual discussion over the years had had some effect. He wrote: 'Elevated as man is above all other animals by his intellectual faculties, it is not to be supposed that the physical laws to which he is subjected should be essentially different from those which are observed to prevail in other parts of animated nature. . . . Food is equally necessary to his support; and if his natural capacity of increase be greater than can be permanently supplied from a limited territory, his increase must be constantly retarded by the difficulty of procuring the means of subsistence. . . . Whatever temporary and partial relief . . . may be derived from emigration . . . (it) may be fairly said not in any degree to touch the difficulty. And whether we exclude or include emigration—whether we refer to particular countries, or to the whole earth—the supposition of a future capacity in the soil to increase the necessaries of life every twenty-five years by a quantity equal to that which is at present produced must be decidedly beyond the truth.

'But if the natural increase of population, when unchecked by the difficulty of procuring the means of subsistence or other peculiar causes, be such as to continue doubling its numbers in twenty-five years, and if the greatest increase of food, which, for a continuance, could possibly take place on a limited territory like our earth in its present state, be at the most only such as would add every twenty-five years an amount equal to its present produce, then it is quite clear that a powerful check on the increase of the population must be almost constantly in action.'

From these extracts it can be seen that Malthus felt that the preventive checks would result in far less misery than the positive checks of 'epidemics, wars, infanticide, plague and famine' and were, therefore, to be preferred. But even after all the argument, 'prudential restraint on marriage' was the only morally acceptable preventive check in his opinion. In the conditions of his day, he doubted if the preventive checks, which he observed to be operating to some extent through 'all ranks of society in England', would ever be sufficiently strong to eliminate the positive checks which arose mostly from the pressure of population on food supplies.

MALTHUS AND CONTRACEPTION

One question remains unanswered. Why did Malthus reject birth control as a means whereby man could marry yet avoid having children? Birth control was not unknown, coitus interruptus was practised, vaginal sponges had been recommended. Malthus must have heard of both methods. Yet he considered them 'vices'. Perhaps this was because he confused coitus interruptus with onanism, as many others have done, and Onan was condemned in the Bible. Perhaps Malthus condemned birth control because he feared public opinion. But he had rejected Condorcet's conception control as a method of limiting population growth in the first edition of 1798, long before he was famous.

More likely it was his fear that if the poor used birth control —and it was the poor with whom he was most concerned—

their fear of want would diminish. And from his middle class, secluded viewpoint, the labouring poor were indolent, dangerous and deceitful. Unless a man was forced to work to maintain his family, he would not exert himself. Consequently he should not marry until he could support a family, but at the same time he should eagerly desire marriage as a spur to induce him to work harder. Contraception would remove that spur.

Malthus' rejection of birth control ignored the surest, and the most humane, way of reducing the population growth below the geometrical growth ratio of which he was so enamoured. This is particularly strange for he must have heard of Francis Place. In 1822 Place wrote a book *Illustrations and Proofs of the Principle of Population*, intended as a reply to Godwin's reply to Malthus. The book is remarkable for two reasons. Firstly, although Place accepted Malthus' postulates and analysis, he rejected, almost completely, Malthus' solutions as inappropriate and unacceptable to the working class; and secondly, he openly advocated birth control. Place had good reason to know that Malthus' solution was unacceptable to the poor. He had had a miserable poverty-stricken childhood. His father had been a gambler and a drunkard, and he knew from bitter experience how the poor lived, which Malthus did not. Place did not question Malthus' sincerity, but believed him misguided, and unintentionally hard-hearted. His solutions would only increase the illwill between the proprietors and the labourers. Malthus' belief that poverty was a law of God was erroneous, it perpetuated injustice, and it showed his ignorance about the poor. The majority of the poor made efforts, against terrific odds, to keep up a decent appearance; the dissolute poor who needed fear to keep them at work were a minority. Place suggested that rather than moral restraint, maintained by fear of want, the rich should explain to the poor the economic necessity for control of population growth, which would improve their lot. But more than this was needed, and Place advocated birth control openly. 'If, above all, it were once clearly understood that it was not disreputable for married persons to avail themselves of such precautionary measures as would, without being injurious to health, or destructive to female delicacy, prevent conception, a sufficient check might at once be given to the increase of population beyond the means of subsistence; vice and misery, to a prodigious extent, might be removed from society and the object of Mr. Malthus, Mr. Godwin and of every philanthropic person, be promoted, by the increase of comfort, of intelligence and of moral conduct, in the mass of the population.'

It was a rational call from a man who knew how the labouring poor lived and thought, and it carried Malthus' theory to its logical conclusion. He was, in fact, the first of the Neo-Malthusians, whose thought is currently dominant in population dynamics.

A CRITIQUE OF MALTHUS' THEORY

Modern demographers have pointed out the defects of Malthus' theory. Firstly, his ratio of geometrical increase of population (1, 2, 4, 8, 16) and arithmetical increase (1, 2, 3, 4, 5) in means of subsidence has not proved correct. Malthus either ignored, or failed to understand, the impact of the agricultural and industrial revolutions as means of increasing subsistence, which is strange as they were well in evidence in the early years of the nineteenth century. The revolutions meant that much larger populations could be supported than in the earlier, mainly unimproved, agricultural and cottage manufacturing systems. However, there is no doubt that the standard of subsistence remained low—and misery was widespread—a fact which did not escape Marx. So that although Malthus was wrong in theory, his remarks were true in practice. Secondly, Malthus failed to define subsistence. At times it appears to mean food supply, which is easily defined; at times he appears to hold it to mean a customary standard of living. This confusion mars the understanding of his principle. Thirdly, and perhaps most importantly today, as has been noted, Malthus failed to comprehend the importance of voluntary control of conception on population growth. However, only with hindsight may contemporary demographers condemn Malthus for these opinions. Even today conception control is violently attacked by a significant group of people. Fourthly, and because of the foregoing, Malthus' *Principle of Population* can no longer be accepted as a valid scientific theory: but then it is doubtful if any model theory of population will survive the assault of the hard facts of ill-understood human behaviour.

Malthus was, in fact, substantially correct in his view that in the absence of effective preventive checks, population growth would inevitably be controlled by the positive checks of disease, famine, war and misery, all of which contribute, not to a diminution of natality, but to an increase in mortality, and are associated with undue misery. In the seventh and last edition of his book, he foretold that preventive checks would become increasingly important: 'I think it appears that in modern Europe the positive checks to population prevail less and the preventive checks more than in past times, and in the more uncivilized parts of the world. War, the predominant check to the population of savage nations, has certainly abated, even including the late unhappy revolutionary contest; and since the prevalence of a greater degree of personal cleanliness, of better modes of clearing and building towns, and of a more equable distribution of the products of the soil, from improving knowledge in political economy, plagues, violent diseases, and famines have been certainly mitigated and have become less frequent.'

He had become much more mellow with age and his earlier pessimism had been reduced. In the final pages of the last edition of his *Essay* he wrote: 'From a review of the state of society in former periods compared with the present, I should certainly say that the evils resulting from the principle of population have rather diminished than increased, even under the disadvantage of almost total ignorance of the real cause. And if we can indulge the hope that this ignorance will be gradually dissipated, it does not seem unreasonable to expect that they will be still further diminished. The increase of absolute population, which will of course take place, will evidently tend but little to weaken this expectation, as everything depends upon the relative proportion between population and food, and not on the absolute number of people. In the former part of this work, it appeared that the countries which possessed the fewest people often suffered the most from the effects of the principle of population; and it can scarcely be doubted that, taking Europe throughout, fewer famines and fewer diseases arising from want have prevailed in the last century than in those which preceded it.

'On the whole, therefore, though our future prospects respecting the mitigations of the evils arising from the principle of population may not be so bright as we could wish, yet they are far from being entirely disheartening, and by no means preclude the gradual and progressive improvement in human society which before the late wild speculations on this subject, was the object of rational expectation. . . .

'. . . And although we cannot expect that the virtue and happiness of mankind will keep pace with the brilliant career of physical discovery, yet, if we are not wanting to ourselves, we may confidently indulge the hope that, to no unimportant extent, they will be influenced by its progress and will partake in its success.'

Malthus' prophesies, and his faint beginnings of optimism, that the voluntary control of population growth may be possible, emphasizes the development of his thought. Indeed, what Malthus prophesied in the 1820s is increasingly of concern to us in the 1970s—one hundred and fifty years later—and is a measure of his importance in the development of demography.

Chinese Demographers of the Late Eighteenth and Nineteenth Centuries

In the Eurocentric educational atmosphere of the past 120 years, it is understandable that few European or American demographers have given much thought to China. China had conducted population counts at periodic intervals from the time of the Han dynasty (equating to the first century AD). Since the counts were mainly for taxation purposes it is likely that they were inaccurate, underestimating rather than over-estimating the population. Such information as is available indicates that considerable fluctuations in the population occurred. Natural disasters, wars and epidemics took their toll; the invasion of China in 1280 by the Mongols, and the Black Death about 30 years later made a particular impact and reduced the population from about 140 million to 80 million over a period of 50 years. Between the periods of famine, pestilence and war, peaceful times with good harvests and good administration led to population growth, which appears to have increased steadily to reach 160 million by 1700 and 300 million by 1800. This implies an annual growth rate of 1·0 per cent.

Hung Liang Chi was born in 1744, and in 1793, at the age of 49, wrote two essays, *Region of Peace* and *Livelihood*. In these essays he discussed population problems. He noted from the evidence available to him that whilst a population in 100 years can increase by five to twenty times, food production, because of limitations of land and the vagaries of climate, can only increase from three to five times. With an expanding population he observed that the number of young dependants, who required food and some education, increased more rapidly than those engaged in food production and commerce. He noted also that the larger the population, the smaller was the income per head; but as more people wanted goods, expenditure and consumption increased. At the same time, because of surplus labour and over-demand for the goods, wages fell but the price of the goods rose. In this way, and because of an unequal distribution of wealth, it became increasingly harder for the mass of the people to obtain a livelihood. When natural disasters, such as famine, flood or epidemics swept the country, the undernourished poor were the first to die, but as their deaths 'from natural calamities do not amount to more than 10 or 20 per cent of the population', population growth continued inexorably.

Hung felt that all that could be done to reduce the problems of too rapid growth of population was to open new land, to practise more intensive farming, to check the growth of landlordism and to discourage the consumption of luxuries. And he concluded: 'During a long reign of peace, the government cannot prevent the people from multiplying themselves, yet its remedies are few.'

It was left to another Chinese, Wang Shi To, writing sixty years later, when the population growth rate had diminished somewhat, to suggest a population policy. He accepted Hung's findings but recommended that the marriage age should be raised and preventive taxation be levied on families with more than two children. To this prescription he added that widows should be prohibited from remarriage and the Imperial prohibition against female infanticide should be relaxed. In addition, he believed that drugs which cause female sterility should be sought and administered. It is not known how widely Wang's views circulated. Certainly no administrative action was taken to establish population control, perhaps because the Taiping wars, and floods in the Yang Tze area, reduced the population by more than 30 million, and because virgin lands were still available.

It is interesting, however, that on two sides of the world at about the same time, Malthus and Hung reviewed the demographic evidence and saw the problems of overpopulation.

European Demographic Theorists of the Nineteenth Century

In contrast to Malthus' qualified pessimism, the economists and social reformers who grew up during the early years of the Industrial Revolution tended to qualified optimism. It is true that all were reasonably affluent, reasonably intelligent and reasonably separated from the rigorous poverty which increased as the manufacturing towns grew and spread across the countryside. Not only did industrialization increase productivity, but agricultural reforms improved food production, and better communications expanded international trade. Under these conditions, Malthus' principles were seen to be erroneous: the means of subsistence were increasing more rapidly and population growth less rapidly than he had predicted. It appeared that the natural law he had formulated was erroneous, and man need not be concerned about population growth, for man's manipulation of nature would ensure that the increase in population would be matched by an increased supply of goods and services. This optimistic view was held by Michael Sadler and by Thomas Doubleday.

Sadler (1780–1835) was a contemporary of Malthus, but there is no evidence that they debated their different theories. Sadler based his theory on the population problems of Ireland which at that time had not suffered the disastrous potato famine. He believed that the fecundity (by which he meant the natality) of human beings was, other things being equal, 'in inverse ratio of the condensation of their numbers'. A dispersed and scanty population favoured fertility, whilst as mankind advanced to the 'highest condition of civilisation, labour becomes divided and consequently diminished in its duration and intensity, and many are liberated from its drudgeries, so as to devote themselves to more intellectual pursuits'. In such instances fecundity fell and population growth diminished. The speculation was correct, but Sadler confused fecundity, or the ability to bear a child, with natality, the actual bearing of a child. He ignored the fact that high fecundity can exist with low natality, if couples used preventive measures, and that this could be the reason for his observations, which can only have been very limited in scope.

Writing some twenty years later, Doubleday (1790–1870) believed that there was a general law of population growth which applied to animals and man. The theory held that 'whenever a species or genus is endangered, a corresponding effort is invariably made by nature for its preservation and continuance, by an increase of fecundity or fertility; and that this especially takes place whenever such danger arises from a diminution of proper nourishment or food, so that consequently the state of depletion, or the deplethoric state, is favourable to fertility, and that on the other hand, the plethoric state, or state of repletion, is unfavourable to fertility, in the ratio of the intensity of each state, and this probably is throughout nature universally, in the vegetable as well as in the animal world; further, that as applied to mankind this law produces the following consequences, and acts thus: "there is in all societies a constant increase going on amongst that portion of it which is the worst supplied with food; in short, amongst the poorest". Amongst those in the state of affluence, and well supplied with food and luxuries, a constant decrease goes on. Amongst those who form the mean or medium between these two opposite states, that is to say amongst those who are tolerably well supplied with good food, and not over-worked, nor yet idle, population is stationary.'

Again the observation was not incorrect but the interpretation was. It is a fact that the birth rate in the developed countries of the world today is much lower than that of the developing countries; and this can be plotted against caloric intake. However, the interpretation for this phenomenon is not that the caloric intake (or the protein intake as De Castro has recently suggested) is the main factor operating, but that voluntary control of conception is utilized in the developed countries more readily.

Twenty years later, Herbert Spencer (1820–1909) applied his not inconsiderable mind to the problem. Like Sadler and Doubleday, Spencer believed that a natural law absolved man from any responsibility for population growth. He, like John

Stuart Mill, held that education offered a solution to many social evils, and education would effectively control reproduction. His biological views of woman would be scorned today, but in the climate of mid-Victorian England they seemed remarkably rational.

'That absolute or relative infertility is generally produced in women by mental labour carried to excess, is more clearly shown. Though the regimen of upper-class girls is not what it should be yet, considering that their feeding is better than that of girls belonging to the poorer classes, while in most other respect, their physical treatment is not worse, the deficiency of reproductive power among them may be reasonably attributed to the overtaxing of their brains—an overtaxing which produces a serious reaction on the physique. This diminution of reproductive power is not shown only by the greater frequency of absolute sterility; nor is it shown only in the earlier cessation of child bearing, but it is also shown in the very frequent inability of such women to suckle their infants.'

Arsene Dumont (1849–1902) echoed and expanded Spencer's theory after studying population growth in France. Dumont held that man in society seeks to improve his status and to climb to a higher social level in his environment, rather in the manner in which fluids rise in capillary tubes. In a graphic analogy, he referred to this process as 'social capillarity'. In the effort to rise through the strata of society man's energies are diverted from fornication and family so that fertility falls. In this way societies, where social capillarity is high, tend to have low birth rates, whilst in countries where social capillarity is low, as in India due to a rigid caste system, the birth rate remains high. In individual instances Dumont's theory holds, but in the mass it does not, unless contraceptive measures are used. Furthermore, only a portion of society wishes to reach a significantly higher social status, and this is generally the more intelligent, affluent and motivated group, who even in Dumont's day might be expected to use birth control measures.

The Twentieth Century

In the twentieth century, population dynamics became an acceptable science and accurate data began to replace inaccurate observations. Of the many names, perhaps that of Alexander Carr Saunders in Britain merits mention, as he stressed man's ability to control his population growth, a factor of great importance today.

Carr Saunders (1886–1966) approached population dynamics from two aspects, 'those connected with the quantity and those connected with the quality of population'. He noted that previously few authors had considered these two aspects simultaneously, so that 'the relation between them is seldom appreciated'.

Carr Saunders believed that each society determined its 'optimum number' of people and by manipulation of social factors over a period of time adjusted the population to the determined norm. The optimum number itself varied, depending on the social factors, so that as economic skills increased 'the number economically desirable tended to increase'. Thus in a society the population might be less than the optimum, might equal it, or might exceed it, in which case economic factors would lead to a reduction to the optimum. He stated that the problem was present in all societies and that, in many, alteration by death and migration was insufficient to keep the population at the optimum, so that measures to restrict fertility had to be taken. 'In primitive races these factors take the form of abortion, infanticide, and prolonged abstinence from intercourse.' In modern societies different factors exist, and the 'numbers desirable are constantly increasing'.

'It may be that we are nearing a time when numbers will be again normally stationary, for though increase may remain economically desirable, it may cease to be so from a wider point of view of human welfare, when, that is to say, facts other than income per capita are taken into account. In the second place, there have been frequent failures to attain the optimum number owing to the many disturbing influences at work. Chief among them are the fluctuation in the number desirable, the erratic action of certain causes of elimination, such as war and disease and migration.'

It must be remembered that Carr Saunders' analysis was made in 1922, with the monstrous deaths of World War I much in his mind, and at a time when differential fertility between different classes of society was being increasingly explored. He refers to this:

'No one problem should be considered without reference to its bearing both upon quantity and quality. At the present day, for instance, differential fertility is almost always considered solely from the point of view of quality; it is forgotten that the reduction in the birth rate may be that which economic conditions demand and that it may be of necessity to have to begin among the upper classes.'

The main problem in accepting Carr Saunders' views is that nowhere is the 'optimum population' defined clearly as an economic or as a demographic entity. However, his views are of importance as they stress very firmly that population growth does not follow a natural law but is firmly and unequivocally in the hands of mankind itself, operating through social institutions. It also alerts demographers to the problem of genetic quality as well as physical quantity in population control. Thus demography is a social science with biological attributes.

A Law of Population Dynamics?

The philosophical problem which confronted all the demographic theorists was the need for population to conform to a law or laws. Since demography was a scientific subject it should be subject to laws, just as physical sciences were subject to laws. As each investigator formulated his theory, he did so on the basis of such data as he could collect, such observations as he could himself make or could obtain from reliable sources, and in the context of the prevailing culture and thought of his time. Each acknowledged, to a greater or lesser extent, that his theory might be inexact because of human behavioural inconsistencies, and this factor is most stressed by the late nineteenth- and twentieth-century demographic theorists. That no theory has emerged which has withstood the test of time and the accumulation of new data perhaps emphasizes that demography is a social science, not a physical science, and that a general immutable law of population dynamics in all probability does not exist. Such a belief demands that students of population dynamics remain intellectually curious, with open critical minds.

THREE

The Collection of Demographic Data

Since the purpose of Government is to improve the lot of the people of the country, it is essential for the authorities to know the number of people living in the area, where they live within the country, and their composition with regard to sex, age, education and other characteristics. The questions: what is the size of the population, what is its distribution and what is its composition, form the core of essential knowledge about population. This information is essential for the proper planning of the social and economic, the political and business needs and aspirations of the people. Without these data, accurately obtained, it is impossible for the development of a country, or a part of a country, to proceed with equity and justice for the inhabitants.

It will be appreciated that the questions relating to the size and distribution of the population largely relate to information about *persons*. Information about the composition of the population also relates to persons (such as their age group, their educational attainment, their economic status), but it also relates to *events*. The events of most interest to demographers are birth and deaths (termed vital events); movement of people into and out of the country, or between parts of the country (migration); marriages and divorces. Information on all these matters enables a demographer to make a much better estimate of future trends in the population, its composition and its distribution.

In a perceptive article, Hawley has pointed out that demographers, and presumably Governments, are concerned with the composition of the population they are studying for four main reasons. Firstly, the data constitute an inventory of the human resources of the society under scrutiny. Secondly, the data on the composition of the population enable the demographers to make an elaborate description of the population. Thirdly, the data obtained describe the variables (such as age, sex, marital status, etc.) which are essential for analysing population dynamics. Fourthly, the demographic variables, together with the knowledge of population size, are of great importance in affecting social change in the society under scrutiny.

WHAT IS POPULATION?

The formulation of the questions to be asked presupposes that the questioner has a clear idea of what is meant by the term 'population'. In the demographic sense, a population is an aggregate of the total number of persons, living in a defined area at a special time, who are subject to the dynamic influences of natality, mortality, migration and social mobility. Since the population is subject to the vital events described, it is a living changing organism, and these vital events are constantly affected by its composition and cultural characteristics.

If this definition of population is used, it is obvious that a crowd of 120,000 occupying a football stadium in Rio de Janeiro is not a demographic population, as it is not affected by vital events, although it is a mathematical population. However, a slightly larger number of people living in Western Samoa (143,000) is a population in the demographic sense, as it is a changing organism, subject to additions from births, subtractions owing to death and various influences due to migration.

A population may be further divided into parts, or 'subpopulations'. For example, the Aboriginals in Australia form a subpopulation, as do the Christian population in Indonesia, or the suburban population of New York. These aggregates of people can be treated as a population, because they have children, they die and they move in and out of the area; in short, they fall within the definition of population in the demographic sense.

The Sources of Demographic Data

If a Government, or other authority, is to plan for social and economic improvements, information about the population of the nation must be obtained as accurately as possible, and any projections from the data must be made after careful mathematical analysis. Even then, the projections can be markedly wrong, because of the little understood vagaries of human behaviour. Despite this, demographers require accurate data, and as in computer technology, the aphorism 'GIGO' applies—'garbage in equals garbage out'. In the collection of any demographic data, the methods must be clearly understood by the collectors (or enumerators), who must be trained to communicate with the people they enumerate. The population to be enumerated must also be informed of the need for the collection of the data, and their full cooperation must be obtained during the collection.

Most of the demographic data come from three sources. They come from *national population censuses*; from *national registers* of births, deaths and marriages, and from *sample surveys*.

National Population Censuses

Most countries in the world have realized the need for a periodic accounting of their population, and the majority enumerate the total population at a predetermined moment of time. This is called a population census and it is taken at 10-year or 5-year intervals. In planning to take a census, a decision has to be made regarding the population to be counted. Should the census be of the *total population*, which includes citizens temporarily outside the country; or should it be of the *total home population*, which would exclude the citizens abroad? In fact, some nations tabulate both. A problem arises in the census of members of the armed forces since they are specially mobile. Should they be enumerated as temporary residents of a specific area or, since this might affect planning for that area, should they be excluded, and only the total *civilian population* be enumerated? These questions have to be answered in the early planning stages of the census. Within a country a further difficulty arises. In making the census of a specific area, should the enumerators count all the persons within that area on the day of the census as residents of that area, or should the enumerator try to allocate the persons counted to their regular place of residence? The first method—the *de facto* method—allocates a person to the area where he happened to spend the census night. The second, the *de jure* method, allocates the person to his usual place of residence. The de facto method gives a more complete coverage, and reduces error due to duplication or omission of entries, but may exaggerate the population of certain areas—such as tourist resorts—and invalidate birth and death rates from such areas.

To avoid this problem, the day and hour chosen to make the census is one on which there is likely to be the least movement of people away from their homes.

A nation making a census weighs up the advantages and disadvantages of each method and chooses the one most suitable for its own needs. Australia used the de facto method in the 1971 census, whilst the U.S.A. chose the de jure method in 1970, although de facto statistics were also collected.

HOW A CENSUS IS ORGANIZED

In most of the nations which have had a census in the last decade, a law has been passed which designates a particular department of government to organize the census, although the Government scrutinizes and approves the questions to be asked, and may delete some or add others. The actual census is only taken at 5- or 10-year intervals, but the department continues to operate all the time. This is because governments today require censuses and surveys of agriculture, of industry, of manufacturers, of retail trade, of service industries, of housing and of other social and economic indices as well as population censuses. The experience gained by officials in the department is invaluable in seeking and interpreting data.

In a population census, the basic unit is the individual and the individual household. But for ease of collection and enumeration it is usual to combine a specified number of individuals into groups, which form census collectors' (or enumerators') districts.

The size of the collector's district depends on the method used, the geographical nature of the area and the literacy of the people. Because of literacy problems in many developing nations, collectors' districts tend to be smaller than in the industrialized developed nations.

Problems of the confidentiality of the information given to collectors occasionally arise, particularly as some of the questions asked in a census relate to matters frequently considered private or intimate in nature. In Britain, for example, in the 1971 census, no collector was permitted to live in the census area for which he was responsible. This was to make sure that the information would remain confidential.

The conduct of a census has been considered by the United Nations, who have issued a document entitled *Principles and Recommendations for the 1970 Population Census*. This admirable document sets out the method of planning, organizing and conducting a population census. It also sets out a number of factors which should be considered in determining which topics should be included in a census. These involve a balanced consideration of the information a nation needs with respect to census data, consideration of the degree that this data can be used for international comparison, the resources available to plan, conduct and process the census, and public response attitudes to the census. The considerable experience of the United Nations in population matters has enabled the organization to specify a number of topics which should be included in any census. These are listed in Table **3/1**. It will be observed that certain recommended topics enable other topics to be derived. A detailed discussion about each topic is found in the publication, which deserves careful study.

CONTENT OF THE CENSUS FORM

Perhaps the most difficult and controversial part during the organization of a census is the first step. This is to determine what questions should be asked. The information listed in Table **3/1** is really the minimum required and most nations seek much more information than this. For example, the United States Bureau of Census, with aid from the Bureau of the Budget, requested suggestions from every department of government, from private business organizations and from many individual users of census data, such as Universities, so that a useful census form could be made for the 1970 census (Kaplan).

In Australia, before the 1971 census, user-committees were established made up of groups of people from a wide range of

Table 3/1

United Nations principles and recommendations for the 1970 population census

Recommended and other useful topics	
Topics which appear on the questionnaire	*Derived topics*
Geographic characteristics	
*Place where found at time of census (para. 265) and/or	*Total population (paras. 283–287)
*Place of usual residence (paras. 258–261)	*Locality (paras. 232–234)
*Place of birth (paras. 249–255)	*Urban and rural (paras. 298–299)
Duration of residence (paras. 200–202)	
Place of previous residence (paras. 256–257)	
Place of work (paras. 262–264)	
Personal and household characteristics	
*Sex (para. 276)	*Household composition (paras. 218–221)
*Age (paras. 176–178)	Family composition (paras. 213–217)
*Relation to head of household (paras. 269–270)	
Relationship to head of family (paras. 266–268)	
*Marital status (paras. 238–244)	
Age at marriage (paras. 179–183)	
Duration of marriage (paras. 179–183)	
Marriage order (paras. 179–183)	
*Children born alive (paras. 184–188)	
*Children living (paras. 189–190)	
Citizenship (paras. 191–195)	
*Literacy (paras. 228–231)	
*School attendance (paras. 274–275)	
*Educational attainment (paras. 203–208)	
Educational qualifications (paras. 209–212)	
National and/or ethnic group (paras. 245–246)	
Language (paras. 224–227)	
Religion (paras. 271–273)	
Economic characteristics	
*Type of activity (paras. 288–297)	Socio-economic status (paras. 277–280)
*Occupation (paras. 247–248)	Dependency (paras. 196–199)
*Industry (paras. 222–223)	
*Status (as employer, employee, etc.) (paras. 281–282)	
Main source of livelihood (paras. 235–237)	

* Recommended Topics

The paragraphs in the Table refer to those in the United Nations publication 'Principles and Recommendations for the 1970 Population Census'.

users of census data for demographic, economic and sociological purposes. The committees advised the Bureau of the Census and Statistics of their projected needs, and their suggestions were used in constructing the census form. The census questionnaire was subsequently discussed by the Cabinet and a final form decided upon. One controversial matter which many statisticians hoped would be included was eliminated. This was a series of questions regarding the distribution in the community of income and wealth. The Government felt that such questions intruded too much on an individual's privacy, although it was realized that the questions were essential in order to obtain factual information of the extent of poverty and its distribution in an affluent country.

Once the questions have been determined, they must be tested to be sure that when answered they will yield the required information; that they are clear and unequivocal, both to the questioner and to the respondent; and that they can be answered easily with the minimum of omissions and errors. To make certain that the questions meet these criteria, the proposed questionnaire is pretested on a variety of groups of the population, and revised when necessary. Questionnaires devised for 12 countries are shown in the *United Nations Handbook of Population Census Methods* (Vol. 1) published in 1958, and provide good models.

In the final stages of the preparation of the questionnaire, the form is re-examined to make sure that not only is the layout suitable for being easily filled in by the enumerator or informant, but also can be readily processed for computerization.

THE CENSUS

The purpose of a census is to enumerate each individual within the nation, so that the basic unit of enumeration is the individual. But individuals tend to make arrangements, either individually or in groups, to provide themselves with food and with other social and physical essentials for living. They do this by aggregating into households. A household may be a one-person household or a multi-person household.

For convenience, the household is treated as a primary unit in the collection of census data, and two main methods are used. In the first, paid canvassers (or enumerators) are selected, trained and each is given a collection area. In his area, he has to interview and obtain information from every person in every household living within the assigned boundaries. The canvasser locates the most responsible person in each household, seeking, if possible, the head of the household. He obtains the information from him, or her, about all the other members of the household and enters it on to the census form.

The canvasser (or enumerator) method is essential in nations where many people are illiterate, but it is also used in several developed nations, where literacy is no problem, as the method permits complex questions to be asked. However, the costs are considerable, and in many nations it is difficult to find suitable people who are prepared to act as canvassers, particularly in rural areas.

In the second method, which is called the householder method, a census form is handed, or mailed, to each household. The head of the household is responsible for filling in the form for all members living in the household. This method is less costly than the canvasser method, as fewer official enumerators are required, as their training is less intensive, and as each can be assigned a larger collector's district for which to be responsible. The enumerator collects the completed census forms, and checks them to ensure that all questions have been answered. He returns to any household which has provided incomplete information, and seeks to complete the form.

Both methods have advantages and drawbacks, and in some nations, such as the U.S.A., both methods are used, the one most appropriate to a given area being chosen.

Whichever method is used, the information relates to a specific time on a specific day of the year, which is designated census day. In the canvasser method, the information is collected, of necessity, over a longer period, as each interview takes up to one to two hours. This has the disadvantage that the householder who is interviewed some time after the census day, may have a poor recall of the events of that day, so that memory bias enters. Equally the information provided in the householder method may be spurious, either from misunderstanding, ignorance or misrepresentation.

TABULATION AND PUBLICATION

The completed census forms are returned to the census office where the results are tabulated, obvious errors checked and, if possible, corrected by referring to other items on the form. The information is next coded, in Australia, for example, first by hand, then on to computer cards which reduces the human element and enables the information to be transferred to magnetic tape with the least interference. Computers today do the calculating, prepare the tables, and print out the results. These are checked and edited for publication. The process is complex. For example, after the 1971 Australian census, it took 1,000 trained clerks nearly one year to transfer the information obtained from the census forms on to computer cards. The cards were then fed into a computer which checked them for errors and transferred the bits of information on to magnetic tape.

Table 3/2

Tabulations suggested by the United Nations to be used in a population census

Recommended Tabulations

(An asterisk (*) preceding the number of the tabulation indicates that it is of first priority; tabulations not so marked are of second priority.)

*1. Total population and population of major and minor civil divisions, by sex.
*2. Population in localities by size-class of locality and sex.
*3. Population of principal localities and of their urban agglomerations, by sex.
*4. Population in households and number of family nuclei, by size of household, and number of persons not living in households.
5. Population in households by relationship to head of household, marital status and sex.
*6. Population by single years of age and sex.
*7. Population by five-year age groups and sex.
*8. Population by marital status, age and sex.
*9. Native and foreign-born population by age and sex.
*10. Foreign-born population by country of birth, age and sex.
11. Native population by major civil division of birth, age and sex.
*12. Population . . . years of age and over by type of activity, age and sex.
13. Population not economically active by functional categories, age and sex.
*14. Economically active population by industry, age and sex.
*15. Economically active population by occupation, age and sex.

Once the information was on tape, the Bureau of Census and Statistics was able to print out the first tables of statistical data, and information will continue to be provided for the next four years. The computer programme had taken the equivalent of three man-years to write, but the process has enabled the Bureau to publish, with minimum delay, an increasing amount of important information.

Table **3/2** lists the tabulations suggested for a population census by the United Nations.

THE CONTROLS TO MAINTAIN PRIVACY

One of the characteristics of the mid-twentieth century is the increasing invasion of privacy by an increasing number of governmental and private agencies, such as credit bureaux, security agencies and the like. Evidence from the U.S.A. indicates that the Armed Forces has data on a very considerable number of citizens, and this data is constantly up-dated and added to existing information retained in computer tape information banks from which it can be retrieved. Because of this, many people fear that census information may be used, at some later date, to the disadvantage of the individual, or to identify and persecute a minority group.

These fears are more imaginary than real. Every nation which conducts a census has strict laws about the confidentiality of the information obtained, and this is ensured in several ways. Firstly, the census data is available only as aggregative statistics, not as data relating to actual persons or households. As mentioned, in most censuses the smallest aggregation is the census collector's area, which comprises at least 100 to 150 households. Secondly, census forms are kept secret for a long period, or as in Australia, are destroyed after the information has been coded. Since the information excludes the name of the individual, confidentiality is obtained after the destruction of the questionnaires. Thirdly, in the case of direct enumeration by a trained census collector, most countries ensure privacy by insisting that no collector may work in any area in which he also lives.

That these controls are not sufficiently publicized is shown by the outcry which arose in Britain and Australia before their respective 1971 censuses. In Australia, in 1971, the census form demanded that the name of the respondent and other personal details were written on the form; opponents of this questioned the need for the information. The Bureau of Census and Statistics replied that the information was needed for several important reasons. Firstly, the names and addresses of respondents were required for collection control purposes, to enable the collector to keep his records straight, and so that he could call back at the house if data was missing. Secondly, they enabled the Bureau of Census to check back if the collector had made omissions on the forms. Thirdly, they were used for family analysis coding and help in allocating sex in forms lacking this information. Fourthly, they enabled the Bureau to make a 0·25 per cent post-enumeration survey to check the accuracy of the way in which the census collectors had checked the forms. The Bureau also stressed that confidentiality was maintained, as neither the name or address was transferred to the magnetic tapes.

For census data to be collected accurately, it must be ensured that the people understand the need for the questions to be asked, and can be fully assured that no information given will permit any authority to identify the informant, at any future time.

THE REDUCTION OF ERROR

Since the data is obtained by many enumerators of varying education, training and ability from the residents in the country who have a wide range of educational ability, prejudices, opinions, integrity, honesty and motivation to answer the questions accurately, it can be understood that the census data will not be free from error. A few countries have managed to obtain a very high degree of accuracy and precision, most manage moderate accuracy, and a few national censuses are so inaccurate that they are almost worthless for any purpose.

In evaluating the accuracy of the census data, demographers have noted two main errors: those of coverage and those of classification. Errors of coverage arise from a failure to count all of the population, or from counting some of the population twice. Of the two, failure to enumerate is most common. This is because the enumerator may find difficulty in making contact with every household in his census area, either because he is not well motivated, or because the householder is elusive. He may make contact with the householder, but fail to enumerate the household correctly. In strong patriarchal societies, women members of the household may be forgotten by the informant; in most societies small children, particularly babies, tend to be omitted unless the enumerator follows this questionnaire systematically and accurately. If the form is long, both enumerator and informant may tire and enter inaccurate data. Lest it is thought that such behaviour is found only in developing countries, it is believed that despite checks and other complicated precautions, the 1970 census in the U.S.A. underenumerated the population by about 2·5 per cent. Those omitted were mainly non-white and young adult males.

Errors in classification are even more likely. Age, marital status, occupation and fertility are frequently incorrectly recorded. It has been found that if the question asked is 'How old are you?', the results in developed nations tend to 'heap' at ages ending in 0 or 5. (In Australia, this is minimized by asking for both years and months of age.) In all nations, children under the age of 1 tend to be omitted. If the question is phrased 'When were you born?', it is claimed that the information is more likely to be correct, although there is some doubt. For example, in Australia, it is believed that young people are more likely to know their age, whilst older people have often forgotten their age, but can remember the year of their birth. Thus it is clear that the question 'When were you born?' will only be answered correctly in nations whose population is motivated to know about dates of birth. In addition, the respondent may give false information for reasons of his own, or the enumerator may forget to ask a question and later when checking his form may find the omission and guess the answer. Fertility statistics tend to be inaccurate, as information about abortions, either spontaneous or induced, is not sought, and in many nations stillbirths are neither enquired about nor recorded. In general, only information about live born children who are still alive at the time of the census is sought. Occupation statistics also tend to be erroneous, as low status jobs are up-graded by the respondent in his answer.

There is, yet, no perfect way to determine the amount of error in a national census. As mentioned, one technique is to re-enumerate a sample of the population, using specially selected census collectors for this purpose. These enumerators are highly trained, well motivated and good communicators, and are taught to be very thorough. The sample re-enumeration field check is made as soon as possible after the census, and the degree of error is calculated. The technique is fairly complex. (1) The sample selected must be representative of the whole nation and of all population groups; (2) The re-enumeration is made, usually, a few weeks later, with differently framed questions; (3) The answers in the two census forms are compared, schedule by schedule; (4) If a discrepancy is found, the enumerator returns to the household to ascertain which of the two answers was correct; (5) Finally, he tries to determine why a wrong answer was given. The purpose of this exercise is to measure the error in data obtained, and obtain information so that questions wrongly answered can be re-framed in the next census. Despite the errors, the value of a national census is considerable and trained demographers with access to other data, especially that obtained by accurate registration of births and deaths, can extract valuable information even from censuses of only moderate accuracy.

Registration of Events

National censuses are complicated to organize, expensive to conduct and only give a picture of the population at a specific time. Continuous registration of demographic events—births, deaths, marriages, divorces and migration measure change in population in the period between censuses, and enable trends in population dynamics to be computed. Registration of vital events is fairly sophisticated and requires a well-trained, well-motivated staff and a cooperative population if completeness, accuracy and reliability are to be obtained. Such accuracy is obtained in Australia, the Netherlands, the Scandinavian countries, Great Britain and a few other nations, but in many nations of the world, population registration is inadequate. In most of Africa, Asia and Latin America, between 20 and 35 per cent of births are not registered; infant deaths fail to be notified, and movement over national borders is unrecorded, whilst statistics for marriage and divorce are ignored. If registration of demographic events is to be of any real value, improvement is urgently needed.

In countries where registration is reasonably accurate and complete, certification of the event is made, and a copy of the certificate is given to the informant. The document is of legal importance; a birth certificate giving evidence of citizenship, a death certificate permission for burial, and a marriage certificate confirming a legal change in status.

The high degree of completeness, accuracy and efficiency of registration in the developed countries mentioned earlier is not only because these countries have evolved a highly organized society, but also because the birth certificate is needed to obtain employment, and to obtain social security benefits, including an old-age pension, whilst the death certificate is necessary to settle insurance claims and indeed to permit burial. The copy of the form which is retained by the registrar is usually deposited in a central office, and is retained should the individual's status be queried subsequently.

The information is given by an informant, usually a near relative, or someone well acquainted with the person involved, and a standard form is completed. The content of this form varies, depending whether it is a birth certificate, a death certificate or a marriage certificate, and which nation has devised the form.

Tabulations from the collected certificates are made at intervals. These are published from time to time during the year, and an annual report is produced.

Sample Surveys

Sample surveys are conducted at regular intervals by Census and Statistics Bureaux to obtain information on matters not normally included in a national census, or under regulations controlling registration of vital events. The methods used are those outlined for the national census and the nature of the sample is carefully determined so that the information obtained does, in fact, give a reasonable representation of the entire group sampled.

Problems Associated with Poor Registration

The United Nations population division considered that in 1965 'whilst nearly all the population in the economically more advanced regions of the world is covered by "complete" birth registration statistics, such data are available for countries containing only 40 per cent of the estimated population in Middle and South America, 8 per cent in Asia (outside the U.S.S.R.), and a mere 2 per cent in Africa'. By 1971, the situation had improved somewhat, but registration of vital events was still below 60 per cent in Middle and South America, below 30 per cent in Asia, and below 10 per cent of the estimated population of Africa.

One of the problems which improved registration of vital events has produced is related to the impact of family planning. For example, if a family planning campaign leads, incidentally, to the better registration of births, as rural people become less frightened of the authorities, the data may appear to show that the campaign has been a failure, since the birth rate is not being reduced, and may be increasing. A little thought shows that the increase is due to better registration of births, not to increased natality.

The influence of poor registration may be reduced by carrying out sample surveys, provided these are well planned, and the questions to be asked are well constructed. Sample surveys, usually multipurpose, are being carried out increasingly in many developing nations. One problem of a multipurpose survey is that the large number of questions, to be asked in a limited time, places a heavy burden both on the interviewer and on the respondent with the result that the latter becomes confused or bored and answers inaccurately, and the former, having failed to complete all the sections at the interview, completes it later with inaccurate data. Less elaborate sample surveys, which seek to obtain less information, are more accurate, and this is increased if the same sample is re-surveyed at determined intervals. However, such a scheme is not only difficult to mount, but may be resented by the people surveyed (Maudlin).

The Methodology of Demography

Once the raw data have been converted into computer readable form, a variety of demographic methodological processes can be initiated, so that the answers to the original questions can be obtained. It will be recalled that these relate to (1) the size of the population under scrutiny, (2) its distribution within the country, and (3) its composition. In addition, data from consecutive censuses, and from annual reports of vital events, are used to obtain a vital, dynamic view of the population studies, and to determine the rate of population change. The methodology used by demographers is considered in the next chapter.

FOUR

The Methodology of Population Dynamics

The figures obtained from the national census, and regularly from registration of births and deaths are actual or absolute numbers. From the statistics it is easy to calculate the number of people in the population aged 65 and over, or the number of births in a given year. Whilst such information is valuable for planning social security pensions, or school facilities, it is often far more informative to know how many elderly people there are in the population *relative* to its total numbers. Relative numbers are the stuff of population dynamics, for in the form of ratios and rates they enable the demographer to compare the behaviour of one population, or part of a population, with that of another.

Ratios

In many nations, births are not registered consistently or are not reported to a central bureau of statistics so that measures of the fertility (natality) of the nation cannot be computed. In such nations it may be easier to obtain counts of the number of children aged 0 to 4, and of the number of women aged 15 to 44 or 15 to 49. The number of young children per 1,000 women of childbearing age, is a ratio. The example just given is, in fact, used in demography if more precise measures of natality are not required, or are not available, and is termed the child–woman ratio. The higher the child–woman ratio, the higher the natality.

The child–woman ratio =

$$\frac{\text{The number of children aged 0–4 on a specific date}}{\text{The number of women aged 15–49 on the same date}} \times 1{,}000$$

A ratio can be defined as a single term which indicates the relative size of two numbers. If a is one number and b is the other, a ratio between the two is a/b, which is the same as saying a divided by b. This ratio measures the size of the first number in terms of the second, and is one way of saying that there are so many a per unit of b.

The child–woman ratio in Britain according to the 1971 census was 336. This means that there were 336 children under the age of 5 for every 1,000 women aged 15 to 49. In Table **4/1**, the child–woman ratio of several nations is shown. It will be observed that the ratio is much higher in the developing nations, and amongst women living in rural areas in most nations.

Table 4/1

Child–woman ratios

	Nation	*Year*	*Urban*	*Rural*	*Total*
Developing	Nigeria	1963	554	683	662
	Egypt	1960	706	700	702
	Colombia	1960	547	826	619
	Mexico	1960	676	783	726
	India	1961	617	668	659
	Iran	1966	746	921	851
Developed	France	1968	288	325	298
	Ireland	1966	503	542	521
	Sweden	1965	303	300	303
	U.K.	1971	329	361	336
	Australia	1966	399	565	423

Child–woman ratio =

$$\frac{\text{Number of children 0–4 in the population}}{\text{Number of women aged 15–49 in the same population}} \times 1{,}000$$

Source: *Demographic Yearbook*, 1969. U.N., New York.

Another important ratio in population dynamics is the *sex ratio* of a nation. This is defined as the number of males in a population divided by the number of females. Since the result of this calculation is usually a number just above or below 1, it is usually multiplied by 100 to make the ratio easier to comprehend.

The sex ratio can then be stated as:

$$\text{Sex ratio: } \frac{\text{Number of males in the population}}{\text{Number of females in the population}} \times 100$$

Proportions and Per Cents

A proportion is a particular kind of ratio, and can be defined as showing the ratio of one part to the whole. It is found by dividing the whole number into the part number. For example, it is of some interest in determining the population dynamics of a particular nation to know the number of women aged 15 to 49 to the total population, as this will give a crude index of the fecundity (or biological ability to bear children) of the population. The value of this ratio is always between 0 and 1, so for easy comprehension it is multiplied by 100. The proportion is then termed a *per cent* value.

In the 1971 census in Australia, there were 3,023,700 women aged 15 to 49, and the total population was 12,728,461. The proportion of women aged 15 to 49 can be calculated as 0·239. If this proportion, 0·239, is multiplied by 100, it indicates that 23·9 per cent of the total population of Australia were women of reproductive age. In algebraic terms, a proportion has the form $a/(a+b)$.

Per cent values and distribution

Per cent values are much more easily understood than proportions, and similarly per cent distribution may make the study of a population more intelligible.

For example, the 1966 Fijian Census showed that the population was just over 450,000. Apart from small European and Chinese communities, the Fijian population was divided into 190,288 Fijians of Polynesian origin, and 240,960 Fijians of Indian origin. The two races tended to be separated by culture, by religion and by attitudes during colonial rule. If the population of two racial groups is divided into age groups, as in Table **4/2**, it will be seen that the Indian–Fijians have 2·3 per cent more children in the 0–14 age group than the Polynesian–Fijians. This implies that if population growth rates continue, the Indian–Fijian population will grow at a faster rate than the Polynesian–Fijian population: a matter of some concern to politicians and sociologists alike. However, Fiji has embarked on a birth control campaign with considerable success, so that potential discord may be averted. The information derived from this Table is obtained by analysis of the composition of the population and has several practical uses, which are considered in later chapters.

Table 4/2

Age distribution of the two main racial groups in Fiji

	Numbers		*Percent*	
	Fijian	*Indian*	*Fijian*	*Indian*
0–14	89,680	119,156	47·1	49·4
15–65	95,144	119,092	50·0	49·4
65–	5,464	2,712	2·9	1·2
	190,288	240,960	100·0	100·0

Source: Fijian Census, 1966.

In the analysis of the characteristics of a population, the demographer has to decide what question he intends to ask. He may, for example, want to know the marital status of the female population over a certain age as this will affect the fertility of the nation. To obtain this information he has to divide the female population over that age into appropriate categories, such as single (or never-married), still married, married but separated, divorced and widowed. From these data he can construct a table, and derive the percentage distribution of women. If he wishes, he can separate women who live in urban areas from those who live in rural areas, as the U.S. Bureau of Census has done in the 1970 census. This procedure gives an additional refinement to the information and is known as a '*spatial differential*'. As can be seen in Table **4/3**, the original census statistics are difficult to understand and compare, since the totals in the columns and rows are of considerable magnitude and are all different. The interpretation is made much easier by dividing the total in each sub-group by the total of the group and multiplying by 100. This gives the percentage distribution. In Table **4/3** it can be seen that there are fewer single women in rural areas, that marriages appear more stable (as fewer women are separated or divorced), and perhaps last longer (as there are fewer widows). But it must be remembered that percentage distribution only gives proportionate or relative size. For accurate understanding the total numbers must also be stated in any table. In Table **4/3,** nearly three times as many married women lived in urban areas as in rural areas, merely because so many more of the U.S. population are urban dwellers. However, when the percentage distribution of married women is obtained, there are proportionately less married women in urban areas as might be expected.

Table 4/3

Marital status of the female population, aged 14 or more, in urban and rural areas of the United States in 1970
(*in thousands of persons*)

Marital status	*Total*	*Urban*	*Rural*
Total	77,915	58,395	19,520
Single	17,459	13,562	3,896
Married (except separated)	45,964	33,188	12,776
Separated	1,799	1,547	252
Widowed	9,624	7,456	2,168
Divorced	3,069	2,641	428
Percentage distribution			
Total	100·0	100·0	100·0
Single	22·4	23·2	20·0
Married	59·0	56·8	65·4
Separated	2·3	2·6	1·3
Widowed	12·4	12·8	11·1
Divorced	3·9	4·5	2·2

Source: *United States Summary: General Population Characteristics.* Table 54, 1970 Census.

PERCENTAGE POINT DIFFERENCES

If the tables of percentage distribution become complex, as may happen, the reader may find it difficult to remember the comparisons and the table may lose its value. This problem can be overcome by calculating *percentage point differences.* In this technique the *differences* in the distribution of each group are compared with the percentage distribution of the total group. In Table **4/4** (which is based on Table **4/3**), it can be seen that the number of single women comprised 22·4 per cent of the total females aged 14 or more. The plus or minus difference between this percentage, that of the total urban single females (+0·8 per cent) and the rural single females (−2·4 per cent), enables a new table of percentage point differences to be constructed. From this table it can be established that a woman living on a farm is more likely to be married, and if married more likely to remain still married, than her sister living in the city.

Table 4/4

Percentage point differences and index of relative composition between total and urban or rural residence, United States 1970

Marital Status	*Urban*	*Rural*
Percentage point differences		
Total	0·0	0·0
Single	+0·8	−2·4
Married (except separated)	−2·2	+6·4
Separated	+0·3	−1·0
Widowed	+0·4	−1·3
Divorced	+0·6	−1·7
Index of dissimilarity	−2·2	+6·4

There are several major conceptual problems in the use of percentage point differences. One is that the differentials are influenced by the size of the percentage from which they were derived. Thus Table **4/4** fails to show that there is a much lower incidence of divorce amongst rural than amongst urban women as the percentage point difference appears small, but the actual number of divorced women is much higher amongst the 58·4 million women living in urban areas than amongst the 19·5 million rural women. There were 2·6 million divorced women in the urban areas, and only 0·4 million in the rural areas.

RATES

A rate is a ratio, which has the additional characteristic of relating what has happened *during a certain unit of time*, which in population dynamics is usually one year. The most commonly used rates relate to births and deaths, and since these are vital events, the rates are called 'vital statistics rates' or 'vital-rates'. Vital-rates answer the question: how much per unit of what per year. In other words, they measure the frequency of occurrence of demographic events over a period of time. The first computation is a crude one, so called because it shows the frequency of a demographic event throughout the entire population, without regard to smaller groups which might sometimes give a more accurate picture of what is happening (see Chapter 6).

The crude birth rate is calculated as:

Crude birth rate =

$$\frac{\text{Total births registered during the calendar year}}{\text{Total estimated population at mid-year}} \times 1{,}000$$

Thus, the crude birth rate in Australia in 1971 was 21·67.

The crude death rate is computed in a similar manner, by merely replacing the total births registered by the total deaths registered.

This calculation demands that the demographer computes the mid-year population. If registration of births, deaths, migration is accurate and reported annually, the calculation is made by the formula

$$P_1 + \tfrac{1}{2}(P_2 - P_1).$$

In this formula P_1 is the number of people recorded as living in the country at the beginning of the year; P_2 the number at the beginning of the next year.

If vital statistics registration is less accurate, the rate of population change can be calculated and examples are given in G. W. Barclay's 'Techniques of Population Analysis' (see Bibliography).

AGE-SPECIFIC RATES

In many cases the crude rates are not adequate for demographic analysis and more precise measures are required. One measure is to calculate the rates for subgroupings of the population. For example, since only women aged 15–49 are likely to conceive, a more accurate measure of the fertility of the population would be to calculate the general natality rate. (It should be mentioned that some nations take the upper age limit to be 44 years.)

General Natality (Fertility) Rate =

$$\frac{\text{Births to women aged 15–49}}{\text{Mid-year female population 15–49}} \times 1{,}000$$

Within this overall fertility, it might be valuable to know at what age natality (i.e. the actual bearing of children) was highest. This information can be obtained by calculating age-specific natality rates.

Age-specific birth rate =

$$\frac{\text{Births to women aged } x}{\text{Mid-year female population of age } x} \times 1{,}000$$

Usually age-specific rates are calculated for 5-year grouping of ages. The age-specific birth rate of two countries reporting in 1967 is shown in Table **4/5**. The two nations chosen are Sweden, which is a developed nation where birth control is widely accepted and used, and the Philippines, a developing nation with a low acceptance of contraception. The effects of these events are shown in the different age specific birth rates, and it will be observed that the purpose of the calculation is to compute the incidence of a particular demographic event.

It can be stated generally,

The rate of incidence of the event =

$$\frac{\text{Number of events occurring during a time interval}}{\text{Population exposed to the risk of the event during that interval.}}$$

It will be appreciated that age-specific death rates, age-specific migration rates, and age-specific marriage rates can be calculated in just the same way as age-specific birth rates.

Standardized Rates

Specific rates, although more precise, make understanding more complicated, as there are many small groups to compare.

Table 4/5

How the age-specific birth (fertility or natality) rate is calculated (Sweden and the Philippines, 1967)

Sweden 1967

Age group	*Births to women of age*	*Females of age*	*Age-specific birth rate*
Total 15–49	121,360	3,700,473	58
15–19	13,823	608,423	25
20–24	43,254	632,182	135
25–29	35,956	490,430	146
30–34	17,855	442,285	82
35–39	8,133	468,312	35
40–44	2,177	522,300	9
45–49	162	536,541	0·6

Philippines 1967

Age group	*Births to women of age*	*Females of age*	*Age-specific birth rates*
Total 15–49	828,015	7,574,000	86
15–19	73,854	1,802,000	19
20–24	204,427	1,472,000	185
25–29	230,432	1,208,000	194
30–34	164,795	996,000	141
35–39	112,480	822,000	139
40–44	35,675	689,000	52
45–49	6,352	585,000	11

On the other hand, although crude rates give a much clearer picture of the dynamics of the population, they are too inaccurate for research purposes. For example, the difference in the crude birth rate of two nations may be due to differences in the composition of the population, rather than to the effect of a specific measure.

It may be of interest to compare the natality of two or more nations. Since their age composition differs, the difference in natality may be that in one there is a preponderance of old people and children compared with the other, rather than any biological difference in natality. In order to control this variable of age, the age-specific birth rates of the populations are compared by using an age structure of a 'standard' population. The standard population used (in the example) is a total of one million females (known as a 'standard million') distributed according to the estimated age composition (in 5-year age groups) of the world in a specific year (at present 1960 is usually chosen). The total number of births this standard million would have in a specific year if it had the age-specific birth rates of the populations under study can then be calculated. This is done by multiplying the age-specific birth rates of the populations by the number of women of each 5-year age group in the standard population. The result is then divided by 1,000,000 and multiplied by 1,000 (or, more simply, divided by 1,000), to obtain an age-standardized birth rate per 1,000 for the populations studied. The differences between the standardized rates for the two populations are differences in pure natality, and not the differences of the age distribution of women in the populations. The procedure is termed direct standardization.

This may be clearer with an example shown in Table **4/6**. If one wishes to compare the natality of Singapore, which by 1968 was introducing family planning on a large scale, with that of Scotland, which had some voluntary family planning, and Ireland, where birth control measures are prohibited, the mean general natality rate in Singapore and Ireland is almost identical, whilst that in Scotland is lower. However, when direct standardization is applied, it is found that, in fact, the general natality rate of Singapore is 133·6, that of Ireland 109·2 and that of Scotland 80·7. In other words, the population in Singapore is growing faster than that of Ireland, despite the fact that Ireland does not permit contraception, and Singapore encourages it. In the same year the crude birth rate for Singapore was 23, for Ireland it was 22 and for Scotland it was 17. It can be seen that standardized rates give more real information of population dynamics than the crude birth rates since they enable the demographer to analyse the factor of natality in two or more nations, whilst holding constant the factor of age.

Table 4/6

Direct standardization

Age group	*Standard Population world* (1960) (1)	*World Age-specific birth rates* (2)	*Singapore Age-specific birth rates* (1968) (3)	*Scotland Age-specific birth rates* (1968) (4)	*Ireland A.S.B.R* (1968) (5)	*Age Standardized Births* *Singapore*	*Scotland*	*Ireland*
15–19	195,827	78·5	14·5	22·7	6·7	2,839	4,445	1,312
20–24	174,139	246·0	170·1	168·5	135·2	29,621	29,342	23,544
25–29	153,801	283·3	243·5	176·8	22·1	37,450	27,192	3,399
30–34	139,763	212·3	153·5	102·3	197·0	21,454	14,297	27,533
35–39	125,761	132·1	85·7	48·5	133·9	10,778	6,099	16,839
40–44	111,878	56·1	36·3	12·1	48·4	4,061	1,354	5,415
45–49	198,231	10·9	7·2	0·7	4·1	1,472	139	813
General Natality Rate		155·7	82·8	68·3	81·0	133,675	80,768	109,255
			Singapore	Scotland	Ireland	133·6	80·7	109·2

Ratio: Singapore $\frac{133{\cdot}6}{155{\cdot}7} = 0{\cdot}85$ Scotland $\frac{80{\cdot}7}{155{\cdot}7} = 0{\cdot}51$ Ireland $\frac{109{\cdot}2}{155{\cdot}7} = 0{\cdot}70$

The standardized birth rates can also be compared by expressing them as a ratio of the rate for the standard population. In Table **4/6**, it can be seen that the sum of the age-specific birth rates (which is termed the general natality rate) in Singapore is 0·85 times that of the world, that of Scotland is 0·51 as large and that of Ireland 0·70 times as large.

Table 4/7

Indirect standardization, using Cambodia as an example

Age group	*Age Composition of Cambodia* (1)	*Standard Age-specific rates for world* (2)	*Expected births* (1 × 2 ÷ 1,000) (3)
15–19	238,613	78·5	18,731·1
20–24	213,548	246·0	52,532·8
25–29	190,122	283·3	53,861·6
30–34	172,967	212·3	36,720·9
35–39	143,712	132·1	18,984·3
40–44	118,602	56·1	6,653·6
45–49	102,977	10·9	1,122·4
Total	1,180,541	155·7	188,606·7

The expected indirect standardized general natality rate for Cambodia is:

Col. 3 ÷ Col.1

or

$$\frac{188{,}607}{1{,}180{,}541} \times 1000 = 160$$

Source: 1962 Census. *Demographic Yearbook*, 1970. U.N., New York.

From the example given it will be seen that direct standardization requires that a table of age-specific rates is available. Unfortunately, age-specific rates are unavailable for some nations, and are unusual for different parts of a nation, for example, specific rural areas, or industrial towns. Since natality may be influenced by factors relating to domicile or to occupation, another method has to be adopted. This is *indirect standardization*. The method is (1) to determine the age composition of the area under study, (2) to calculate age-specific birth rates for the 'standard million', (3) to calculate the expected age-specific births for the area under study by multiplying the number in each age group by the standard age-specific birth rate, and by dividing the result by 1,000. This will give the number of expected births in each age group. If these are totalled and then divided by the number of women aged 15–49 in the population, an indirect standardized general natality rate will be obtained.

This will be clearer if an example is given. The population of Cambodia was determined in a census held in 1962, and from tables available it was possible to compute the number of women between the ages of 15 and 49 in five-year groups. However, since there is no effective birth registration in Cambodia, no information about age-specific natality rates is available. If the demographer is anxious to obtain some indication of the natality in Cambodia he can carry out the calculations shown in Table **4/7**. Although this calculation is not too accurate, it does give some indication of natality and enables some projections to be made.

Rate of Population Change

One of the most important pieces of information in population dynamics is the rate of growth of the population. In population growth there are two components, the reproductive change, which is the difference between births and deaths, and the increase due to migration. If births exceed deaths, the reproductive change is positive, whilst if deaths exceed births it is negative. Since in the past three decades of this century at least, births have usually exceeded deaths, the reproductive change is positive, and this can be referred to as the *natural increase*. The term has been validly criticized by Bogue, since it implies that migration is less natural than reproductive growth. In this book it will be referred to as the *reproductive change*.

Migration may be positive or negative. The difference between immigration (or in-migration) and emigration (or out-migration) is termed *net migration*. In countries attracting migrants such as Australia, Brazil, Canada and the U.S.A., net migration can make a significant positive change to population growth, whilst in countries encouraging out-migration, such as Greece, or condoning it, such as Yugoslavia and Italy, it can reduce the rate of population growth significantly. This is considered further in Chapter 8.

The measure of the rate of population change can be expressed:

Rate of population change =

$$\frac{\text{Births less deaths plus net migration}}{\text{Mid-year population}} \times 1{,}000$$

FIVE

The Composition of Population

The composition of populations varies very considerably, particularly in regard to sex and age. In the years after World War I, the sex ratio in France was well below unity, indicating that the loss of young men during the war years had markedly affected the sex ratio. Similar demographic events occurred in Germany and the U.S.S.R. after World War II. In the 1956 census of West Germany, the sex ratio was 88·3, whilst that of the U.S.S.R. in 1959 was 81·9. By contrast the British census of 1961 showed a sex ratio of 93·7, and that of the U.S.A. in 1960 of 97·1.

The effect of age on a population is also considerable, and the age composition of far-reaching consequence. With good preventive medicine, which eliminates or reduces infectious disease; with good nutrition throughout life, which increases the resistance of the individual to infection; and with good curative medicine, which deals effectively with acquired disease, people are living longer. In most countries there is a tendency for people to cease work at about the age of 60 to 65, so that an increasing number of old people, who are now dependent on others, continue to live and require goods and services. The proportion of old people in the population will obviously affect the socio-economic objectives of the nation, as will the proportion of young people in the community.

These two variables in the composition of the population, sex and age distribution, influence each other. These and the variable of marital status are considered in this chapter.

From conception to birth the ratio between the sexes of the embryo and fetus is about unity. In the first years of life more females die than do males, but by puberty this has been reversed. From puberty onwards, at every stage of life, more males than females die, at least in nations where the female is given as much medical attention as the male. The effect of this becomes most marked after the age of 50, and in old age there are more women alive than men (Figure **5/1**). The sex ratio of a population describes these facts, and the ratio for selected countries and at selected ages can be seen in Table **5/1**. It will be observed that what has been just written applies particularly to Western type countries; it does not appear to apply so well to Asian nations. This may be factual, or may be due to under-reporting of female births, or to a relatively higher female mortality due to neglect because of the inferior status of women.

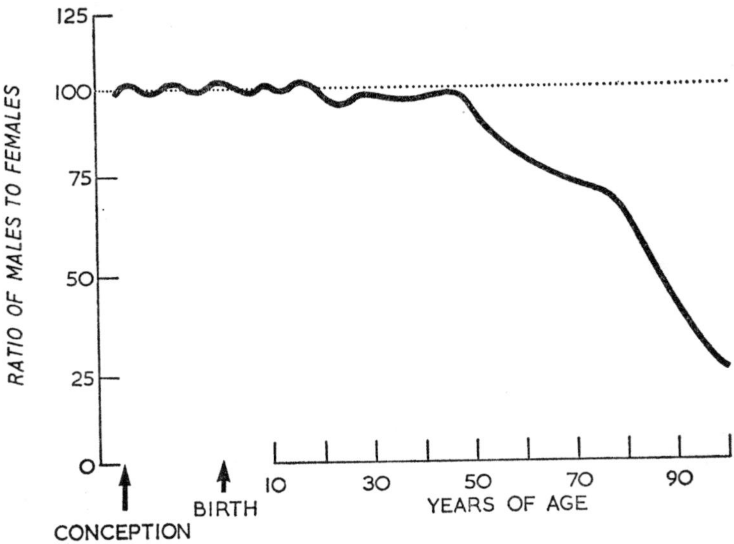

Figure **5/1** The changing sex ratio with age.
Source: Stevenson, A. C., and Bobrow, M. *J. Med. Genet.*, **4**, 190, 1967.

The sex ratio at birth in most countries is about 105; by the age of 15 it has fallen to between 98 and 102, and it remains about this until the age of 45, when it tends to fall progressively. Variants from this pattern will be found in countries after wars have eliminated large numbers of young men, in countries where the maternal mortality is high and sick women are neglected, and in countries where migration of males is common.

In the examples shown in Table **5/1**, the changes in the sex-ratio in the U.S.A. are typical for most developed nations in

Table 5/1

The sex ratio related to age, for four nations, 1967 statistics

All ages	*U.S.A.*	*Australia**	*India*	*Chile*
0–4	104	105	105	100
10–14	104	105	104	100
20–24	94	106	106	98
30–34	96	106	105	99
40–44	96	108	107	98
50–54	95	100	115	92
60–64	88	98	112	90
70–74	64	72	96	79

$$\text{Sex ratio} = \frac{\text{Number of males in the population}}{\text{Number of females in the population}} \times 100$$

* Affected by migration.

which migration is limited. The pattern for Australia shows the effect of encouraged migration, particularly of single men in the 20 to 40 age groups, whilst that of India shows how the relative neglect of the health care of women can maintain a high sex-ratio into the older age-groups. In most nations the sex ratio is sufficiently close to 100 to ensure that prevalent cultural patterns are not markedly distorted by a shortage of one or another sex. In fact, the sex composition of a population does not appear to influence its so-called ‘national characteristics’. The sex ratio in the aggressively oriented Germany of the 1930s, was not markedly different from that of peace-loving Switzerland. This is of course merely saying that masculinity *per se* does not necessarily denote aggressiveness, which is an acquired, not an inherited, characteristic, and is not necessarily a solely male characteristic.

Age Composition

The social and economic structure of any society is obviously influenced by its age composition. In a society where the birth rate is high and the death rate low or decreasing, there will be a considerable proportion of the population dependent on the others. Those too young to work will require food, shelter, care, health services and education; those too old to work will also require support. The cost of this dependency will be borne by those who are economically active. In a society where the birth rate is low, and the age of death is rising, because of good nutrition throughout life, the absence of communicable disease and good health care, ageing of the population occurs with its attendant problems. For example, the present cohort (or population group) of old people can be supported by their children; but when the latter become old, will *their* children be sufficiently numerous to support them? Both types of society described exist today. The former is typical of the developing countries, the latter of the developed nations of the world. It is obvious that the age composition of a society is a fundamental demographic variable, and one which is of considerable importance when plans are made for social and economic change. Unless reasonably accurate data can be obtained, proper planning is impossible.

Age-Composition Data

1. *Five-year categories*

The age composition of a nation is usually obtained on asking a question on the national census, and in the intercensal years by adjusting the composition with statistics supplied by the reports of the registration of vital events. The accuracy of the data will depend on the way in which the question is put and on the reliability of the informant. If the informant is asked: 'How old were you last birthday?', experience has shown that the ages reported 'heap' considerably at ages ending with 0 or 5. Greater accuracy will be obtained if the questioner asks, 'In what year were you born?', but even so errors are likely. The effect of the errors is far less if the age classification is based on five-year categories rather than single-year categories, and such a classification is more than adequate for many demographic purposes.

2. *Median age*

If a demographer wishes to compare the age structure of several nations, the simplest, but least informative method is to find the median age of each nation. The median age is that age which divides a population into two equal parts, half lying above the median age, and half below it. In more developed countries there has been a steady rise in the median age over the past 100 years, mainly because of the reduction of the effect of communicable diseases. In the developing countries, the higher birth rate and lower infant death rate of recent years has reduced the median age, and in most the median age is below that of the developed nations. In fact it is possible to relate the degree of development to the median age. Developing countries will be found to have a median age below 25, whilst developed countries will have a median age above that figure.

3. *Dependency ratio*

The median age is a poor way of describing the age distribution of a population. Much more useful is the 'dependency ratio', which itself is derived from a percentage distribution of the population. If the total population is divided into age groups, and the percentage falling into each is calculated, a table can be produced comparing the developed and the developing nations. However, although all the population are consumers, requiring food, shelter, clothing, health care and some education, not all are producers. In most countries very few children younger than 15 are full producers, and only a few people aged 65 or more are fully employed. These two groups, the young aged 0 to 14 and the old aged 65 and over, are dependent (for most things) on the population aged 15 to 64. The dependency ratio measures the impact of age composition on the economy and is:

$$\text{Dependency ratio} = \frac{\text{Population under 15} + \text{65 years and over}}{\text{Population 15 to 64}} \times 100$$

Examination of the definition of dependency shows that the ratio has two parts, each of which can be calculated separately. The first measures the dependency load of youth, and the second the dependency load of the aged.

The youth dependency ratio is calculated by dividing the number of people aged 15 to 64 into the number of people under the age of 15 and multiplying the result by 100. Similarly the aged-dependency ratio is calculated by dividing the percentage of the population aged 65 or more by the percentage of the population aged 15 to 64, and multiplying the result by 100. These ratios are shown in Table **5/2** for certain selected countries.

In a way, the decision to call the lower limit of economic activity, 15 and the upper, 64 is arbitrary. In many developing

Table 5/2

Dependency ratios of representative nations
(*latest available year*)

Nation	*Population percentage distribution by age*			*Dependency ratio*		
	0–14 *years*	15–64 *years*	65 *and over*	*Youth*	*Aged*	*Total*
Africa						
Kenya	46	49	5	94	10	104
Nigeria	43	55	2	78	4	82
U.A.R.	43	54	3	80	6	86
Americas						
Canada	34	58	8	60	13	73
Chile	40	56	3	71	5	76
Colombia	47	50	3	94	5	99
Mexico	44	52	4	85	7	92
U.S.A.	29	61	10	47	16	63
Asia						
Iran	46	51	3	92	6	98
India	41	56	3	73	5	78
Malaysia	44	53	3	85	6	91
Thailand	46	52	3	88	6	94
Europe						
France	25	63	12	40	19	59
Hungary	24	66	10	36	15	51
Italy	24	66	10	36	15	51
Sweden	21	66	13	32	19	51
U.K.	23	64	13	39	17	56
Oceania						
Australia	30	62	8	48	13	61

Source: *Demographic Yearbooks*, 1969–70. U.N., New York.

countries, children younger than 15 are economically active, but in such countries the upper age of work is often no more than 59 years as nutrition is poor, debilitating diseases such as hookworm and anaemia are common, and life is hard. In other countries, the control of infections, the relief of degenerative diseases, and active rehabilitation services permit people to work after the age of 65. However, in such countries the desire for education prevents many young people from seeking work under the age of 16 or 17. If these factors are taken into account, the arbitrariness of the definition is greatly reduced.

Study of Table **5/2** shows that the countries with the low youth dependency and high age dependency rather tend to be the developed industrial or post-industrial nations, which are mainly in Europe, North America and Australasia. On the other hand, countries of Asia, Africa and Latin America, which are developing economically, have high youth-dependency ratios, and low age-dependency ratios. Since the youth-dependency ratio is very high, it over-compensates for the low age-dependency ratio, and causes a much higher total dependency ratio than is found in the developed countries. The effect of this in retarding development of Asian, African and Latin-American nations is quite obvious. With increasing emphasis on preventive medicine, people are living longer, so that the numbers of old people in these countries is rising, at the same time as rising birth rates and lowered mortality in the economically active years are occurring.

In economic and social terms, aged-dependency is of much less consequence than youth dependency. The aged may have made savings during their working lives, or be in receipt of a pension; often they are taken into a family unit, and may have few needs apart from food and health care. The young, on the other hand, are more of an 'economic drag' as they require food, shelter, education, health care—and their expectations are greater. The minimum dependency load is that obtained by a society which is just replacing the deaths of the aged by the births of infants. In other words, there is a slight positive balance between natality and mortality. This leads to a slow population growth, which will not strain social or economic progress.

Currently, the developing countries, particularly, and the

developed countries to a lesser extent, have too high a birth rate and now that health care has advanced the age of death, the well-being, and perhaps survival, of all people will depend on fertility control.

It has been argued that such control will lead to an ageing population with a reduced youth-dependency rate, but a greatly increased age-dependency rate, and that this will impose severe economic and social strains on the population. However, the aim of population control is not necessarily to eliminate population growth (which in many countries would be almost impossible) but to create a better balance between births and deaths so that population growth is slow.

Age and Sex Composition

The difference in the age distribution of a nation and its sex composition can be determined by reading two sets of tables. In many cases, however, the demographer requires to know the age and sex composition of a population. Although by scanning the tables he can obtain this information, it is tedious work, and the information can be more clearly demonstrated in graphic form. One commonly used representation of the age and sex composition of the population is the 'population pyramid' or population profile.

Population profiles are of two kinds, being based either on absolute number or on percentage proportions. Profiles based on absolute numbers are more useful for comparing populations of similar size (Fig. **5/2**).

The proportional population pyramid is constructed by calculating the percentage distribution of the population simultaneously classified by age (in five-year age groups) and by sex. This pyramid is most useful for comparing the age and population structure of nations of different sizes, for whatever the *shape* of the pyramids their areas are identical.

In both forms of population profile, it is conventional to record age on the vertical axis, and to plot the numbers or percents of the population of each five-year age group along the horizontal axis. Male age groups are conventionally plotted on the left and female age groups on the right.

Although it is affected by past demographic events the

population profile gives a static picture of the age and sex composition of a population at a fixed point in time. To observe the effects of health control, of famines, of wars, of fertility

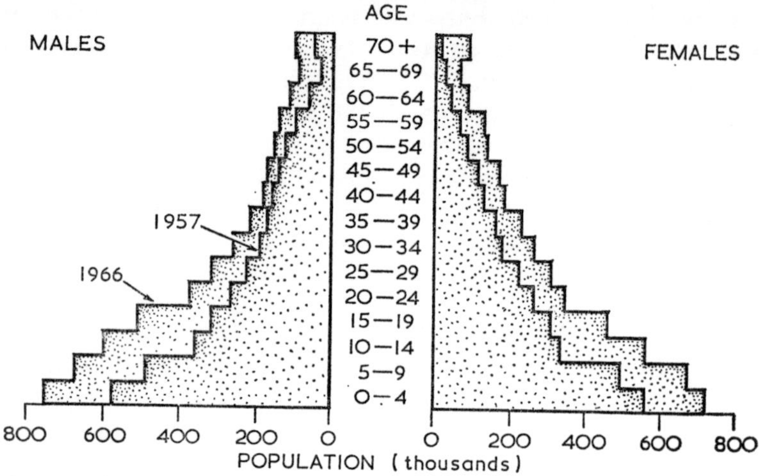

Figure **5/2** The population profile (or pyramid) of Malaya in 1957 and 1966.

control, of pestilence, a series of population profiles for a nation needs to be constructed and then compared. Without knowledge of the historical events, an explanation of the different shapes of the pyramid is hardly possible.

The Shape of the Population Pyramid

The shape of the pyramid will depend on the past and current natality and mortality patterns in the country. When the birth rate and death rate are high, as is usual in the developing countries, the pyramid has a broad base and gently sloping sides (Figure **5/3**). As preventive health measures are instituted, with purification of water supplies, improved infant nutrition and inoculation against infectious disease, the base of the pyramid becomes even broader and the slope eventually steeper (Figure **5/4**). If a campaign for fertility control is now started and is successful, the birth rate will fall, with the result that the base of the population pyramid will become pinched in the 0 to

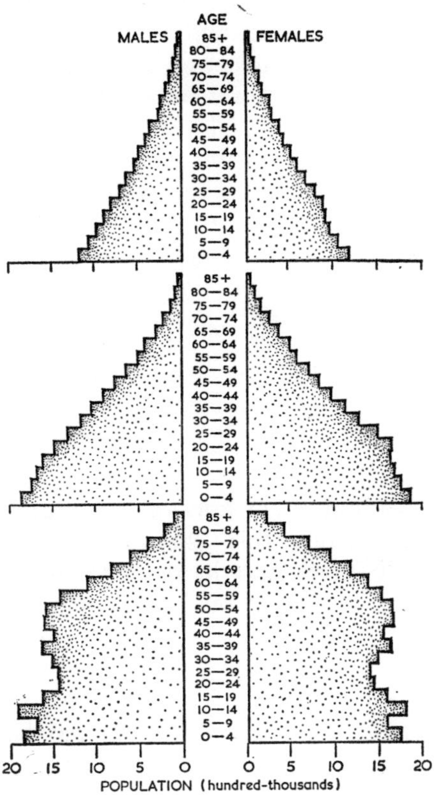

Figure **5/3** This population profile, or pyramid, is typical of developing nations with a high birth rate and a high death rate. It could be any one of a number of nations in Africa. In fact, it is that of England and Wales in the year 1851.

Figure **5/4** This population profile is typical of nations which have reduced the deaths of infants and children but have not yet controlled fertility, so that they are beginning to increase rapidly. A number of developing nations fall into this category, particularly in Latin America. In fact, this profile is that of England and Wales in 1901.

Figure **5/5** This population profile is typical of nations which have done much to control both fertility and mortality in the years before 65. It is typical of most developed nations. It is, in fact, that of England and Wales in 1961.

4 age group cohort. However, the 5 to 9 and the 10 to 14 cohorts will not be affected and will overhang the base. As health care becomes more effective, the age of death is delayed and the upper steps of the population pyramid become proportionately wider (Figure **5/5**). The effect of the health measures on control of mortality in infancy also means that more children reach the reproductive age, which will increase natality —more children being born with a resulting broadening of the base of the pyramid. These findings are illustrated in the accompanying population pyramids, and show the use of the technique in the study of population dynamics.

Marital Status

The 1960s have been characterized in Western countries by an apparent increasing permissiveness in sexual matters, a greater openness in discussion of sex and an apparent increase in consensual unions. Despite this changed attitude in Western countries, both in them and in the rest of the world, most conceptions which end in the birth of a child, lead to, or occur within, marriage. In studies in Australia, Britain and the U.S.A., it has been found that between 6 and 10 per cent of babies are born to single women, although it is likely that between 15 and 35 per cent of conceptions occur outside marriage, the couple marrying before the child is born. Other cultural patterns are found in other areas. In Central and Southern Africa, child marriage (before the age of 16) is usual. In India most girls are married between puberty and the age of 18; in Islamic countries early marriage is usual and conceptions outside marriage exceptional. In the Caribbean and South America, a married category in which the partners live together without a formal marriage is not uncommon, and between 5 and 20 per cent of marriages fall into this category. It is termed consensual union or 'conviviente', and is similar to de facto or common-law marriages of Anglo-Saxon nations.

It is apparent that marital status has a considerable influence on population dynamics. In fact, the key-index to population growth is not the number of fecund females, but the number of cohabiting fecund females. It is for this reason that marital status is studied here.

CLASSIFICATION OF MARITAL STATUS

In most countries census and registration forms require the informant to declare marital status.

When they analyse these data, demographers classify marital status into further groups, so that the effects of marriage may be studied more readily. These categories are:

- Never married (i.e. single)
- Ever married
  - Still married (or now married)
  - Separated (or married but permanently separated)
  - Divorced
  - Widowed

It must be admitted that many of the statistics gathered are inaccurate, as informants who have formed a consensual or common-law union may be reluctant to have this known, and will usually admit to marriage, implying that it is a legal union.

Since this book deals with population problems, only the never married, or the single, and the ever married (legally or de facto) who are living with their spouse will be considered at length. As far as population dynamics is concerned, divorce has little influence, as in most nations the divorce rate is only between 4 and 8 per cent of all marriages, and widowhood is a decreasing factor in population dynamics. However, both of these require consideration.

DIVORCE

Cultural attitudes and fashion have a considerable influence on a nation's attitude towards divorce. For example, in the U.S.A., the divorce rate is rising, and between 1960 and 1970 the rise was about 40 per cent. In Australia, the divorce rate rose by 37 per cent between 1966 and 1970: in 1966, about 8 per cent of marriages ended in divorce, and this had risen to 14 per cent by 1970. In Britain, and other developed industrial countries, a similar rise has occurred. There is a belief that divorces tend to occur most in the early years of marriage, but this is not found generally. For example, in Australia in 1970, only 10 per cent of marriages ending in divorce had lasted less than 5 years, whilst in the U.S.A. the figure was 35 per cent. In both countries divorcees were prone to remarry and to have children in the new marriage. It is also of interest to note that the Australian data showed that 34 per cent of divorces involved childless couples. The combined effect of these two factors is to reduce the effect of divorce on fertility. In non-Christian cultures, divorce statistics are difficult to obtain. In Islamic nations, for example, a man may divorce his wife with relative ease. In Buddhist and Hindu cultures, divorce, except because of infertility, is relatively uncommon.

It will be appreciated that in most societies, cultural behaviour either discourages divorce, or prevents the divorced person from remarrying. These attitudes are weakening, and in Western developed countries today about 20 per cent of divorced women remarry, and others form a de facto relationship. There are no reliable statistics for separation, whether permanent, or temporary, but in the U.S. separation appears to be as common as divorce, but a higher proportion of separated men and women have found other partners.

Widowhood

The effect of widowhood on population dynamics is also difficult to calculate. As general health measures improve, mortality of males (between the ages of 15 and 55) tends to fall, so that fewer fecund women are widowed. As an example of this trend India may be chosen, where for cultural and religious reasons a widow, since she may not remarry, is removed from childbearing. In the census of 1901, 18·5 per cent of Indian women aged 30, and 25·8 per cent of those aged 35, were widowed. By 1961, the proportion of widows aged 30 had fallen to 6·4 per cent, and of those women aged 35 to 11·2 per cent. In the developed countries of North-west Europe and North America, the proportion of women widowed in their reproductive years is very much lower and many widows remarry. For example, in 1960 in Britain only 0·8% of women aged 30 were widowed, and this pattern applies to other developed countries (Table 5/3). The conclusion is that with improvement of nutrition and health fewer women aged 15–49 are widowed, and that this has a positive effect on population change.

Table 5/3

The proportion of women aged 30* who are widowed (*per cent*)

	1920–30	1960–70
Developed Nations		
France	1·5	0·8
Japan	3·7	1·5
Sweden	1·5	0·6
U.K.	1·5	0·8
U.S.A. (white)	1·9	0·9
Developing Nations		
Ceylon	10·0	3·5
India	16·0	6·4

* The age of 30 has been chosen as it is half-way along the reproductive period.

The Never-Married

A certain proportion of the population never marries. As far as population growth is concerned, the number of females not marrying is a far more important variable than is the number of males. Examination of data available from several countries indicates that with the exception of Ireland, between 5 and 15 per cent of women living in the developed countries of the world do not marry. In the Islamic countries of Asia and Africa, only 2 to 5 per cent and in India less than 0·5 per cent of women remain single. In the African countries south of the Sahara, little reliable information is available, whilst in the predominantly Roman Catholic countries of South America, probably less than 10 per cent of women never marry, although as noted, a significant proportion continue in consensual unions.

The Ever-Married

Age and marital status

Age at marriage is considerably influenced by cultural attitudes. In India it is customary for Hindu girls to be formally married at puberty, although the first coitus is usually delayed for two to four years. In Central and Southern Africa, child marriage is usual (that is marriage when the girl is less than 16). In these societies coition is not delayed as in India, and the girl's fertility is proved whilst she is still less than 18. In Islamic countries, custom encourages an early age of marriage for females. In the industrial or post-industrial nations of Europe and North America, the age of marriage has become earlier for both males and females in the past 50 years, and this has been most marked since 1940. In part this is due to the greater affluence of the country, with higher wages being obtainable by men of 18 years and over; in part it is due to a relaxation of sexual prohibitions and taboos; in part it is due to a consumer society and the availability of many goods on time-payment. The necessity to save to purchase furniture is thus reduced, and marriage becomes economically feasible at an earlier age. There is also a factor of imitation: if other members of the peer group tend to marry earlier, the custom spreads. In China, it would

Table 5/4

Marriage of females, mean age and cumulative percentage married at various ages in representative nations

Country	*Year*	*Median age*		*Cumulative percentage females married at*					
		Female	*Male*	18	20	25	30	35	40
Czechoslovakia	1961	20·6	24·4	13	47	87	93	94	94
England and Wales	1961	23·2	25·7	6	25	72	84	87	89
France	1962	21·6	25·1	9	33	73	88	90	91
Ireland	1961	24·7	27·8	2	8	45	66	75	77
Bolivia	1950	21·2	23·0	21	38	69	81	86	87
Egypt	1960	19·2	24·7	37	58	90	96	98	98
Turkey	1955	18·0	19·6	58	80	94	95	96	98
India	1961	17·2	18·9	—	94	98	99	99	99
Japan	1960	24·3	27·0	1	16	62	89	94	96

Sources: Mertens W., *World Nuptiality Patterns*, Community and Family Study Centre, Chicago.
Also: *Demographic Yearbooks*, U.N., New York.

appear from the limited information available, that early arranged marriages are discouraged and that the age at first marriage is rising, partly in deference to the wishes of the Government and the Chairman of the Communist Party.

In Table **5/4** and Figure **5/6**, the cumulative percentages of married females for several countries are shown. In most it will

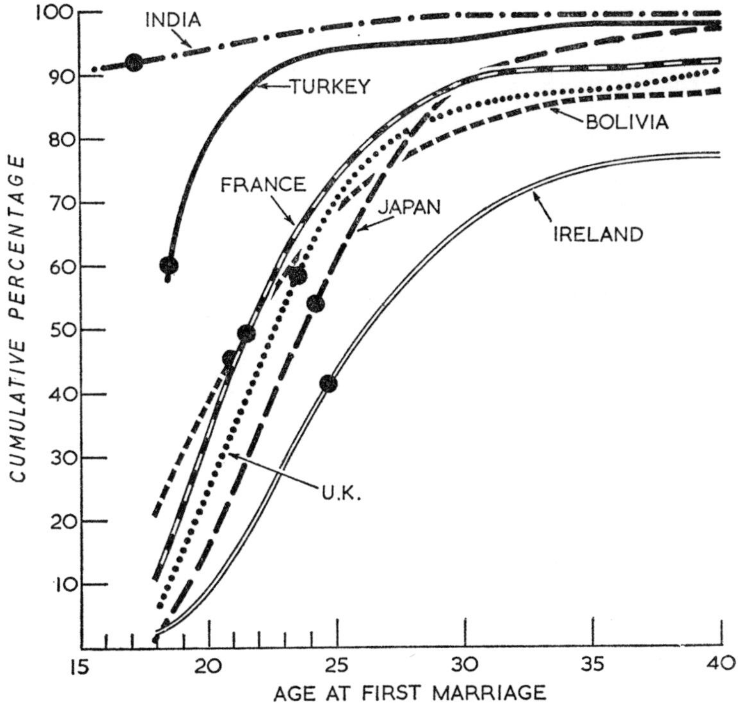

Figure **5/6** The cumulative percentages of married women in various nations. The median age at first marriage is indicated by the solid circle on each line.

be observed that whilst only between 2 and 25 per cent are married at 18, by the age of 25 the cumulative percentage has risen to over 60 per cent in all except Ireland. The reason for the low percentage there is that Irish men tend not to marry until they have inherited land. Consequently, many seek employment in Britain, as do many females, and marriage tends to be delayed amongst those remaining in Ireland.

It will also be noted that despite differing percentages of women married at different ages, the shape of the curves is very similar. If the data available are studied, a general pattern emerges. A nation which has a low level of industrial development, a high incidence of communicable diseases and a low literacy level tends to practise early marriage, whilst in developed nations the age of marriage has tended to be later, but recently

Table 5/5

The secular changes in the percentage of women married at various ages

Country	*Year*	*Age*		
		20–24	25–29	45–49
England and Wales	1871	34	63	87
	1911	24	56	83
	1931	26	58	83
	1951	47	78	82
	1961	62	87	95
Ireland	1891	14	41	83
	1936	14	36	75
	1946	17	43	74
	1951	18	45	66
	1961	22	55	88
Sweden	1870	16	46	84
	1910	20	49	78
	1930	20	48	77
	1950	40	78	74
	1960	43	79	89

Sources: Hajnal and others.

is becoming earlier. This does not necessarily mean that with industrialization, increased literacy and better health care the age of marriage will rise. Hajnal investigated this hypothesis by obtaining data from several European countries which have reliable statistics. He found that in Northern Europe, prior to the Industrial Revolution, the age of marriage was relatively late, and that it did not change substantially in the 250 years between

1790 and 1940, although there was a slight downward drift, which suddenly has accelerated in the past 35 years. In both the developed and the developing nations, early marriage is becoming more frequent, and this is likely to be followed by a higher birth rate, unless fertility control is encouraged (Table **5/5**).

The trend to earlier marriage is particularly marked in the

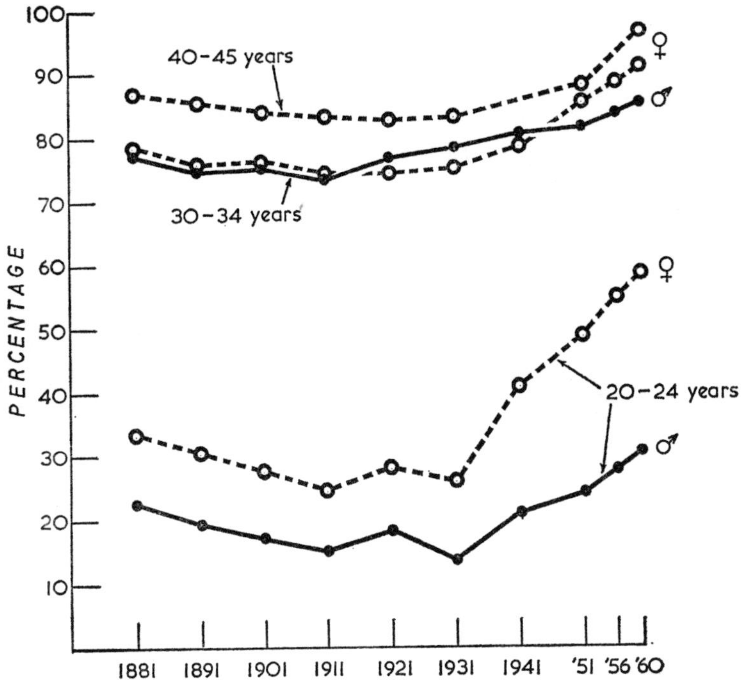

Figure **5/7** The percentage of persons ever-married at various ages for various years in England and Wales.
Source: Registrar General.

U.S.A. and recently in the U.K., where there has been a rapid rise in 'teenage marriages' in the past 15 years. This change is due to increasing teenage affluence and to fashion, but currently appears to have certain social consequences. Studies both in the U.S. and in Europe indicate that teenage marriages are more likely to be followed by divorce than are later marriages; and in such divorces the woman is left with one or more small children. It has also been found that the degree of sexual and marital satisfaction is much lower in such families, as their emotional maturity is less, even though on average the husband is two or three years older than the wife. Further observations show that a high proportion of teenage marriages are due to premarital conception, that the couple are of below average educational level, that they tend to come from the lower socio-economic groups, and that they work in an unskilled or semi-skilled job.

Socio-Economic Influences on Nuptiality

In the developed countries of the world there is a general belief that men and women of the lower economic groups marry earlier and have more children than those of the higher socio-economic groups. This has led some critics to complain that this is lowering the intellectual content of humanity. The socio-economic variables affecting fertility are considered in Chapter 6. Here the effect of socio-economic status on age of marriage is discussed. Unfortunately objective data are scarce. Information from Britain has been reported by Grebenik and Rowntree, from Australia, Sweden and Switzerland by Hajnal, and from the U.S.A. by the Bureau of the Census.

These studies show that in all the nations reviewed, persons

Table 5/6

The median age at marriage in U.S.A. and U.K. by husband's socio-economic group

Class	*Classification*	*U.S.A.*		*U.K.*	
		Males	*Females*	*Males*	*Females*
I	Professional and Managerial	24·0	21·3	25·3	23·3
II	Officials, etc	24·0	20·6	25·0	23·0
III	Clerical	22·8	19·8	25·0	23·0
IV	Skilled craftsmen	23·8	20·1	24·2	22·2
V	Unskilled labourers	21·5	19·0	24·2	21·9

Source: Grebenik, E., and Rowntree, G. (U.K. figures relate to people born between 1925 and 1929).

higher in the socio-economic scale, whether this is decided by parental occupation, educational attainments or income, marry at a later age than those in the lower socio-economic groups. This finding is most marked for males, but applies to females, although to a lesser extent (Table **5/6**). The studies also show that those groups which were previously inclined to delay marriage are now marrying earlier, and the effect of the socio-economic differences is much less than prior to 1960.

Measurement of Marriage Rates

The general marriage rate can be calculated for all persons, or for males and females separately. In population dynamics, it is the female marriage rate which has the greatest influence on population growth, and for this reason this rate will be computed.

General marriage rate (females) =

$$\frac{\text{Number of marriages of unmarried females aged 15 to 49}}{\text{Number of unmarried females aged 15 to 49}} \times 1{,}000$$

The ages of 15 and 49 are taken, as few women marry before the age of 15, and even fewer conceive, whilst after the age of 49 marriage is unusual and almost none of the women become pregnant.

The calculation can also be made for age-specific general marriage rates and this gives useful information.

The general marriage rate relies upon an accurate reporting, in the population under examination, of marriage registration data. Where such data are inadequately collected, the resulting calculations will be markedly biased. Unfortunately this is the situation in most developing nations, and in a few developed nations.

THE EFFECT OF THE VARIABLES ON POPULATION DYNAMICS

The effect of the variables of age composition, sex composition and marital composition on a population's growth is considerable. The aggressive health measures adopted in all countries have increased the number of females and of males entering the reproductive years and have led to an increased fertility of the population. As well, a significant reduction in the age of marriage in the developed countries, and in the number of widows in both the developed and the developing countries, has increased the potential fertility of the population. These factors have combined with other factors to be considered later to increase the population growth of all countries of the world in a spectacular way.

SIX

Natality

The desire of man and woman to reproduce is embedded deep in their subconscious. Animals copulate in response to physiological stimuli, but in certain species these are controlled by environmental factors. The human animal has the same instinctive urge to copulate in response to physiological stimuli, but has added an intellectual desire for children. Children on growing added to the labour pool for agriculture and hunting. Children provided security, food and shelter for their parents when they became too old and feeble to work. Children added to the strength of the family or tribe in war. These intellectual needs were mythologized and, in almost all religions, children—particularly male children—became needed to ensure that the parents were given succour after death. The rites, duties and prayers of children ensured a safe passage into another world and a comfortable sojourn there. Since the rituals could only be made by blood relatives, children were needed to provide further children, so that the rituals might continue for all time.

The fertility of woman, therefore, has been a matter of vital concern to all peoples, particularly as it is only in the last century that it has been accepted that barrenness could be caused by the male. Previously this concept seemed ridiculous. If the male copulated, and on reaching orgasm ejaculated, it was obvious that he had introduced the necessary ingredient to ensure a child would result. If the child failed to appear, it was obviously the fault of the female. Since between 5 and 15 per cent of women in a society failed to become pregnant, rites were devised, diets instituted, astrologers and wise men consulted to ensure fertility, and to render the barren woman fertile. And in the society the pregnant woman was given special consideration, and the birth of the child surrounded by ritual.

Despite this glorification of fertility, in many tribal and peasant societies, at specific times, practices were evolved which aimed at controlling fertility, so that the available supply of food, and land, could be more readily shared. These practices were related to need, and after war, famine or pestilence, might be dropped. In many societies abortion was permitted. In some, infanticide, especially of multiple births and of female infants, was encouraged. In some societies, segregation of women after childbirth, for prolonged periods for ritual purification, was adopted. Other societies observed that breast feeding reduced fertility and encouraged prolonged lactation. Still other societies encouraged the belief that copulation was 'weakening' to the male, and that ejaculation removed from him a vital essence, so that coitus should only take place at infrequent intervals.

But despite the restraints, the fertility and natality of the woman was of vital concern to the society in which she lived. This concern is even more marked today, particularly as we have now entered an era of death control. Medical science and sanitary engineering, by reducing drastically infant and childhood deaths, have enabled more and more children to reach the reproductive years. In their turn they are conceiving and bearing children who live to reach the reproductive years with a multiplying effect on childbirth.

The bearing of children is termed fertility or natality by demographers. Uncontrolled natality, allied with a markedly reduced infant and childhood mortality, occurring today, is the cause of the sudden spurt in population growth. In other words there is an imbalance between premature death control and birth control.

In this chapter natality is considered so that the reader may have some idea of the methods of measurement of natality, problems connected with this, and may consider factors influencing natality. One factor may be eliminated at once. That is the theory that different races have a different biological potential to become pregnant. There is no evidence that the fecundity of any racial group is different from that of any other. In other words, all women, whatever their racial or ethnic origin, have an equal ability to conceive children. What does vary from group to group is their ability to bear a live child. In other words, the natality of different ethnic, racial and socio-economic groups does differ. It is this difference which is considered in this chapter.

Fecundity, Fertility and Natality

In any discussion of natality, the problem of definition arises. This is most marked when the term fertility is used in place of natality. To the biologist and gynaecologist, the term fertility means the ability to *conceive*, and even if the woman subsequently aborts, she has proved her fertility, although she has no child in her arms to prove it. By contrast, to the demographer the term fertility means that the woman has actually given birth to a live child. Because of this ambiguity, and the fact that most readers of this book will be health workers rather than pure demographers, the term *natality* is used to refer to the actual bearing of a child.

The term *fecundity* also causes confusion. To most English-speaking scientists, fecundity means the biological ability to conceive and bear children. However, to some European demographers, fecundity means the production of a live birth. Amongst English-speaking demographers, a woman who has no ovaries or no uterus, or whose oviducts have been irreparably damaged by disease or removed by surgery, is obviously unable to conceive or bear children, as is a woman who is post-climacteric. In the reproductive years, such a woman is termed infecund, but to avoid confusion, she might be better called sterile. A woman who has attempted to conceive for a reasonable time (usually one year) and has failed to achieve a pregnancy is said to be infertile and investigations are initiated to see if she can be helped. In these investigations, the *couple*—man and wife—are investigated, as about one-third of infertility problems are due to faults in the male. Faults in the male may be due to ignorance about coition, but are generally due to defective or absent spermatozoon production and delivery. In the remaining two-thirds, the fault lies with the wife, or there are multiple problems affecting both partners. Investigations and treatment will enable about 40 per cent of infertile couples to have a live baby, but in the others, infertility remains a problem. Studies throughout the world show that childlessness is a not inconsiderable problem (see p. 126).

The Measurement of Natality

Demographers consider that six measurements may be of value in analysing the natality of the country under examination. The degree of sophistication of the calculations increases with the more complex measurements, but each is related to the others to a greater or lesser extent.

THE CRUDE BIRTH RATE

The crude birth rate is obtained by dividing the number of live births registered in a population during a year by the total number of the population at mid-year or the mean population. Since the result is a fraction, it is multiplied by 1,000, to give the rate per 1,000 of population. Since this calculation ignores the number of men in the population and ignores the age-structure of the population, which may contain a disproportionate number of people under the age of puberty or past the age of the climacteric, it is a crude measure. But it has several considerable advantages. Firstly, the data required are relatively simple to obtain and, therefore, likely to be accurate. Secondly, the calculation is easy to make, so that the information is generally available within a few months of the end of each year. Thirdly, the rate can be used to express the effect of natality on population growth. If the effect of migration is ignored, the annual rate of population growth can be readily computed by subtracting the crude death rate from the crude birth rate. Despite its simplicity, it is likely that no more than 60 per cent of births occurring in the developing world are registered.

If a birth rate of 25 or less is taken as a dividing line, it can be seen that no economically 'developed' nation has a crude birth rate above this, whilst very few developing nations have a birth rate below this level. (Table **6/1**).

GENERAL NATALITY (FERTILITY) RATE

Because of the inadequacy of the crude birth rate for a particular investigation, a more sophisticated index is often used. This is the *general natality rate*. It is obtained by dividing the number of live births by the number of females biologically able to bear a child. These are usually taken to comprise all women aged 15 to 49, though some nations take the fertile age range as 15 to

Table 6/1

Crude birth rates for 1965–70 per 1,000 population, for nations of 5 million or more in 1970 in order of population size

Continent	*Natality Level*				
	Less than 20	20–29	30–39	40–49	50 *or more*
Africa				U.A.R. 44 Ethiopia 46 S. Africa 40 Zaire 44 Sudan 49 Morocco 49 Algeria 46 Tanzania 47 Ghana 47 Uganda 43 Cameroon 43 Rhodesia 48	Nigeria 50 Kenya 50 Madagascar 50 Zambia 50 Upper Volta 50
America	U.S.A. 19 Canada 19	Argentina 23 Cuba 27	Brazil 38 Chile 33	Mexico 43 Colombia 47 Peru 42 Venezuela 41 Ecuador 45 Guatemala 42	
Asia	Japan 19		China 33 S. Korea 36 N. Vietnam 37 S. Vietnam 37 Taiwan 30 Sri Lanka 33 W. Malaysia 34	India 42 Indonesia 48 Bangladesh 48 Pakistan 46 Philippines 45 Turkey 40 Thailand 43 Burma 40 Iran 45 Nepal 44 Iraq 49 Cambodia 45 Syria 47	Afghanistan 51 Saudi Arabia 50 Yemen 50
Europe & U.S.S.R.	U.S.S.R. 17 W.Germany 18 U.K. 18 Italy 18 France 17 Poland 17 Yugoslavia 19 Czecho-slovakia 16 Netherlands 18 Hungary 15 Belgium 17 Greece 17 Bulgaria 16 Sweden 15 Austria 16 Switzerland 17 Denmark 14	Spain 20 Romania 21 Portugal 24			
Oceania	Australia 19				

44 years. Although it is accepted that some girls under the age of 15 conceive and deliver children, as do a few women over the age of 49, the number of never-married women between those ages more than offsets this omission. The result of the calculation is then multiplied by 1,000 to avoid the decimal point for better understanding.

General natality rate =

$$\frac{\text{Total births in the year}}{\text{Number of women aged 15–49 in the population at mid-year}} \times 1{,}000$$

As an example, in Ceylon in 1963, there were 364,472 births and 2,347,786 women were aged 15 to 49. The general natality rate was:

$$\frac{364{,}472}{2{,}347{,}786} \times 1{,}000 = 155$$

AGE-SPECIFIC BIRTH (NATALITY) RATE

Age-specific birth rates are one of the most valuable refinements made in the study of natality. Without this refinement, most of the other, more precise, measurements could not be made. Age-specific birth rates are calculated for any year by dividing the number of births to women of each age group (usually five-year age groups) by the total number of women in that age group in the population at mid-year, and multiplying the result by 1,000.

The rate can be stated as:

Age-specific birth rate =

$$\frac{\text{Total births to women aged } x \text{ years}}{\text{Mid-year population of women aged } x} \times 1{,}000$$

In Table **6/2**, the method of computing the age-specific birth rates for Ceylon is shown. This Table also shows several other rates which will be mentioned later. Age-specific birth rates enable demographers to study the population in greater detail (Table **6/3**). It is known that fertility (and natality) is not uniform throughout the reproductive years. Age-specific birth rates permit this factor to be studied and to measure more accurately the impact of birth control measures on fertility. It also enables a demographer to calculate the next natality index —the total natality rate.

Table 6/2

How natality rates are calculated (using the births in Ceylon (Sri Lanka) in 1963 as an example)

Age group	*Number of women in age group* (1)	*Number of births* (2)	*Age-specific birth rate* (3)	*Cumulative natality rate* (4)
Total (*age* 15–49)	2,347,786	364,472	981·5	4907
15–19	503,551	26,273	22·9	114
20–24	441,443	100,569	228·7	1258
25–29	368,454	102,575	279·4	2655
30–34	314,595	75,332	240·4	3857
35–39	310,129	48,694	157·6	4645
40–44	212,641	9,731	45·9	4874
45–49	196,973	1,298	6·6	4907

$$\text{Crude birth rate} = \frac{\text{Total births}}{\text{Total population}} \times 1{,}000 = 34{\cdot}4$$

$$\text{General natality rate} = \frac{\text{Total births}}{\text{Total women aged 15–49}} \times 1{,}000 = 155$$

$$\text{Age-specific natality rate} = \frac{\text{Entries in Col. 2 in age-group}}{\text{Entries in Col. 1 in age-group}} \times 1{,}000$$

Cumulative natality rate = A.S.N.R. × 5, cumulated by age (see Col. 4)
Total natality rate = Sum of A.S.N.R. × interval = 981·5 × 5 = 4,907

Even more informative than comparisons between nations, are secular changes in the age-specific birth rates in a single nation. In Figure **6/1** the age-specific birth rates for Australia for the years 1921 to 1971 are shown. It can be seen that throughout the period the age-specific birth rates of women aged 35 and older have tended to fall, those of women aged 30 to 34 have remained reasonably unchanged, whilst the age-specific birth rates of women aged 15 to 19 have risen spectacularly since 1941. The age-specific birth rates of women aged 20 to 29 rose steadily from 1931 to 1951, levelled off between 1951 and 1961 and then began to decline. In summary, Australian women are marrying earlier, having their children at a younger age (and having fewer children) today than they did 40 years ago.

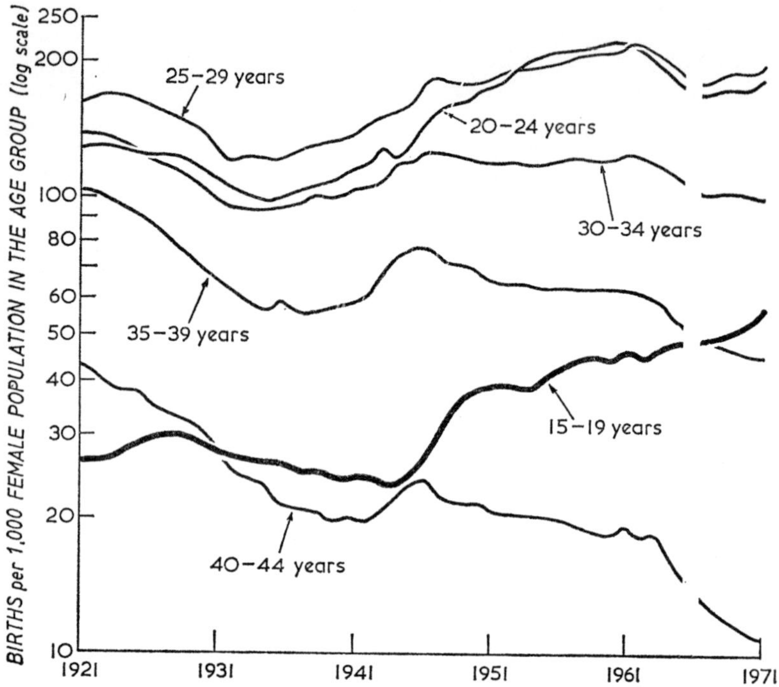

Figure **6/1** Age-specific birth rates, Australia 1921–71.
Source: Bureau of Census and Statistics, Canberra, ACT, Australia.

CUMULATIVE NATALITY RATE

The cumulative natality rate estimates the number of children an age cohort of 1,000 women would deliver from the time they began childbearing until they reach a specified age, if they were exposed to the age-specific birth rates in effect at a given time. It can be calculated up to any age, but the most common calculation is up to the age of 49, when the result is referred to as the *completed or total natality rate*. To make the calculation, the age-specific birth rate of each 5-year age group is multiplied by 5, and added to the age-specific birth rate multiplied by 5 of the next five-year age group. The cumulative natality rates for Ceylon are shown in Table **6/2** (Col. 4), and it will be seen that the total natality rate was 4,907.

THE TOTAL NATALITY (FERTILITY) RATE

The total natality rate is an estimate of the number of births, both male and female which 1,000 women of a specific age (known as a cohort) will have through their reproductive life if the age-specific rates of a given year remain constant, and if no woman entering the reproductive years dies before reaching the age of 49. It is calculated by adding the age-specific birth rates and multiplying the result by the interval into which the ages are grouped. This index is independent of mortality and is not influenced by differences in age composition of the population. If the total natality rate is 2,000, which means that each woman has two children, it indicates that each couple is just reproducing itself, and that the population will eventually become stable.

Table **6/3** shows the age-specific natality rates and total natality rates for various nations in 1967.

Table 6/3

The age-specific natality rate of seven representative nations, 1967

Age group	*Australia*	*Chile*	*Indonesia*	*Philippines*	*Sweden*	*U.K.*	*U.S.A.*
–20	49	33	46	19	25	49	33
20–24	173	196	217	185	135	165	174
25–29	184	191	176	194	146	165	143
30–34	105	147	143	141	82	92	79
35–39	15	115	159	139	35	43	38
40–44	14	47	40	52	9	11	11
45–	<1	8	14	11	0·6	0·8	0·7
General natality rate	95	96	104	86	58	66	63
Total natality rate	2,843	3,685	3,975	3,705	2,163	2,509	2,399

Source: *Demographic Yearbook*, 1968. U.N., New York.

THE GROSS REPRODUCTION RATE

The total natality rate can be refined still further by ignoring male births. This calculation gives the *gross reproduction rate.*

It shows how many female infants are born to the cohort of 1,000 women. It is calculated by multiplying the total natality rate by the percent of all births that are female in the index year (Table **6/4**). Since only girls are potential mothers, the gross reproduction rate gives a truer index of the reproductive performance of a population. The rate can be refined still further by applying the mortality rate of the same time. This gives the *net reproduction rate*. It estimates the number of female children who would survive to the reproductive age to replace their mothers assuming the continuation of the current natality and

Table 6/4

Gross and net reproduction rates

		Reproduction rates	
Country	*Year*	*Gross*	*Net*
Australia	1970	1·394	1·349
Chile	1967	1·874	1·498
Sweden	,,	1·148	1·110
U.K.	,,	1·276	1·243
U.S.A.	,,	1·255	1·213
Japan	,,	1·082	1·050
Malaysia (west)	,,	2·554	2·316
France		1·288	1·252
U.S.S.R.		1·171	1·114

Source: *Demographic Yearbook*, 1969, Table 31. U.N., New York.

mortality schedules. If the net reproduction rate is above unity it means that more fertile women will be living in the next generation and the population is likely to increase, unless measures are taken to control population growth.

The net reproduction rate is calculated by multiplying each age-specific birth rate by the life table mortality of that age group. This is obtained from a life table, and is the ratio of ${}_5L_x/l_0$ (see Chapter 7).

The net reproduction rate rests on assumptions about the natality and mortality of hypothetical cohorts, in particular that the mortality of the year of the construction of the life table will persist. Since this is unreal, it is currently out of favour as a measure of natality.

The Relationship Between the Various Natality Rates

The relationship between the crude birth rate, the total natality rate and the general natality rate is shown in Table 6/5, so that if one is known a rough estimate can be made of the other two.

Table 6/5

Relationship between crude birth rate, general natality rate and total natality rate

	Crude birth rate	*General natality rate*	*Total natality rate*
Developed post-industrial countries	13–14 15–19 20–24	50–65 60–85 75–100	1,900–2,300 2,200–2,800 2,800–3,600
Underdeveloped countries at take-off point	30–34 35–39	120–145 145–170	4,000–4,600 4,500–5,500
Underdeveloped countries	45–49 50–54	200–215 215–240	5,800–7,000 6,500–7,400

Source: Bogue, D. J. and Palmore, J. A. 'Some Empirical and Analytical Relations Among Demographic Fertility Measures'. *Demography*, **1**, 219, 1964.
Lee, J. C. 'Estimated Refined Measures of Fertility'. *Demography*, **1**, 359, 1964.

It must be pointed out that the crude birth rate, although easy to compute, is indeed crude, and its acceptance as an index of the secular trend in natality can be misleading.

In the U.S.A. between 1946 and 1957, the crude birth rate was almost unchanged, after an initial post-war jump due to returning servicemen. In fact, up to 1957, the total natality rate increased by 23 per cent, whilst the crude birth rate increased by a mere 6 per cent. This indicated a changing age distribution of births. Women were having children at an earlier age. Between 1957 and 1966, the crude birth rate and the total natality rates both fell, the former by 26 per cent, the latter by 27 per cent. Since both indices fell, the cause must have been something other than the changing age distribution of women becoming pregnant (Figure 6/2). Evidence from Ryder and Westoff indicates that that something was an increased acceptance of family planning by women, and, in particular, the in-

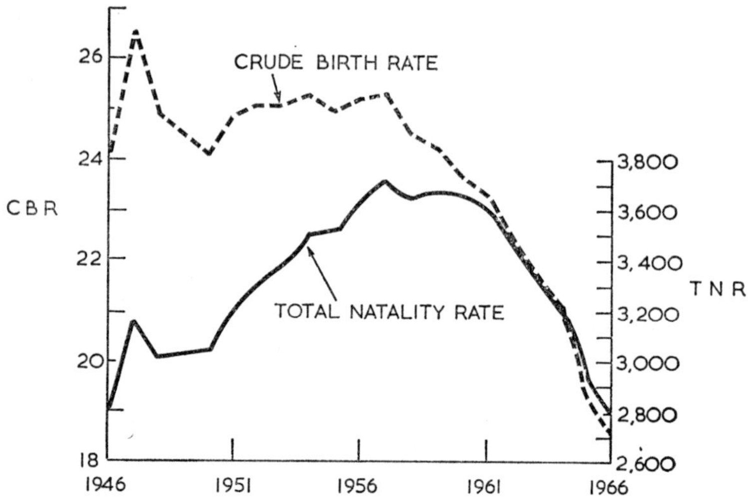

Figure 6/2 Crude birth rate and total natality rates, U.S.A. 1946–66.

creasing adoption of oral contraception. This would not have been revealed had not both the crude birth rate and the total natality rates been computed simultaneously and compared.

Standardized Natality Rates

It is known that certain social and demographic differences in two populations will influence their birth rates. For example, if most of the young men are away at war, the birth rate is likely to fall, and on their return after the war there is likely to be a 'baby boom'. Similarly the age composition of a population has some effect on natality. The natality of females varies according to their age, and age-specific birth rates show that natality is lower under the age of 20 and over the age of 35. If two populations differ markedly in the way the ages of their females are distributed in the five-year age groups between 15 and 49, the general fertility rate is likely to be affected considerably. The population having a greater proportion of women aged 20 to 35 is likely to have a higher general natality rate, although in fact the difference may merely be transient. However, it prevents the demographer from measuring the effects of pure natality (i.e. the natality without reference to other variables, such as age distribution, income level or whatever).

This statistical difficulty can be overcome by comparing the populations under study with a 'standard' population, such as a 'life table' population. The method of obtaining standardized rates was described in Chapter 4. As I have mentioned, standardization can be made to exclude the influence of other variables such as socio-economic group, husband's occupation and place of residence; but the method of calculation becomes increasingly complex.

Factors Influencing Natality

Any examination of the effect of the social status, educational attainment and economic level of a couple in relation to their desire for children and the natality of the wife is defeated, in large measure, by two facts. In the first place, the data from all except a few developed countries are scanty and often inaccurate; in the second place, the dissemination of modern contraceptives has coincided, in time, with the investigations by interested demographers into socio-economic factors influencing natality. This has resulted in a considerable bias. However, some facts are available.

SOCIO-ECONOMIC STATUS

In countries which divide their population into social classes, as does Britain, it has been found that the higher the social class the fewer the number of children in each family. This applies in Western countries irrespective of income and place of residence. It is not so obvious in developing countries. In one study in

India, it was found that in rural areas, women of higher socio-economic status had a higher natality than women of lower status. This difference may have been due to better health and nutrition of the former group, or to longer breast feeding by women of the latter group, the absence of their husbands seeking work elsewhere, or to 'debility' of both partners reducing fertility, although the evidence for this last is very debatable.

PROPORTION OF POPULATION LIVING IN RURAL AREAS

The United Nations has been unable to obtain agreement on what constitutes an urban area. Of the many definitions, by many nations, the most generally accepted is that an aggregation of at least 20,000 persons shall constitute an urban area and all other areas are designated as rural. Countries which have a majority of their populations living in rural areas are likely to have a high natality, and the larger the proportion of the population which is rural, the higher is the natality likely to be. But in this, too, there are very considerable variations, and several nations with a large rural population have achieved considerable fertility control. Further analysis of the data from these countries shows that, in most, an active government-supported campaign for family planning has been in progress (as in Hungary, Romania, Korea and Taiwan), or the nations are small and have a close relationship between town and country (e.g. Israel, Puerto Rico).

AGE AT MARRIAGE

It is generally believed that the earlier the age of marriage, the greater is the natality. That this is so in the developed nations is shown by evidence from Britain and the U.S.A. In Britain, for example, an average of 2·47 live births occurred for each uninterrupted marriage which had lasted at least 10 years, if the wife was under 20 years of age at marriage. This fell to less than half that figure if the wife's age at marriage was 30 to 34, and even lower if she was aged 35 at marriage (Table **6/6**). Deficiencies of data in most developing countries prevent any such statement, and since the introduction on a wide scale of contraceptives, the impact of this factor has diminished to some extent.

Table 6/6

Number of live births per marriage after ten years of uninterrupted marriage (England & Wales)

	Age at marriage (years)					
Date of marriage	*under* 20	20–24	25–29	30–34	35–39	40–44
1940	2·08	1·73	1·50	1·16	0·61	0·24
1950	2·41	1·89	1·66	1·32	0·68	0·22
1957	2·47	2·04	1·94	1·48	0·80	0·22

Source: *Registrar General's Statistical Review of England and Wales* 1967, Part II Population Table QQ(b). London, 1969.

EDUCATIONAL ATTAINMENT

Throughout the world there appears to be a strong inverse relationship between educational attainment and the degree of natality. The higher the proportion that is illiterate, the higher is the natality of that nation, although there are considerable variations. If a cut-off point can be postulated, it can be stated that when more than 20 per cent of the population is illiterate, natality is likely to be high, whether measured by the crude birth rate, or one of the more refined measures. Conversely, the higher the educational attainment, the lower is the natality. This applies when different nations are examined, or when different groups within a single nation are considered. In the United States, for example, in 1969 the number of children born to women who had completed the reproductive era, fell from 2·42 in white women who had only elementary education, to 1·30 amongst white women who had had a university or tertiary education. Amongst non-white women, the figure for women who had completed elementary education was 3·95, and this fell to 1·23 children per non-white woman who had been to 'College'. It would appear that in the U.S.A. at the present time, the increased natality of the non-white population is associated with differences in educational attainment. Whether educational deprivation is associated with a lower acceptance of modern contraceptives, or with ignorance of their availability, is unclear from the data available.

More important, this investigation shows that there is a progressive lowering of the level of natality from one educational attainment group to the next (Figure **6/3**).

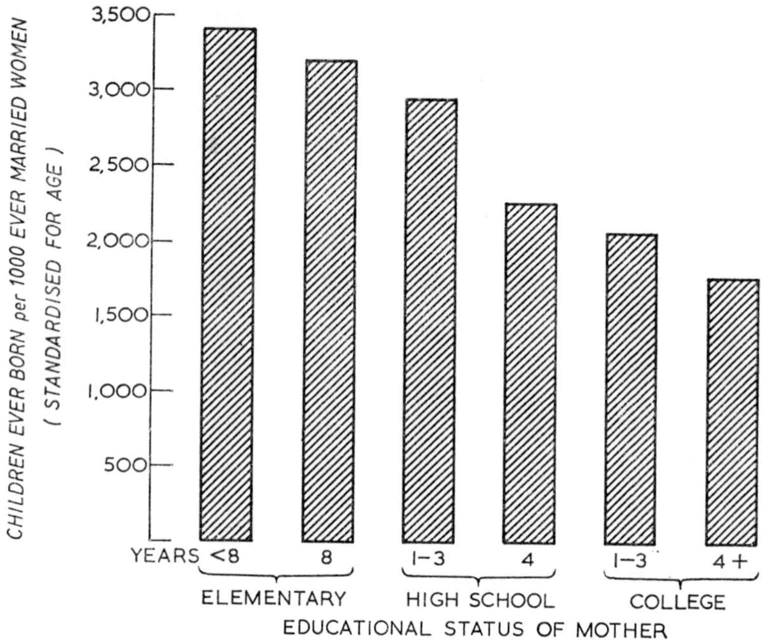

Figure **6/3** Number of births related to educational status of the mother, U.S.A. 1960.

Source: U.S. Department of Commerce, Bureau of the Census. 'Fertility of the Population', Table 4, Series 8–20, No. 203.

BREAST FEEDING

When breast feeding is not practised, ovulation recommences within 10 weeks in over 50 per cent of women. Breast feeding delays considerably the onset of ovulation, and in one investigation more than 40 per cent of lactating women were not ovulating 36 weeks after childbirth. In many developing countries, it is customary to continue breast feeding for up to 2 years. It is not known if this custom developed in an attempt to reduce infant mortality from malnutrition and infectious disease, or from the observable fact that natality was reduced; but the custom has the effect of spacing births in a considerable number of women. It might be argued that lactating women avoided coitus—but there are no data to support this, whilst there are many data that the prolonged anovulatory interval in lactating women is the critical factor. It is true that conceptions may occur during the period of breast feeding (when amenorrhoea is usual), but probably such conceptions occur to less than 5 per cent of women. In a study in the Punjab, Potter found that in 11 villages studied, amongst lactating women the median length of postpartum amenorrhoea was 11 months, and the mean interval between births was 30 months. If lactation was not practised, postpartum amenorrhoea had a median length of 2 months, and the birth interval was reduced to a mean of 15 months. A similar study in Taiwan showed that in the absence of contraception, lactating women took an average of 16 months to conceive again, and amenorrhoea lasted for a mean of 11 months. When the woman did not breast feed, menstruation resumed on average in three to five months postpartum (Jain).

Unfortunately, the incidence of breast feeding is diminishing both in developed and developing countries. In the U.S.A., Britain and Australia, less than 30 per cent of women are lactating six weeks after delivery. The practice of bottle, or formula, feeding is increasing in developing countries as well, particularly amongst urban women, so that the effectiveness of lactation as a measure of fertility control is reduced.

INFANT MORTALITY

It is noticeable that nations which have a high infant mortality rate tend to have a high birth rate. Since in many of these nations the family unit remains strong, and it is considered the duty of the children to provide for their parents in old age, the advantage of having many children is apparent. This applies particularly to the more traditional, conservative, rural population, where children are also a means of cheap labour. But much variation occurs. For example, East European countries, such as Czechoslovakia, Hungary and Romania have over 50 per cent of the population designated as rural, yet they have crude birth rates and infant mortality rates well within the range of highly urbanized countries. The reasons are that these countries offer a comprehensive free health service with a considerable bias towards preventive health care. In addition they have adopted liberal abortion laws and have encouraged the use of contraceptive measures.

Investigations amongst several populations, by Henry, show that the mean interval between confinements is longer if the preceding child lives to the age of one year than if the child dies during the first year of life. The reason may be that the loss of a child induces a desire to replace the loss quickly, or it may be due to the contraceptive effect of breast feeding.

Childlessness

The number of married couples in any population who have no children, despite their desire to have a child, is an index of the prevalence of childlessness in that community, and this will affect the natality of the population. Childlessness may be involuntary, or in certain circumstances may be voluntary. Studies in several countries show that voluntary childlessness is relatively uncommon, and fewer than 5 per cent of all married couples decide to have no children. It would seem from this that if the couple are childless the reason is an involuntary one in most cases.

As was mentioned earlier in this chapter, the husband is responsible for the childlessness in about one-third of cases, the wife in one-third, and there are factors affecting both partners in the remaining one-third. If the husband has no spermatozoa, or if infection (usually gonococcal) has damaged his vas deferens, the couple will remain childless. If the wife has previously developed infection of her genital organs, because of gonorrhoea or tuberculosis, she may have residual, irreparable damage to her oviducts and will be permanently childless. Even more unfortunate and sinister is pelvic infection following an induced septic abortion, which may cause permanent childlessness. These factors may well be the reason for the different proportions of barren women in the nations of the world. In countries where natality statistics are reliable, the proportion of women aged 40 or over who have borne no children varies from country to country (Table 6/7). In Western industrial nations between 12 and 18 per cent of women aged 45 to 49 have never had a child. These figures include never-married women

Table 6/7

The proportion of women aged 40 or more in selected nations who have had no children, 1965

Nation	*Childless (per cent)*
America	
Canada	13·1
Chile	24·7
Peru	11·8
Jamaica	19·8
Mexico	21·8
U.S.A.	13·9
Asia	
Japan	8·1
Malaysia	9·0
Thailand	6·5
Europe	
Czechoslovakia	15·4
Hungary	18·7
Ireland	12·5
Netherlands	14·2
Switzerland	19·7
U.K.	11·7

Source: *Demographic Yearbook*, 1965, U.N., New York.

and ever-married women who have voluntarily accepted childlessness. It would be of interest to analyse the data available further to determine the amount of involuntary childlessness amongst ever-married women. This is possible by studying the census reports of the U.S.A. In the 1960 census, 18·3 per cent of women aged 50 or over at the time of the investigation (i.e. whose reproductive life was complete) were childless. Further analysis of the statistics showed that the proportion of childlessness was related to the level of education of the woman. Only 14 per cent of women who had ceased to attend school at the end of the elementary period (i.e. at about the age of 12) were childless, whilst 27 per cent of those who had been to college had had no children. It is certain that most of the childlessness amongst the better educated was voluntary. In the same census it was found that only 11 per cent of women aged 35 to 39 were childless. In this age group the influence of educational attainment again related directly, although the difference between the educational groups was much less. In the study, less than 9 per cent of those who had only been to elementary school were childless, whilst about 11 per cent of those who had attended college had had no children at the time of the census.

By the age of 35 the majority of these ever-married women will have either decided to remain childless, or will have failed to become pregnant. This is because the median age of marriage for women in the U.S. is 20·3, and even in the group with higher educational attainment, the median is 21·6, so that by the age of 35 any women wishing to conceive should have been able to do so. In addition, if late marriage were a factor, it would be minimal, as only 10 per cent of women had not married by the age of 30.

Investigations into infertility show that over 90 per cent of those wishing to conceive become pregnant within one year of trying, and treatment of infertility produces the highest rate of conceptions (about 40 per cent) within one year of starting therapy. Thus by the age of 30, those women who had remained childless had either chosen this voluntarily or had not achieved pregnancy. The rather small difference between the educationally privileged and the educationally deprived suggests that voluntary infertility in both of these groups is small, and that about 10 per cent of women in a developed industrial country are involuntarily childless. Studies in other developed countries give similar results. In 1946, the Family Census of England and Wales showed that 12 per cent of women, whose reproductive history was complete, were childless, and investigations in Sweden confirm this finding.

In the developing countries it might be assumed that poor childhood nutrition, a higher incidence of infectious disease and overcrowding might increase the proportion of childless women in the community. Statistics from Asia fail to confirm this assumption. In 1965, for example, the date of the publication of the statistics in Table **6/7**, little progress had been made in family planning in Malaysia or Thailand, yet the percentage of childless women was less than in the developed nations of the West. The higher incidence in South America and in the Caribbean area could be accounted for by the known increased use of induced abortion to terminate unwanted pregnancy in Latin America, and the greater likelihood of the spread of gonococcal salpingitis due to the more flexible sexual liaisons practised in the Caribbean.

The Sociology of Natality

It will be apparent from the discussion thus far that although many factors have been thought to influence natality, by far the most important are not biological (as in primates and other animals) but psychological ones. In closed societies, such as those found in the rural areas of Asia, in tribal societies such as those found in Africa, in the peasant societies of rural Latin America, tradition is of great cultural importance. The wisdom of the family, of the village, of the area, lies in the hands of the older people; changes are slow and are only made after long deliberation; the people hold the attitude that 'what was correct for my father is correct for my descendants'. The oral tradition of many of these subcultures holds certain things to be self-evident. A large family is an insurance against childhood mortality and against a shortage of labour. It is a hostage for the preferential treatment of the parents in the next world. There is evidence that in villages studied, the death in infancy of a first-born child is a strong incentive to have a large family. Perhaps the Gods were angry and so took the first-born child; to appease them the woman should bear as many children as possible. In this type of family too, the influence of the grandmother is strong, and it is likely that she will believe that many grandchildren is a desirable aim.

In an attempt to introduce family planning into such communities, certain authorities have used the approach that uncontrolled population growth limits the land available for inheritance, and that, therefore, a reduction in natality would help the family unit. This proposition has not met with much success, as the hazards of famine, pestilence and war are well known to the listeners, and it is in their tradition that high natality will correct possible deaths from such 'natural' events. In such a

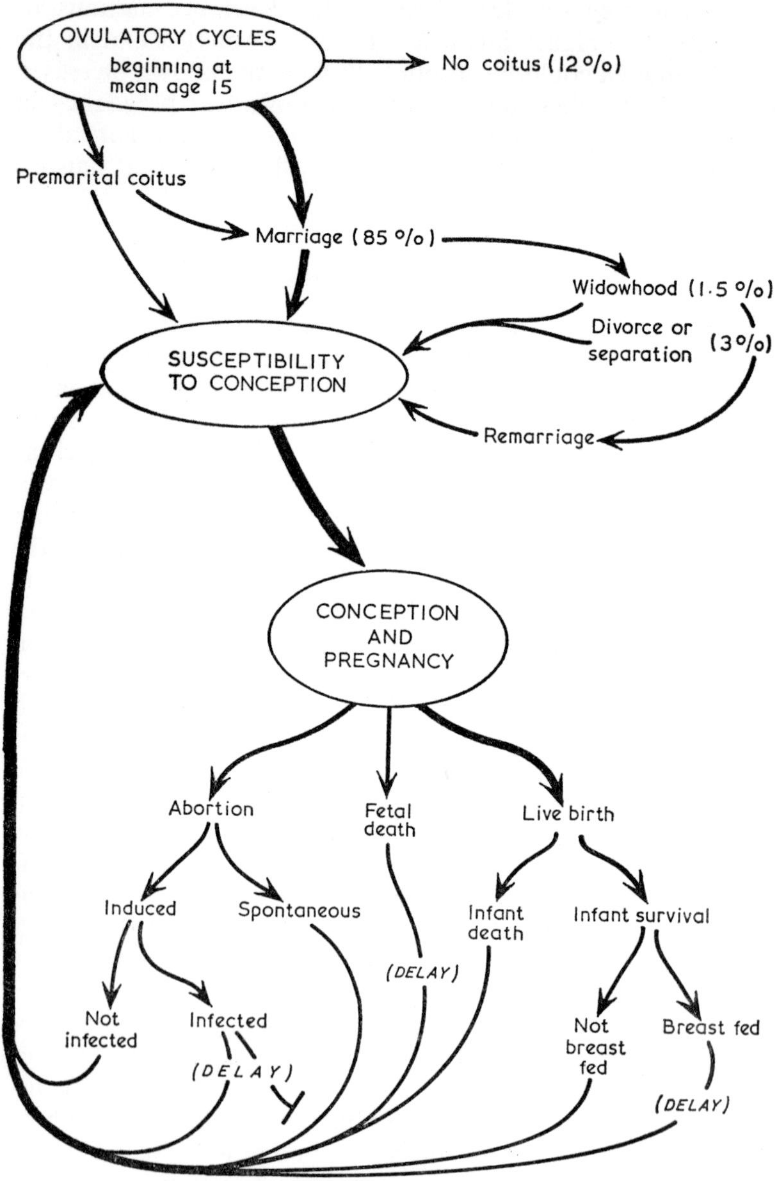

Figure **6/4** The fecundity cycle in a fertile Western woman who uses no contraceptive methods.

society where fertility is relatively uncontrolled, a fecundity cycle can be delineated, and such a cycle is also applicable to Western women who use no family planning (Figure **6/4**).

The behavioural attitudes of rural societies, especially towards natality, reduce the impact of measures introduced to limit population growth. But with persistence and the right approach, attitudes change. Change is more likely as traditional values are eroded by better roads, by better communications and by the mass media. However, the greatest agent for change in village society is human. If a key person within the community accepts natality control, his (or possibly her) attitude to this will influence others. In this process, education appears the key.

Long before today's highly efficient, easily utilized contraceptives were available, the more educated couples limited the size of their family. Amongst the better educated women, usually of a higher social status, family limitation was practised throughout the nineteenth and early twentieth century in almost all Western countries, even when the methods available were much less aesthetic than today. The decision was a psychological one based on social and economic pressure. If social custom induced women of the subculture to limit family size, the aspirant to that social group, who sought the status implicit in the group, also limited the size of her family by using the vaginal sponge, or by inducing her husband to use contraceptive measures. If the husband considered that the cost of education of children hindered his own social mobility, he was careful—practising coitus interruptus or using a condom rather than risking a pregnancy. In other words, for both sexes a conscious decision to reduce natality was made, and the method of achieving this was concordant with the rules of the society and within the canon of the religion to which they belonged. Abstinence from coitus, or primitive birth control (by the man) was permitted; abortion probably frowned upon and infanticide condemned.

In the context of today's world, where increasing numbers of people are concerned with uncontrolled natality, but where preventive measures are available, it is prudent to list the characteristics of those families which currently have a low natality and those having a high natality. Clearly any programme seeking to reduce natality, or to reduce fertility, must focus on the populations with a high natality. The main factors detected are shown in Table **6/8.** Of these factors, by far the most important is education. The better educated the husband and wife, the more open and receptive will their minds be to new and often disturbing ideas, and the better their chance of making a decision for themselves without the constraints of traditional or religious beliefs. The more educated they are the

Table 6/8

Socio-economic characteristics of families with a low or a high natality

Low Natality	*High Natality*
Urban dweller	Rural dweller
Area of low infant mortality	Area of high infant mortality
Good education	Poor education
High, or moderate income	Low income
High social class or occupation	Low social class or occupation
High rent dwelling	Low or no rent
High age at marriage	Low age at marriage
Protestant-Christian	Catholic-Christian, Moslem, Buddhist, Hindu

Factors with variable effect on overall natality

Employment of wives
Breast feeding of infants
Age of husbands
Duration of marriage

less are ignorance and poor motivation likely to play a part in rejecting family limitation. The more educated they are, the better can they appreciate that the cost of rearing an extra child may diminish the health or educational opportunities of existing children. In other words, the better can they perceive the economic aspects of natality control, which may more than offset the possible economic gain in having additional hands for a family agricultural or business venture.

SEVEN

Mortality

Inevitably a person dies. The inexorable journey from birth to death goes on, and all that may be done is to delay the moment of death. Good nutrition, good sanitation and good medical care help; but despite such aids, death occurs at all ages. In the past 75 years, in the developed countries, the mortality associated with pregnancy and childbirth, and that of infants and children, has fallen dramatically. Good obstetric care has reduced the deaths of parturient women; whilst better nutrition of children, reduction of overcrowding, the general availability of safe water and good sanitation, have led to the control of infectious disease, which was the great killer in infancy, childhood and adolescence. Civilization has given these benefits to one group, but has increased the mortality in other groups. Deaths from accidents, particularly those involving motor vehicles, are increasing and affect mainly the 17 to 35-year-olds; deaths due to coronary artery disease are increasing, and are probably the result of an overabundant diet in the under-exercised male. They affect the 35 to 55-year-old group particularly. Deaths from lung cancer, whether due to tobacco pollution or environmental pollution, and from other respiratory diseases, are increasing and affect the 55 to 75-year-olds particularly.

On balance, however, the twentieth century has witnessed a startling reduction of the death rate, with a considerable prolongation of life. This reduction in the death rate has been particularly of infant, childhood and adolescent deaths, with the result that increasing numbers of children are now reaching the reproductive years and are now producing children of their own. This is the cause of the rapid population growth which is occurring at present, and which is causing so much concern to thinking people.

The second effect of death control has been to increase life expectancy, that is the number of years a person may expect to remain alive. Unfortunately the only reliable statistics over a long period, are those obtained from Oceania (Australia and New Zealand), North America (Canada and the U.S.A.), and North Western Europe, as accurate registration of deaths before 1920 has only been possible in these countries. The registration of deaths has been most accurate in England and Wales and in Sweden. In England and Wales, for example, the expectation of life at birth in 1850 was 42 years; in 1900, 50 years, and in 1960, 72 years. This means that life expectancy at birth has increased by 71 per cent between 1850 and 1960.

Table 7/1

The mortality per 1,000 conceptions for various age groups in England and Wales in 1860 and in 1960

Age period		1860*	1960
Prenatal	Prenatal	250	180
0–1	Infancy	150	19
1–14	Childhood	70	5
15–44	Reproductive years	150	30
45–65	Middle age	140	124
65+	Old age	240	642
		1,000	1,000
Life expectancy at birth (years)		43	72

* Partly estimated. 'Prenatal' includes abortions and stillbirths.

When the decrease in mortality is calculated between different age groups for these years, a clearer picture appears. In Table **7/1**, it can be seen that in a hundred years the mortality in infancy has been reduced sevenfold, that of childhood, fourteen-fold and that during the reproductive years, fivefold. It can also be seen that even in 1860 if a child reached the age of 20, it had a fairly good chance of living into old age. It follows that the main reduction in the death rate has been to eliminate those deaths due to infectious disease occurring in infancy and childhood, and to a lesser extent in the reproductive years.

The study of mortality, particularly of deaths occurring in

infancy, childhood and the reproductive years, is clearly of importance in population dynamics. However, it is likely that fewer than 50 per cent of deaths occurring in the developing nations are recorded.

Measurement of Mortality

The data for the measurement of mortality are obtained from information on death certificates which are required by law in many countries before burial or cremation is permitted. In most of the developed nations, registration of death depends on a certificate issued by a medical practitioner on which the age, sex, race and cause of death are also usually stated. Because of shortage of physicians in developing countries, particularly in the rural areas, certification of death where required is made by a Government official, a village headman, or a policeman, and the cause of death is speculative. This, of course, limits the study of the *causes* of death, but does not necessarily interfere with the other indices.

CRUDE DEATH RATE

The crude death rate is the total number of deaths that occur during one year per 1,000 of population.

$$\text{Crude death rate} = \frac{\text{Deaths in a given year}}{\text{Mid-year population}} \times 1{,}000$$

AGE-SPECIFIC DEATH RATES

As was noted in Chapter 6, crude vital rates hide information which may be of great significance in social and economic planning. For example, the death of an infant or of a child has a much greater social, economic and demographic effect than the death of an elderly person. The death of an elderly person has little demographic influence, other than that the population is reduced by one. The death of an infant or child means a reduction not of one person, but of the many descendants which the child might have had. The death of a person in late adolescence or the early reproductive years is the loss of a person in whom an economic investment has been made (by the cost of care and feeding, by that of schooling and further training) but who has barely begun to give an economic return.

To make allowance for the different demographic influences of the age at death, age-specific death rates have been introduced, and are essential for the study of population dynamics. Age-specific death rates are not complex, they are merely the crude death rate calculated for each age group. For much demographic research, five-year age groups are adequate, and since the mortality differs between each sex, the age-specific death rates are usually calculated separately for each sex.

In most nations of the world, males have higher age-specific death rates than females. Exceptions to this general rule are decreasing and relate to those countries where females tend to be neglected and do not receive medical care when they become ill, as the available resources for the payment of medical care are reserved for the male members of the family. This cultural pattern was usual in India and Pakistan until recently, but is diminishing as medical and health services reach out to more and more rural areas. It is also found in Africa where the disparity persists, especially in tribal societies.

In most countries of the world, the life expectancy of females is considerably higher than that of males, and the difference increases as age-specific death rates decline. For this reason the difference is greatest in the developed countries, females having 2 to 9 years greater life expectancy at birth than males (Table **7/2**).

Because of the high mortality in the first year of life, two further subdivisions of the age-specific death rates in the age group 0 to 4 are often made. These are firstly, the *neonatal mortality*, or the number of deaths occurring in the first 28 days of life per 1,000 live-born children, and the *post-neonatal mortality*, which is the number of deaths of infants aged 29 to 365 days per 1,000 live-born children. Both are included in the *infant mortality* rate, which computes the number of deaths in the first year of life per 1,000 live births.

The age pattern of mortality follows a 'U' shaped curve, both in the developed and the developing nations. Mortality tends to be high in the first year of life, but then falls rapidly and it reaches the bottom of the trough between the ages of 10 and 14, remaining low until about the age of 30 to 40, when an increase occurs, which accelerates earlier in the developing than in the developed countries. Using age-specific death rates, it is pos-

Table 7/2

Life expectancy at various ages in selected nations related to the sex of the individual

Nation	*Year*	*Sex*	*Age of individual*					
			0	5	15	30	45	60
Africa								
Egypt	1960	Male	52	60	52	39	26	15
		Female	54	66	57	44	31	18
N. America								
U.S.A.	1968	Male	67	63	54	40	26	16
		Female	74	71	61	47	33	19
S. America								
Chile	1961	Male	54	59	45	37	25	15
		Female	60	64	60	41	29	18
Peru	1960–61	Male	53	58	49	37	25	15
		Female	55	60	52	39	27	16
Asia								
India	1951–60	Male	42	49	41	29	19	12
		Female	40	47	40	28	20	13
Malaysia	1966	Male	63	60	54	40	27	16
		Female	66	65	56	42	30	18
Japan	1967	Male	69	65	56	42	30	20
		Female	74	70	61	46	31	23
Europe								
Czechoslovakia	1966	Male	67	65	55	41	27	15
		Female	74	70	60	46	32	19
France	1968	Male	68	65	55	41	28	16
		Female	75	72	62	48	33	20
Sweden	1967	Male	72	68	58	44	30	18
		Female	76	72	63	48	34	20
U.K.	1965–67	Male	69	65	56	41	27	15
		Female	75	71	62	47	33	20

Source: ***Demographic Yearbook***, 1970, Table 20. U.N., New York.

sible to compare the patterns of mortality between two countries and within a country (Figure **7/1**).

An example of intra-national difference in age-specific death rates comes from the U.S.A. In 1964, the crude death rate for the white population was 9·4 per 1,000 and that for the black population 9·7 per 1,000—an insignificant difference. However, when age-specific death rates were calculated, a considerable differential in the mortality between whites and blacks appeared. In Table **7/3** it can be seen that at all ages below the 75 and over group the age-specific mortality of the black population is 1·4 to 2·5 that of the white population. Infant mortality (0–1 age group) is 90 per cent higher, childhood mortality (1–4) is 100 per cent higher, and deaths in the 5 to 15 age group are

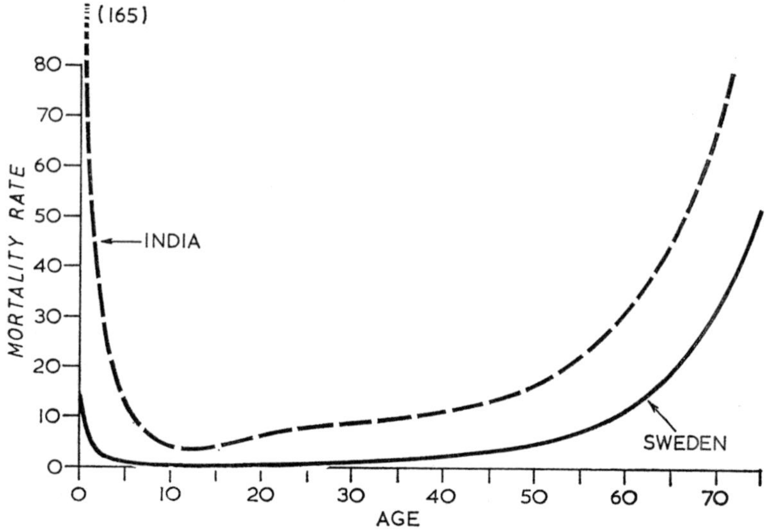

Figure **7/1** Age pattern of mortality, India and Sweden, 1960–61.

50 per cent higher amongst non-whites. In the age group 25 to 44, the mortality for blacks is 150 per cent higher. At all ages the differential between females of the two ethnic groups is more marked than that of the males. These differences could be explained by a worse genetic inheritance, implying that the blacks were biologically less fit, or by differences in environmental health. There is no evidence whatsoever for the first hypothesis, so that the increased age-specific mortality must be due to a lower educational standard, a reduced level of environmental sanitation, worse nutrition and a lower standard of preventive and medical health care available to the black people.

Table 7/3

Age-specific death rates and differentials between white and black U.S.A. citizens, 1964

Age	*White*	*Negro*	*Differential* (*white* : *black* = 1 : *x*)
0–1	21·5	40·9	1·90
1–4	0·8	1·6	2·00
5–14	0·4	0·6	1·50
15–24	1·0	1·6	1·60
25–34	1·3	3·3	2·54
35–44	2·6	6·6	2·54
45–54	6·8	13·2	1·94
55–64	15·9	27·1	1·70
65–74	36·7	50·6	1·38
75–	82·8	69·9	0·84
All ages	9·4	9·7	1·03

Source: U.S. Public Health Service: *Vital Statistics of the United States*, 1964 Report.

Although this differential exists, it should be stressed that compared with the citizens of the developing countries, the black population of the U.S.A. has relatively low age-specific mortality rates. But this should not obscure the fact that within the richest nation of the world, these differences do exist. This emphasizes the problems facing less wealthy nations, who are currently seeking to reduce death rates and increase longevity.

Standardized Death Rates

For the better comparison of the mortality in different nations, the age composition of the nations being compared needs to be related to a standard population. Standardization has been considered in Chapter 4. To recapitulate, if the age composition of two populations is markedly different (as, for example, India and Sweden) a comparison of age-specific mortality between the two will fail to demonstrate the differences. However, if the age-specific death rate of each country is related to the standard million (see page 83) a much clearer picture of the level of mortality is obtained, without the bias imposed by different age compositions in the two populations. The method used is identical to that used in calculating standardized natality rates. In Table **7/4** an example is shown comparing India and Sweden.

Table 7/4

Standardization of the death rates of India and Sweden, using the composition of the world's population in 1960 as the standard population

Age	*Standard population (world in mid-*1960)	*Age-specific death rates*		*Expected deaths per* 1000 *of the standard population*	
		India	*Sweden*	*India*	*Sweden*
	A	*B*	*C*	$A \times B = D$	$A \times C = E$
Under 1 year	30	164·9	15·3	4·947	0·459
1–4 years	111	23·1	1·0	2·564	0·111
5–14 years	226	4·4	0·4	0·994	0·090
15–24 years	181	6·2	0·7	1·122	0·127
25–44 years	261	9·8	1·3	2·558	0·339
45–64 years	146	23·3	7·7	3·402	1·124
65–74 years	32	64·8	32·7	2·074	1·046
75 years and over	13	159·6	119·9	2·075	1·559
Total	1,000	18·5	9·7	19·736	4·855

India Actual rate 18·5 Standardized rate 19·7
Sweden Actual rate 9·7 Standardized rate 4·8

Source: *Population Bulletin* No. 6. U.N.

The Life Table

The life table is a mathematical model for estimating the probability of dying, or conversely, of surviving to any specific age in a given population (Table **7/5**). Modern life tables arose when life insurance became a business. Since it was not unreasonable to assume that individuals would be prepared to insure their lives so that at death—whether natural or accidental—a sum of money would be available for their surviving relatives, the business of life insurance began. But to function, and to make a profit, which is the main objective of any business, life insurance companies had to calculate the probability of a given individual living or dying, so that they could more accurately estimate the premium he would need to pay. In other words, the insurance companies needed to measure the probable longevity (or mortality) of an individual as a member of a group whose age-specific mortality rates over a short period of time were known. Once this information was available, the company could calculate the annual sum of money, or premium, an individual as a member of the group would need to pay in order to guarantee each member of the group a specific sum of money at a determined age, or his heirs a specific sum of money at his death. For example, a group of 100,000 people are all 20 years old and it is known that they will all live an average of 40 years; it is possible to calculate how much each would need to pay annually to provide a specific sum at death for all members of the group. Whilst some individuals would die before the age of 60, and would pay fewer premiums, others would live much longer than 60 and pay more premiums. The deficit payments of the former would be balanced by the excess payments of the latter.

The life table is a life history of an imaginary, or hypothetical group, or cohort, of people as they grow older, and are diminished gradually by death. The record begins at the birth of each member and continues until all the cohort have died. At each age the cohort loses a number of people, this number being predetermined by the actual mortality in the region, or nation, under study at the time the table is constructed. It is, therefore, an artificial measurement and relies on several assumptions. The first assumption is there is no migration, therefore the only reduction in the size of the cohort is due to death. The second assumption is that people die at each age according to a schedule which is fixed in advance and never alters. The third assumption is that the cohort has a specific size. Usually 100,000 is chosen, so that the proportion surviving at any age can be seen by looking at the table, and without any further calculation. Since the age-specific mortality rates of the two sexes differ, it is usual to construct a life for each. This means that the female life table starts with the birth of 100,000 females who are then followed throughout their lives. The fourth assumption is that at each age, or in each age group, the deaths are distributed equally throughout the age interval.

In the study of population dynamics, life tables have proved useful models for the study of mortality. They can be used to calculate the probability of an individual of any specified age dying in any particular interval. The life table also indicates the average number of years a newborn infant can expect to live, and the number of years remaining to a person of any specified age. These and the other functions of the life table can be better appreciated if an actual life table is shown and the various factors in the table are considered. For insurance purposes, a *complete life table* dealing with the chances of dying at intervals of single years is used, but in demography, an *abridged life table* which deals with mortality over five-year age-groups is sufficient (Table **7/5**).

Age interval (Column 1, notation x to $x + n$)

The age interval in a life table is that between two birthdays n years apart. In the abridged life table, the interval n is usually taken as 5 years. Throughout the table the notation x denotes the person's age at the birthday beginning the interval, or put another way, x equals the number of complete years which have elapsed since birth. A person reaches the age x on his xth birthday. For a year afterwards he remains in the age interval $x + 1$, until his next birthday when $x + 1$ is his exact age. Algebraically he has been in the age interval x to $x + n$. For example, an Indonesian girl is exactly 5 years old. In the next year she remains in the interval $5 + 1$ until the day of her next birthday when her exact age becomes $5 + 1$, or 6.

Proportion dying (Column 2, notation ${}_nq_x$)

Since people die at every age, this is illustrated in the life table. The term q is used to indicate the probability of dying and the full notation ${}_nq_x$ describes the probability of dying in the interval between the exact age x and the exact age $x + n$. For example, to determine the probability of the girl dying in the 5-year interval between her 5th and 10th birthday, the notation would

1970 provisional life table—white female

Age interval	Proportion dying	Of 100,000 born alive		Stationary population		Average remaining lifetime
Period of life between exact ages stated in years (1)	*Proportion of persons alive at beginning of age interval dying during interval* (2)	*Number living at beginning of age interval* (3)	*Number dying during age interval* (4)	*In the age interval* (5)	*In this and all subsequent age intervals* (6)	*Average number of years of life remaining at beginning of age interval* (7)
x to $x+n$	${}_nq_x$	l_x	${}_nd_x$	${}_nL_x$	T_x	$\mathring{e}_x$
00–01	0·0149	100,000	1,494	98,659	7,542,381	75·4
01–05	0·0025	98,506	246	393,436	7,443,722	75·6
05–10	0·0015	98,260	146	490,902	7,050,286	71·8
10–15	0·0015	98,114	145	490,226	6,559,384	66·9
15–20	0·0028	97,969	274	489,197	6,069,158	61·9
20–25	0·0032	97,695	313	487,711	5,579,961	57·1
25–30	0·0037	97,382	361	486,042	5,092,250	52·3
30–35	0·0049	97,021	471	483,995	4,606,208	47·5
35–40	0·0080	96,550	774	480,949	4,122,213	42·7
40–45	0·0116	95,776	1,107	476,313	3,641,264	38·0
45–50	0·0183	94·669	1,733	469·308	3,164,951	33·4
50–55	0·0278	92,936	2,587	458,577	2,695,643	29·0
55–60	0·0396	90,349	3,574	443,394	2,237,066	24·8
60–65	0·0592	86,775	5,135	421,878	1,793,672	20·7
65–70	0·0946	81,640	7,722	390,077	1,371,794	16·8
70–75	0·1495	73,918	11,048	343,494	981,717	13·3
75–80	0·2356	62·870	14,810	278,813	638,223	10·2
80–85	0·3512	48,060	16,878	197,955	359,410	7·5
85 and up	1·0000	31,182	31,182	161,455	161,455	5·2

Source: Department of Health, Education & Welfare, National Center for Health Statistics, Rockville, Maryland 20852.

read $_5q_5$. The accuracy of the estimate of the probability of dying depends on how efficiently the information from death certificate records has been collected and analysed by the actuaries who prepare the life table. Efficient, accurate life tables require careful construction. An illustration of the use of Column 2 can be taken from the life table. In the 30 to 35 age interval, the proportion of women expected to die has been estimated to be 0·0049. This can be multiplied by 1,000 to give a life table mortality rate. In this example, of every 1,000 women who are alive on their 30th birthday, 4·9 will die before reaching their 35th birthday. The calculation can be made more accurate by considering Columns 3 and 4 of the life table. Column 3 uses the notation l_x to indicate the number of persons alive l on their xth birthday. Column 4 shows the number dying in the age interval x to $x + n$. In the column the notation d indicates the number dying, whilst x and n continue to have the meanings already given. Thus for the age interval 30 to 35, the notation can be translated as $_5471_{30}$, when x is 30 and $x + n$ is 35. This indicates that in the five-year period from the age of 30, 471 of the 100,000 born alive will die.

In Column 2, it will be seen that all the values lie between 0·0000 and 1·0000. In other words, this indicates that the proportion dying in the interval ranges from an impossibility of anyone dying (0·0000) to an absolute certainty of all of the cohort dying (1·0000). It therefore estimates the chances (or risk) of dying in each age interval. Clearly the first number is absurd for someone will die, and the second equally absurd until the last row of the table, when it becomes certain—for eventually everyone in the cohort must die. For this reason the values lie between 0·0000 and 1·0000 for each age group.

An example from the life table may help to clarify this concept. In the life table of the 100,000 females born alive, 1,494 will die before reaching the age of 1. This is shown in Column 4 ($_nd_x$). This means that the probability of any one person dying in the interval is 1,494/100,000 or 0·0149. It will be noted in this example that although the abridged life table is divided into 5-year intervals, the exception is the age interval 0–1. This is because of the very great importance of this interval, which is termed the neo-natal interval.

The Stationary Population

The stationary population is shown in Columns 5 and 6 of the life table and this concept requires some consideration as it has major applications in demographic theory.

These two columns make use of the concept of a stationary population, and enable the demographer to compute the population pyramid of a population in which the natality and mortality rates do not alter. Instead of following a single cohort of 100,000 through life, the stationary population concept computes the age-structure of a population as if its natality and mortality were those of the cohort *at the time the table was constructed.* It also assumes that the number of live births during a year must be equal to the number of deaths during that year. It supposes that a group of 100,000 people is born each year, and each such group has the mortality rates shown in Column 2 (that is those of the cohort previously considered). Thus a stationary population shows the number of persons who would be alive at any given time until all the 100,000 members of the original cohort had died. With the fixed number of births each year (100,000) and the predetermined probabilities of dying in each age applied, a stationary population would eventually be reached, when the birth rate exactly equalled the death rate. The stationary population gives information of the number of survivors at the midpoint of each age interval. This is shown in Column 5 of the life table. The number of survivors is given the notation L, and the column heading has the notation ${}_nL_x$, where x is the age at the beginning of the interval, and n the number of years in the designated age interval. For example, the figure in the 55–60 age interval is 443,394. This means that in a stationary population of American women, to which are added 100,000 female births each year, but which are subjected to the rates of mortality shown in Column 2, a census taken on any date would show that 443,394 women were between 55 and 60 years old. The notation for the example given would be ${}_5L_{55}$.

Column 6, which is designated T_x, shows the total number of persons, in this case women, in the stationary population (Column 5) in the age interval studied and in all subsequent age intervals. For example, in the stationary population of white females, just referred to, 2,237,066 would have passed their

55th birthday, and the total white women in the stationary population would be 7,542,381.

LIFE EXPECTANCY

The rather ponderous calculations in Columns 5 and 6 are the means of providing the very useful calculation of the mean expectation of life of members of the population. This has the notation $\mathring{e}_x$, and is shown in Column 7 of the abridged life table. Once the Column T_x has been completed it is easy to calculate the average number of years lived by the cohort after each age ($\mathring{e}_x$).

The concept and the calculation of $\mathring{e}_x$ may be easier to understand if the second meaning of T_x is considered. In this, T_x is the total number of man-years expected to be lived by the l_x survivors of the original births (l_0). It can then be stated that if l_x are alive at the exact age x, and if they can expect to live, in total, T_x years, then the average number of years each individual of the cohort will live is

$$\frac{T_x}{l_x} = \mathring{e}_x$$

Thus $\mathring{e}_x$ is the average life expectancy at age x.

This mean life expectancy at birth ($\mathring{e}_0$) is obtained by dividing the total years lived by the cohort (T_0) by the number in the cohort (l_0). Similarly the life expectancy at the age of 25 is obtained by dividing the total number alive at the exact age of 25 and over (T_{25}) by l_{25}.

Column 7 shows how long, on average, persons of a given age may expect to live, if conditions of mortality remain unchanged throughout their life. In recent years certain gynaecologists have recommended the use of oestrogenic hormones to 'maintain femininity' in women aged 50 and over claiming that it is only since 1910 that women survived longer than 45 years of age. The protagonists of this belief claim that in the past women reached the age of 45 and 'exploded like sky rockets', and therefore there was no need at that time to prescribe hormones. The truth of this claim can be determined by calculating life expectancy at specific ages in Sweden in 1828 and 1968 (Table **7/6**). Whilst it is true that there are proportionately more women aged 45 and over alive in 1968, if a woman reached the age of 45 in 1828 she had a life expectancy of 23 years, only 10 years less than in 1968. So that to say that women in the past 'exploded like skyrockets' at the end of the reproductive era is nonsense. Of greater importance than justifying or condemning the use of hormones from climacteric to death, the life tables do show that in 1828 only 72 per cent of live-born girls reached childbearing age, and only 65 per cent reached the midpoint of the reproductive era. By 1968, 98 per cent reached childbearing age and 97 per cent were still alive at the age of 30. The consequences of this additional infusion of women of childbearing age on the birth rate, if birth control were not used, can be readily imagined, and is a model demonstrating one of the reasons for the current rapid population growth.

Table 7/6

Life expectancy at birth of Swedish females in 1828 and 1968, computed from life tables

	Number alive at year		*Difference*	*Life expectancy in years*		
	1828	1968		1828	1968	*Difference*
0	100,000	100,000	—	43·6	75·2	+31·6
15	71,940	98,127	+26,187	44·7	61·6	+16·9
30	65,230	97,418	+31,897	33·4	48·1	+14·7
45	55,320	95,543	+40,223	23·0	33·8	+10·8
60	40,890	89,089	+48,199	13·2	20·4	+ 7·2

The table also emphasizes the high death rate of female infants and children in 1828. The life expectancy at birth was 43·6 years, by the age of 15 it had risen to 44·7 years. In other words, if a girl could escape death in childhood, she had a good chance of living to the age of 60. By 1968, this appalling wastage of infant and childhood deaths had been largely eliminated in Sweden, and the life expectancy falls progressively from birth.

THE VALUE OF LIFE TABLES

Once age-specific mortality rates are available (Column 2, q_x) the remainder of the life table is related to this column and the values in the other columns can be computed and can give considerable information about a population. Thus mortality and survival rates for any age,* or age group, can be obtained and since they are the only alternatives they must add up to unity. For example, in the table, by the age of 15, there were 97,969 female survivors. Therefore, there must have been 2,031 deaths. A quick glance at the total deaths before the age of 15 in Column 4 (${}_nd_x$) will prove this to be so.

SURVIVAL RATIOS

Survival ratios can also be calculated. It may be of value to calculate the probability of a girl in the 10–14 age group surviving to the age of 42½ as this will give an indication of the possible natality in a population. This probability can be obtained by making use of Column 5 (${}_nL_x$) of the table. The number of females in the stationary population in the 40–45 age group is divided by the number in the 10–14 age group. The result shows the probability of the girl surviving to the age of 42½ in that population. Survival ratios are of great value in estimating how much mortality has occurred in a population for which no death statistics are available.

AGE PATTERN OF MORTALITY

Perhaps it is even more useful to use life tables to compare the age patterns of mortality by comparing the values in Column 2 (${}_nq_x$) or by comparing life expectancy at any specific age in two populations.

POPULATION PROJECTIONS

If age-specific mortality patterns are known, the projected population of a country at a specific date in the future can be computed from life tables. Since censuses only take place at 10-year intervals (if they are made at all), there are gaps in the statistical records of every country. In planning an educational programme, or in estimating future food requirements of a nation, the information can be obtained from a life table provided there is a reasonably accurate registration of births. This is considered in detail by Shryock and Siegal in *The Methods and Materials of Demography*.

* Mortality rate is: ${}_nq_x = 1 - \left(\frac{l_{x+n}}{l_x}\right) = \frac{{}_nd_x}{l_x}$ and survival rate is $p_x = 1 - q_x$.

INFANT MORTALITY RATES

It has already been pointed out that the effect of death in the 0 to 1, and 1 to 4 age groups, influences considerably the pattern of mortality in a population. Of the two, the period 0 to 1 is the most influential. The infant mortality rate is calculated from the formula:

$$\text{Infant Mortality Rate} = \frac{\text{Deaths in the first year of life}}{\text{Total live births in that year}} \times 1{,}000$$

This, in fact, gives the infant death rate, but the infant mortality rate (q_0) of the life table is difficult to compute and, of course, relates to the number who will probably die during the first year, as a proportion of the number (100,000) *starting* the year. In most populations which are growing fairly uniformly, the two values are very close, and the infant mortality rate is used interchangeably with the infant death rate by human biologists, to the irritation of pure demographers.

The measurement of infant mortality is not without problems. The first is that the definition of a live birth is not clear. Recently the World Health Organization has considered this and an expert committee has recommended the following definition be adopted by member nations in order to bring about some uniformity. The World Health Assembly in 1959 agreed that a '*live birth is the complete expulsion or extraction from its mother of a product of conception, irrespective of the duration of the pregnancy, which after such separation, breathes or shows any evidence of life, such as beating of the heart, pulsation of the umbilical cord, or definite movement of the voluntary muscles, whether or not the umbilical cord has been cut or the placenta is attached; each product of such a birth is considered live born*'.

This definition has occasioned considerable argument as it may include infants whose weight is less than 400 g and who have been delivered when the gestation period is less than 20 weeks. By definition such a conceptus is an abortus, so that the two definitions overlap. This raises the question, can an abortus be a live birth?

Studies from several centres indicate that if the fetus weighs less than 500 g at birth, the mortality is 100 per cent, whilst if the birth weight lies in the range 500 to 999 g (i.e. approximately

20 to 27 weeks gestation) the mortality is 85 to 95 per cent, so that an excess of such births might adversely influence the infant mortality. However, investigations in Sydney, Australia, and in other countries indicate that fewer than 1 per cent of all births fall into the range 500 to 999 g.

The second problem in the World Health Organization's definition is how to separate live births from stillbirths. A personal investigation in several countries indicates that medical attendants tend, whenever possible, to designate the births as dead-born, even if some signs of life as defined above are present. This is because custom, religion and the law of many nations treat a dead-born baby differently from a live-born baby. Far less ritual and administrative details are required for burial if the baby is designated as still- or dead-born. This problem is considered in greater detail in Chapter 18.

The third problem is that statistics on infant mortality (especially statistics on infants weighing less than 1,000 or 1,250 g at birth) tend to be inaccurate, and under-reporting is frequent in most developing nations and in several developed nations.

An example of under-reporting can be deduced from Indonesian data, according to Ruzicka. In 1967, the Indonesian National Social and Economic Survey recorded infant deaths by age of death. The infant mortality rates for the urban and rural areas of Java–Madura were reported to be 40·6 and 78·4 respectively. These rates were only half those expected when other data were examined. When the infant mortality rate was divided into neonatal and postneonatal deaths, the proportion of neonatal deaths was 36 per cent of all infant deaths in urban areas, and 26 per cent in rural areas. Since in most developing nations whose socio-economic conditions are similar to those of Indonesia, neonatal deaths are equal to, or exceed, postneonatal deaths, Ruzicka considers that 'some 35 per cent of neonatal deaths in urban areas and about 50 per cent in rural areas were missed'. This suggests that they were not reported, although the infants did die.

This is because in many societies, the death of a new-born infant—particularly if very premature—is not felt to concern anyone but the parents, and is not reported. To many of the people, both in urban aggregations and in rural areas, it seems ridiculous if the child has lived only for a few hours, or days, to have to fill in a birth certificate form simultaneously with a death certificate form. In such cases the dead infant is disposed of by the midwife, or buried quietly by the father.

Although the death of an infant may fail to be reported to the authorities, it does not fail to have a psychological effect on the parents, and particularly on their desire for further children. For example, in France, Henry concluded that 'the mean interval between confinements is greater when the preceding child survives to the age of one year than if the child dies before this age'.

Despite the limitations of infant mortality statistics, the study of infant mortality is of great importance in population dynamics. In nations which have a high mortality, deaths in the age group 0 to 1 constitute the largest single age-specific mortality. It is also the group which is most readily influenced by preventive health measures and specific health programmes. If such programmes successfully reduce the infant mortality, an increasing number of children will reach the reproductive age and will tend to reproduce with a resulting increase in natality.

Trends in most nations show that in the past 30 years, infant death rates have fallen considerably and that the effect of improvement in environmental and sanitary care, allied to increasingly effective health measures, have been dramatically successful.

Such information as is available shows that in North-West Europe the infant mortality between 1750 and 1800 ranged around 200 per 1,000 live births. Swedish statistics confirm this, and indicate between 1820 and 1900 the rate fell to about 100 per 1,000 live births. From the year 1910 when the infant mortality rate was 100, until 1970 the fall has been dramatically steep, and in 1970 had reached a low of about 13 per 1,000 births (Figure **7/2**). The infant mortality rates of other North–West European countries show similar patterns.

In the years prior to 1900, advances in the medical care of infants were rudimentary and the decline in mortality cannot be related to better medical care. Over the period improvements in living conditions, in the sanitary control of infectious disease and the provision of pure water, were the main factors in the reduction in the infant mortality rate. Only after 1910 did preventive

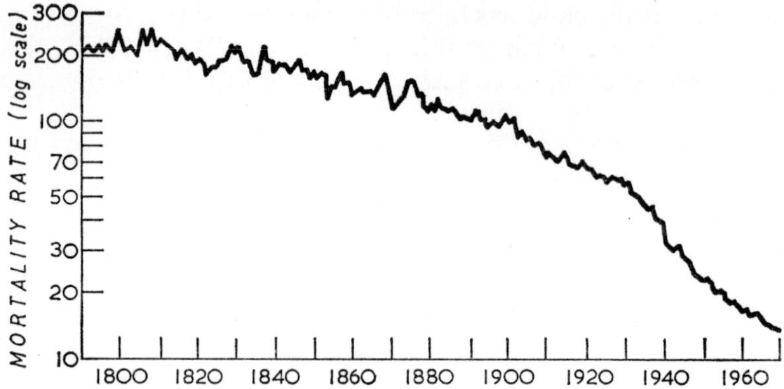

Figure **7/2** Infant mortality in Sweden from 1800 to 1970.
Source: Statistiska Centralbyran, Sweden.

and curative medicine have an impact. In the first 35 years of the century this was largely limited to better maternal nutrition and to the availability of protective inoculations. The steeper decline after about 1935 can be attributed to the availability of potent chemotherapeutic and antibiotic drugs and to the better training of physicians in child health.

In many developing countries, such infant mortality rates as are reasonably accurate (and most are understated), show rates resembling those of North-West Europe in the mid-eighteenth century (175 to 225 per 1,000 live births), some have rates resembling those of developed countries in the mid-nineteenth century (125 to 174 per 1,000 live births), a few show the rates of the developed countries in the first 25 years of the twentieth century (75 to 124 per 1,000); and the smallest number have the rates of the developed countries in the second quarter of the twentieth century (35 to 74 per 1,000). In each group of nations listed in Table **7/7**, there has been a tendency in the period 1950 to 1970, for the majority of them to reduce their infant mortality to that of the next lowest group.

In the state of our present knowledge, there is probably a lower limit to infant mortality rates. It can be calculated that an infant mortality rate of 8 to 12 represents the lowest obtainable. This is because between 4 and 6 babies per 1,000 are born alive with congenital defects, due either to chromosomal abnormalities or to environmental causes, such as infection, which are

Table 7/7

Infant mortality rates in nations of 5 million population or more, 1970–71
(*Latest year reported*)

Very high		*High*		*Moderately high*		*Intermediate*		*Low*	
250–150		149–100		99–50		49–25		24 *or less*	
Angola	230	Morocco	149	Rhodesia	95	Venezuela	45	Canada	21
Mali	190	Malawi	145	Algeria	86	Caribbean		U.S.A.	20
Zambia	190	Cameroon	140	Tunisia	84	Islands	40	—	
Upper Volta	180	Kenya	130	—		Cuba	40	Japan	16
Ivory Coast	180	Nigeria	130	Guatemala	94	—		—	
Uganda	160	Sudan	120	Chile	92	Taiwan	25	Austria	24
Tanzania	160	Zaire	120	Ecuador	86	—		Germany (W.)	23
Ghana	156	Malagasy	120	Colombia	78	Poland	35	Czechoslovakia	23
—		Egypt	115	Mexico	65	Hungary	34	Belgium	22
Brazil	170	—		Peru	65	Bulgaria	31	Germany (E.)	20
—		Haiti	130	Argentina	54	Greece	31	U.K.	19
Bangladesh	180	Bolivia	110	—		Italy	30	France	16
Pakistan	150	—		Philippines	80	Spain	30	Switzerland	15
Indonesia	150	Turkey	155	Thailand	70	U.S.S.R.	25	Denmark	15
		India	140	Malaysia	70			Finland	14
		Cambodia	140	Korea (S.)	60			Netherlands	13
		Korea (N.)	135	Sri Lanka	55			Sweden	13
		Iraq	120	—				—	
				Portugal	56			Australia	18
				Yugoslavia	55				
				Romania	54				

Source: *Demographic Yearbook*. U.N., New York.

It should be noted that some of the infant mortality rates of the developing nations are noticeably and grossly underestimated.

incompatible with life (Table **7/8**). In addition, a proportion of apparently normal low birth weight babies (less than 2,000 to 2,500 g at birth) fail to survive despite advances in neonatology. This adds a further 2 to 4 deaths per 1,000 live births to the total. Finally, a few infants will die from the effect of disease in pregnancy or from birth trauma (2 per 1,000).

Table 7/8

Major congenital defects per 10,000 births

Congenital defect	*Total conceptions*	*Estimated percentage born alive*	*No. born alive*	*Estimated percentage dying in year 0–1*	*Estimated no. dying in first year of life*
Down's syndrome	10	90	9	30	3·0
Anencephaly + spina bifida	10	80	8	100	8·0
Hydrocephaly + myelocele	15	80	12	100	12·0
Spina bifida	10	100	10	50	5·0
Heart	6	90	5	20	3·0
Gut	15	80	12	40	4·8
Hare-lip, cleft palate	12	100	10	0	0·0
Talipes	20	100	20	0	0·0
Congenital dislocated hip	5	100	5	0	0·0
Urogenital	10	60	6	30	2·0
Multiple defects	15	50	7·5	100	7·5
	128	—	104·5	—	45·3

Source: World Health Organization. *Congenital Malformations*, 1966.
Note: The calculated rate of 4·53 per 1,000 live births is similar to the actual rate of 5·8 per 1,000 determined in the Perinatal Survey in U.K. (1955), Table 74.

The lesson which may be drawn from a consideration of infant mortality trends is that the main impact upon the high rates in many developing countries will come from a multi-pronged attack. This approach to family welfare includes the provision of pure water, the control of insect-borne disease (such as malaria), the availability of preventive inoculations against common infectious diseases, the education of mothers during schooling and in pregnancy in the care and nutrition of their children, the limitation of large families by properly organized family planning campaigns, and the availability of curative medical care, although this is the least important factor from a demographic viewpoint.

Factors Influencing Mortality

That there are differences in mortality between urban and rural areas has been demonstrated in many investigations in developed nations, but the reasons for these differences are many and often contradictory. In the nineteenth century, urban mortality rates were higher than those of the rural areas surrounding the towns. But at that time, piped, pure water supplies were unusual, sewage disposal primitive, housing congestion considerable, and air pollution beginning. By 1900, most urban areas in North-West Europe and North America, and many in other areas of Europe, had piped water and proper sewage. The differentials now diminished, and often became reversed. These are most clearly demonstrated when age-specific death rates are studied. In many recent investigations, infant mortality has been found to be lower amongst urban than amongst rural dwellers, but that of children and young people shows no statistical difference, and only after the age of 45 is the mortality lower amongst rural dwellers. This finding is not absolute, however. In Scotland, between 1911 and 1968, there was a tenfold reduction in postneonatal mortality (1 to 12 months) whilst neonatal mortality (0 to 1 month) had fallen only threefold and this pattern is typical of most developed nations.

The reduction in the neonatal mortality has been due to better care of the newborn, that of postneonatal mortality to a reduction in the deaths from respiratory infections and diarrhoeal diseases.

Despite the reduction in infant mortality in Scotland (to 19·6 per 1,000 in 1970), there is a pronounced socio-economic gradient both in the overall infant mortality and when specific diseases are considered. For example, the mortality from respiratory and diarrhoeal diseases was five times as high when the father was a semi- or unskilled labourer as when he was in professional or higher clerical employment. When the socio-economic factor was analysed further, it was found that the highest infant mortality rates were in the Glasgow region, where housing is poor, room-density is high and where families tend to be large.

Thus certain urban conditions can be productive of as high an infant mortality as is found in rural areas in developed nations. Unfortunately, no accurate information is available for developing nations. It would be of great interest to know if urban-rural differentials in mortality occur and of their magnitude.

This has been investigated to some extent by Ruzicka. He noted that in India, for example, the range of infant mortality rates can be as wide as from 50 (in Kerala) to 197 (in Uttar Pradesh). When the rates in urban and rural areas in individual states were examined, he found that the rural rate was higher in most instances. For example, in Uttar Pradesh in 1964–65, the infant mortality rate in the urban areas was 131, and that in the rural areas was 197.

It seems that in most developing nations at least 10 per cent of live-born children die before their first birthday, and that a larger proportion of infants in rural areas may be expected to die. In the developing nations, in contrast to the developed nations, the neonatal mortality is as high as, or may exceed, the postneonatal mortality rates. Clearly many of these deaths could be prevented by the better provision of health care in pregnancy, during delivery, and just after birth.

SOCIO–ECONOMIC STATUS

Investigations in Britain, the U.S.A., France, Japan and other countries indicate clearly that the higher the socio-economic group, the lower the mortality. From an analysis of cause of death statistics in Britain by Logan, the increased mortality in the lower socio-economic groups is not due to occupational hazards, but to poor childhood nutrition, worse environmental living conditions, and a lack of knowledge of preventive health measures. From this analysis it would appear that any reduction will be brought about by better 'social engineering' rather than better curative medicine.

FAMILY SPACING

The relationship between high infant and child mortality and socio-economic status in the developing regions is not so clear, and there is little objective data available. A study in Taiwan, by Rutstein, confirmed that a higher infant and child mortality was found amongst older women of high parity who lived in poor environmental conditions, and had low incomes. This is what would have been expected. However, Rutstein found that actual deaths of children, or the fear of mortality amongst young children, had a minimal influence on natality, or on attitudes to family size.

MARITAL STATUS

Studies in past years show that at every age the married have lower death rates than the single, the divorced or the widowed. The differences in all groups are greater for men than for women. Despite a multitude of theories, no factual data have yet been obtained to explain the finding.

TRENDS IN MORTALITY IN THE NATIONS OF THE WORLD

The improvement in infant mortality due to preventive health measures and better nutrition has reduced crude death rates and increased life expectancy in the past 30 years. As well as this, there has been a reduction of the age-specific mortality in other age groups, at least those through the reproductive years. This has the effect that the life expectancy at birth is increasing in most countries of the world. This improvement is not uniform and the world can be divided in three groups.

GROUP 1—LOW MORTALITY, HIGH LIFE EXPECTANCY

This group contains all European countries, the U.S.S.R., North America, Australia, New Zealand, Japan, Israel and Uruguay. Although the actual crude mortality rates vary, in most they lie below 10 per 1,000, and in all the countries the life expectancy at birth is 65 years or more. In most of these nations the infant mortality rate is below 40. These countries all have a high level of environmental sanitation, relatively good supplies of pure water and a reasonable level of expenditure on social services, including health care and education.

GROUP 2—MEDIUM MORTALITY, MEDIUM LIFE EXPECTANCY

This group contains nations whose crude death rate lies between 10 and 20. Occasionally because of a favourable age structure the death rate is less than 10, and life expectancy at birth is between 55 and 65 years. The infant mortality rate generally lies between 40 and 99. In these nations expenditure on economic and social projects is increasing and an effort is being made to initiate or implement family planning programmes. These countries include most countries in Latin America, Asia and some African nations.

GROUP 3—HIGH MORTALITY, LOW LIFE EXPECTANCY

In these nations the crude death rate exceeds 20 per 1,000 and life expectancy at birth ranges from 35 to 54 years. The infant mortality exceeds 100. These nations are beginning to institute death control measures, particularly to reduce their high infant mortality, but family planning measures, in general, have not been adopted as government policy.

These crude figures fail to emphasize the change which is currently taking place throughout the world. Over the past decade the infant mortality has dropped in most nations, and childhood mortality is also falling. In 1955, when the United Nations suggested classifying nations in the groups mentioned, there was a fourth group. This comprised those nations which had very high mortality and very low life expectancy. No nation now lies in Group 4.

EIGHT

Migration

The earliest information that we have about man is that he was a nomadic hunter. He lived by collecting roots and fruits and by hunting animals. He had few possessions, but was able to endure extremes of heat and cold. He was a prey of other animals, and because of his defencelessness probably hunted in bands of 10 to 15 men. With high infant mortality, and a low life expectancy, this would suggest that the size of a hunting tribe was never more than 50 people. When his traditional hunting grounds were invaded by another tribe, he became aggressive, but because of the low population density such contact was usually avoided by all tribes (Ardrey). His way of life was nomadic, although it is likely that the range of his migratory journeys was limited in most cases. He followed the animals wherever they ate: if they moved, because of drought, he moved; if they stayed grazing on the lush grass, he stayed. A few tribes moved on into unknown lands, where sexual liaisons between them and tribes living in the new lands took place, so that the variants in the genetic pool spread and found phenotypic expression in the offspring of the unions. This type of nomadic society exists today amongst the Australian aboriginals, the Kalahari bushmen, and the Sakai peoples of Malaysia.

After at least 2,400,000 years of this kind of existence, a change occurred, about 10,000 years ago. At about the same time in three distinct areas man learned how to cultivate cereals instead of merely gathering the seeds. The areas were the foothills adjoining the valley of the Tigris–Euphrates; the foothills bordering the Hwang-Ho river in North China and an area in Central America.

For the next 5,000 years man continued to obtain meat by hunting so that his diet was better balanced. He ate meat which he hunted and cereals which he grew and such fruits and roots as the women gathered. Over this period he learnt to domesticate wild animals and by so doing became a pastoralist. No longer requiring to hunt to obtain meat, the tribes followed their flocks through traditional grazing areas, and only supplemented their diet by hunting when the opportunity arose. Hunting had become easier with the invention of the bow and arrow, which enabled man to kill at a distance, a matter of some importance for the puny, thin-skinned, light-framed biped. With the better diet, the infant mortality tended to fall, but population growth was slow, and was further slowed by inter-tribal fighting, which now became increasingly common, and by drought and epidemics which decimated the people at unpredictable intervals. To some degree, societies at this stage of development continue to exist in Central Asia, Mongolia and Arabia.

In certain areas where water was plentiful and constant, the pastoralists found that the grass was sufficient for their flocks throughout the year and it was no longer necessary to move to find pasture. In time, too, they developed techniques to cultivate grains for human consumption.

The cultivation of grain and the domestication of animals produced a ready supply of food, so that the necessity to hunt diminished still further.

The settled tribes increased in size, as a more ready supply of food reduced infant mortality. But as the tribes became larger and land became scarcer, it became necessary for some people to leave the tribal lands, which could no longer support the population. It is unknown whether these migrants were the most intelligent and the best physical members of the tribe, or the worst; but whichever it was, man's migratory movement led to the exploration of greater and greater portions of the earth's surface. In the most fertile river valleys, the population pressures leading to migration were slow to develop and migration was delayed. But such rich areas attracted the more warlike tribes from the wilderness, with resulting turbulence, and the forced migration of the weaker tribes.

It can be seen that two factors influenced migration. The first was the necessity to find new land and new food sources when population pressures became too great in a particular area. The second was the forced migration of some or all members of defeated tribes after inter-tribal war. The relative importance of these two influences cannot be assessed, but both are of importance today. In the first, economic, social or political influences induce people to leave their homes and seek better conditions in an alien environment. These may be called the attractive (or pull) forces. In the second, political or military events impel the weakest, the most vocal, or the most fearful out of their homeland into new territories. These are the impelling (or push) forces.

Migration and Population Change

Migration, therefore, may affect population dynamics quite considerably, for the migrant not only brings his physical presence, but his psychological and cultural way of life, which has to be adjusted to fit in with the prevailing norms of the new community. This applies both to internal migration, between regions within a country, or from rural to urban areas, and more forcibly to international migration. But in both forms, it would appear that two groups are most likely to migrate—the intellectually strong and the physically weak. The great majority of people will resist moving from their home, even when conditions there are becoming increasingly unfavourable. The psychological security of living in a familiar society, amongst familiar people, prevents migration—other things being equal. Only when the familiar area ceases to satisfy intellectual or physical needs, or when continuing to live there imposes danger of physical or intellectual discomfort, does the urge to migrate exceed the urge to stay.

This simplistic statement does not tell the whole story. In all nations of the world there is an increasing mobility of people: the increasing influence of radio and television is breaking down the fear of strangers, and the increasing contact between peoples is encouraging mobility. The crude influences of 'push' factors and 'pull' factors are therefore being modified by intervening factors, one of which is the increased information available via the media.

THE IMPELLING OR PUSH FACTORS

The main factors which impel or 'push' people from their familiar territory are twofold. The first are economic and the second political, although the two often interact and influence the individual. Economic factors include (1) lack of opportunity for continued employment because of redundancy; a reduction in demand for a particular commodity or product; or a reduction in the supply of a particular resource; (2) an over-supply of labour, so that the former factors are aggravated, and (3) the inability of the person to adjust to changes in technology (for example, automation), or to remain in a different job. In many cases such economic changes merely lead to internal migration, which has no effect on a nation's population, but does cause problems of urbanization and increasing environmental pollution. The economic change may lead to emigration, either permanently or on a temporary basis, as occurs in Europe today, and as was the way in which the population of the U.S.A., Canada, Australia and Brazil increased so dramatically in the past century.

Political factors include alienation from a community because of different beliefs, or modes of behaviour, and lack of 'cultural' facilities in the area. These two factors may lead to internal migration to another area of the country where facilities are more suited to needs, such as the drift of young unmarried people from the country to the provincial towns, or to the capital. Alternatively they may lead to emigration. A stronger political motive for migration, usually emigration, is oppressive or repressive discrimination because of the ethnic group of the individual and his religious or political beliefs.

ATTRACTING OR PULL FACTORS

The attracting factors for migration operate in conjunction with the impelling factors in many instances. These pull factors include: (1) the lure of greater recreational, cultural, scholastic or intellectual activities in the new area. This is often the reason for migration from rural areas or small country towns to larger centres. (2) The movement because of occupation, or other reasons, of other persons who have a close relationship to the individual. For example, if a man moves, his family usually migrates with him. (3) The superior opportunities for employment, or the acquisition of a larger income, in the new area. (4) The better physical environment of the receiving area. Such environment may be better climatically, or better because of institutions such as educational establishments or other community facilities.

Obviously the attracting factors operate both for internal migration and for emigration and the influence of each is considered when the individual makes his choice.

INTERVENING FACTORS

Lee has pointed out that a decision to migrate is rarely made only after considering the attractions of the new home and the disadvantages of the existing home. The decision is influenced by intervening factors, many of which are difficult to identify, and are related to the psychological make-up of the individual. The same factors which appear insuperable to one individual appear trivial to another. Examples of this are the refusal of one migrant family to leave Britain when they found that in Australia there were no kippers; and the return of another because the wife missed her mother, whom she had always visited three times a week. In both cases the opportunities offered in Australia, on considered thought, far outweighed the intervening factors. It is clear that when migration is voluntary, emotions often replace reason in making a decision. A wet, grey summer in Britain increases by 20 per cent the number of enquiries about migration to Australia.

The importance of intervening factors is not felt only in migration between the developed nations. Java, with 132,000 km^2 of land and 80 million people, has sought to encourage migration to Sumatra, an island of 474,000 km^2 and 18 million people. In the past 20 years only 420,000 have migrated, although land in Sumatra was given to the migrants, there was no real language barrier, and the predominant religion in both islands is Islam.

Trends in Migration

INTERNAL MIGRATION

In the developed countries, the trend in the past fifty years has been from rural to urban or suburban areas. This trend is most marked in the United States, where metropolitan areas (the term includes the city and its ring of suburbs) have gained between 5 and 15 per cent, and the rural areas have lost a somewhat smaller percentage in the past three decades. It has also occurred in Britain since about 1880, when rural depopulation set in on a national scale, mainly as a result of the import of cheap American foodstuffs; but the speed of the migration has also increased in recent years.

Within the metropolitan area itself, the trend in the U.S.A. is from the city to the suburban ring; but this merely aggravates the ecological problems of the metropolitan area.

Similar migratory trends, with comparable percentages, are found in most European countries, Canada and Australia. In Italy, for example, there has been a considerable movement away from the rural South to the industrial North. In France and Germany there has been an annual decrease of about 1 per cent in the population of rural areas since 1950, most of the migrants going to the larger industrial cities. Even in Australia, underpopulated by world standards, the size of the major cities of Sydney, Melbourne and Brisbane is increasing at the expense of the rural areas and country towns. In Australia, over 85 per cent of the population live in urban areas and over 65 per cent in metropolitan areas, making it the most urbanized nation in the world.

Investigations confirm that in the developed countries, since 1940, there has been an increase in the rate of migration from the low-income, recreation-poor, rural areas to the large metropolitan areas, where jobs are more readily available and facilities for non-participating indoor and outdoor recreation are greater. This trend has been marked particularly in people aged 17 to 37, with a peak in the early twenties. In the United States the internal migrants are usually married, or marry soon after migration, with a consequent rise in birth rate, and an increase in the size of the 0 to 4 and 5 to 9 age groups, in the new area. This pattern probably also applies to other developed countries. Older people are less likely to migrate, and have greater psychological problems if they do. After the age of 40, males tend to migrate more than females, and after 65 females more readily than males. The second phenomenon in recent internal migratory trends has been the exodus of people from the city proper to the suburbs. This trend is most marked in the U.S.A., where city centres are becoming increasingly decayed; but it occurs in most other developed countries.

In the developing countries, the trends of internal migration are somewhat different. In many nations in Asia and Africa new agricultural land has been opened up, and has been settled by formerly landless peasants. However, concurrently with this, there has been a movement of people to the major industrial cities. As the industrialization of a developing nation has progressed, this movement has accelerated. But despite internal migration, the urban population of India, Indonesia, Bangladesh, Pakistan, Malaysia, Thailand, probably China, and most African nations, is less than 20 per cent of the total. In Latin

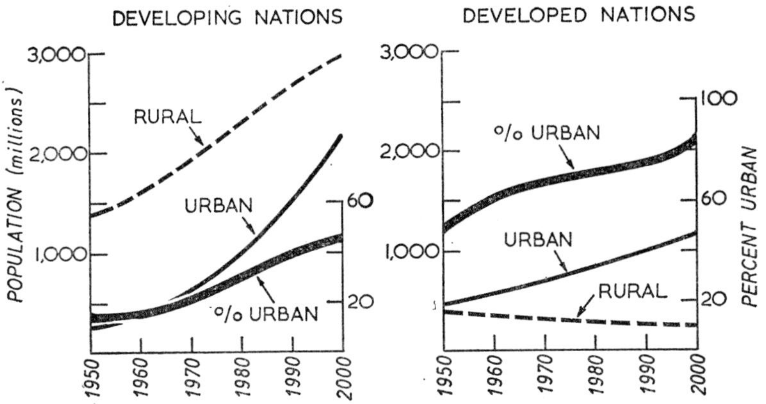

Figure 8/1 Urban and rural population, actual and projected, 1950–2000.

Source: *The World Population Situation in 1970*. U.N., New York, 1971.

America, about 45 per cent of the people are urban dwellers. This means that the people of the world are still predominantly rural dwellers. However, the trend is disturbing as can be seen in Figure **8/1**. In each of the nations listed, the urban population growth rate of the major cities exceeds the high reproductive growth rate of the nation as a whole. The rural areas are losing population to the urban areas, with the resulting problems of environmental congestion. The increasing urban congestion leads to problems of hygiene, housing and sanitation and to the increasing alienation of people, as their traditional rural values are superseded by aggressive urban attitudes.

The question remains: Will increasing industrialization in

the next decade in developing countries increase the rapidity of internal migration to (metropolitan) urban areas, and what will be the sociological effect of this migration with regard to health, education and human reproduction?

International Migration since 1840

Although throughout history there has been a movement of people from one nation to another, or from one continent to another, until the nineteenth century the movement was mainly of families escaping from persecution or seeking better living conditions. The initial colonization of the Western Coast of North America was largely by people escaping from religious persecutions; whilst the Huguenots fled from France after 1560 to settle and to bring their skills in the wool trade to England.

Spain, in the sixteenth, seventeenth and eighteenth centuries, sent migrants and soldiers to South America to exploit the riches found there for Spain's benefit. The numbers migrating permanently probably did not exceed 500,000, but their effect on the cultural development of the area was considerable.

In the nineteenth century, sea transport became safer and more regular across the Atlantic, with the consequent migration of Europeans to the Americas. The United States was the main recipient, and in the early years most of the migrants came from Britain, although after the Irish famine in 1846, increasing numbers of Irish migrated. Towards the end of the century, migrants were leaving Poland, Italy, Greece and Scandinavia in considerable numbers.

The earlier immigrants were mainly ill-educated peasants who had insufficient capital to buy land of their own in Europe, or had been cleared from feudal lands they had tilled. Their main objective in migrating was to obtain the cheap land available in the U.S.A., and to a lesser extent, Canada. The pull effect of cheap land was backed by the push effect of dear, or unobtainable, land in Europe. The migrants had very limited capital but much muscle power. They knew how to clear and to cultivate land, and they cleared and cultivated it. They opened mid-western America, and because their efforts were labour intensive but required little capital, they were readily absorbed. After about 1880, most of the land had been settled, and increasing numbers of migrants went to the cities, where they took the lowest paid, least skilled work. Wage rates were low, and it was possible for manufacturers to use sweat shop techniques, which again limited capital expenditure. The migrants had high natality rates, usually higher than those of the earlier settlers, but this was in part artificial as so many migrants were young and in the peak reproductive ages, and in part due to their abnormally high infant and childhood mortality rates. Health care was rudimentary for the poor; housing conditions inadequate, families crowding into decaying, unsanitary dwellings; public education was elementary and minimal, so that the social costs of absorbing migrants were limited, and were less than the social value of cheap labour readily available. The consequence was that capital accumulated.

Between 1820 and 1920, about 33 million migrants went to the U.S.A., the greatest number migrating between 1880 and 1919. After 1920, immigration quotas were imposed, which favoured migration from North-West Europe and Mexico, at the expense of Southern Europe, West Asia and East Asia, so that immigration slowed, only 3·5 million migrants crossing the Atlantic between 1920 and 1940.

On a reduced scale, migration was taking place from Russia into the relatively empty lands of Siberia. Between 1800 and 1912, 8 to 12 million settlers crossed the Urals, and since that date another 12 to 15 million probably have joined them.

Chinese from the several provinces of Imperial China also migrated to neighbouring countries from the middle of the nineteenth century, and by 1950, 11 million Chinese lived overseas, mainly in Malaya (3·5 million), Indonesia (4 million), Thailand and the Philippines.

As a consequence of the social, economic and political upheavals which convulsed Europe during and after World War II, European emigration increased. With the appearance in Europe of Communist and Non-communist blocs, those who disliked or feared one regime attempted to move to a nation which had adopted the other. Between 1945 and 1960, 4·5 million migrants went to North America; and Oceania (mainly Australia and New Zealand) had a net migration of 1·6 million people, Australia taking more than 85 per cent of the total. Europeans, mainly from Southern Europe, also migrated to South America, particularly to Argentina and Brazil, who had a net gain from migration of about 1 million.

By 1960, the large migrations had diminished. Europe was not only rehabilitated but was booming economically with the result that Central and North-Western Europe were seeking immigrants, although usually only on a temporary and seasonal basis. Between 1961 and 1970, fewer than 1 million migrants have gone from Europe to North America, Australia has had a total net migration of 547,000, and very few migrants (less than 20,000 per year) have migrated to Latin America.

Migration continues in Africa but is largely undocumented. It tends to be seasonal and temporary, as, for example, the workers recruited in Mozambique and Malawi for work in South Africa.

Perhaps the largest movement of people in this century has occurred in the Indian subcontinent. Partition of India in 1947, which established the predominantly Hindu State of India, and the largely Muslim State of Pakistan, led to a movement of people fearing religious persecution and probable massacre. The size of the exodus was gigantic: between 14 and 16 million people moved between the two nations. However, as the immigration to Pakistan was about 7 million and that into India about 8 million, the net migratory movements did little to distort the population dynamics of either country. More serious socially was the migration to India of over 10 million Hindu peasants from Bangladesh following the suppression of the independence movement in 1971 by the Pakistani Government. The addition of 10 million people to India's population negated the effect of about four years' effort in population control. Their return to Bangladesh after the intervention of India and the establishment of the new nation of Bangladesh relieved India, but has imposed considerable strains on the new nation.

Apart from the Indian subcontinent, migratory flow between developing nations has largely ceased since 1960, because of legal restrictions on movement. In 1965–71, for example, only five countries had a net migration (immigrants less emigrants) of 100,000 or more. These nations were the U.S.A., Canada, Australia, Argentina and Brazil.

Most of these migrants are Caucasian, under the age of 40, who bring to the recipient country a number of dependants under the age of 16. For example, in the 1961–65 period, 24 per cent of the 1·4 million migrants to the U.S.A. were under the age of 16, and only 12 per cent over the age of 40. There is increasing doubt of the economic value of migration in a modern technological society and increasing awareness of its adverse effects on population dynamics.

Australia may be used as an example to demonstrate this new concept. Australia is large and relatively under-populated. Up to 1940, a slow net migration, mainly of people from the British Isles, occurred, but the Japanese war stopped this. Suddenly, Australia was physically and psychologically alone—a Caucasian outpost in an Asian sea. The Japanese bombed Darwin and invaded New Guinea. Time, courage and the U.S. Navy saved Australia from an alien occupation. The lesson was learned. In the war years, Australia had changed from a wool-shed, a wheat store and a dried fruit warehouse for Britain into an embryo industrial nation. And she was short of manpower. In addition, humanitarian impulses induced her to accept many European refugees, dispossessed of their homes and goods by the redrawn political map. On three grounds Australia sought immigrants who were to be almost exclusively Caucasian so that they would assimilate more readily. The first was defence. Populate or perish was the cry. More people meant more strength, and God was known to be on the side of the big battalions. The Yellow Peril was in the forefront of people's minds. And even if Japan had been defeated, there were others. China, perhaps; or Indonesia; or even, in the wildest fantasy of some leaders, India. The second reason was economic. Men were needed for the burgeoning factories, and the migrant workers were prepared to take any job. The third was humanitarian.

The policy was encouraged by setting up centres in Britain and other European nations and by offering subsidized passages to the migrants and their families. The scheme worked.

By 1971, net migration was boosting Australia's growth rate to 2·0 per cent, one of the highest in the developed world. And questions began to be asked. Most immigrants had settled in the main cities, adding to the social congestion. Many were employed in labour intensive jobs and, because of high wage rates, many industries sought tariff protection against more cheaply produced equivalent imports. These two factors led to questioning of the economic basis for immigration, which was that 'immigration contributed to the economic and technological base on which national security today depends so heavily'. It was pointed out that a community of 25 million led to no greater economies in production than a population of 12·5 million. The real question was what was the real cost to the community of an immigrant worker. An accepted figure was \$650; the real figure was 10 to 15 times higher, as each migrant cost not only the \$650 to induce him to come to Australia and to bring him to the country, but a much greater sum to provide houses, roads, electricity, water supply, sewage disposal, education for his children, and health care for his family. This was calculated in 1970 to add up to over \$5,000 for each addition to the population. This meant that the total net migration in 1970 cost \$500 million. And this huge sum had to be taken out of the pool of capital available otherwise for national development, for educating existing Australians, and for other social services. Immigrants were needed, but to service the immigrants, more were needed. In other words, the labour shortage which existed was partly caused by the immigration programme itself.

There is no relationship between the conditions in North America in the late nineteenth century and that in the late twentieth century in Australia. In the first place, the migration to North America was proportionately far smaller (to size of the population). In the second, most migrants to America went to open new lands. They were frontiers-men, requiring little capital and demanding few amenities. Australia's immigrants mainly go to the cities. Australia's resources require large amounts of capital, and because of technological progress, only small infusions of labour. Encouraged immigration, therefore, seems to be less advantageous economically, and for defence, than previously thought; in fact, it is a dis-economy, since the migrants are often under-educated.

In recent times, the net effect of migration on the population dynamics of a nation has been minimal, with the exceptions of the U.S.A., Canada, Australia and Brazil which have registered net gains. The fact is that forced massive migration to under-populated countries, were this politically possible, would be logistically impossible. Not only are there insufficient ships to carry the migrants and their household goods, but potential recipient countries have neither the facilities nor the money to make ready the areas for their reception, to construct the roads, to build the houses, to organize schools and extend social services, and to make available jobs for more than a very few. Even those developed countries which have continued to seek migrants in the past decade are currently reviewing their policies, and tending to reduce quotas because of the ecological, industrial and psychological problems involved.

It is clear, therefore, that emigration can do nothing to relieve the population pressures in nations such as those of Asia and Latin America, although it may be possible for such nations to redistribute some of its own population within the boundaries of a single nation.

NINE

The Growth of the World's Population

Analysis of the components of population dynamics leads to the conclusion that the current rate of population growth is the highest that has ever occurred; that its effects are of considerable magnitude; and that, with purpose, man has a chance of avoiding the malignant consequences. In this chapter it is intended to review methods of measurement of population growth, to study trends in population dynamics, to discuss the theory of demographic transition, and to outline possible solutions to the problem.

Measurement of Population Growth

The population of the world on 1 January, 1971, was estimated to be 3,634 million. In 1971 an additional 73 million, and in 1972 an additional 74 million people were added. The population is currently increasing at a rate of more than 74 million persons per year. This is nearly 200,000 persons per day, 8,300 persons per hour and 140 persons per minute. These crude statistics hide the fact that this growth rate is not uniform throughout the world. Amongst the 1,100 million people living in the affluent developed nations of Europe, North America, the U.S.S.R., Japan, Israel and Oceania, the annual rate of population growth is 0·6 to 1·5 per cent, but in the rest of the world, in the hungry developing nations, whose population comprise 2,500 million, or 60 per cent of the world's total, the annual rate of population growth is 2·0 to 3·0 per cent (Table **9/1**).

Table 9/1

The crude birth and death rates, and the annual population growth rate in the developing and developed nations, 1960–1970

Rate	*Developing countries*	*Developed countries**	*Difference in developing countries*	*Difference (per cent)*
Total population 1970 (in millions)	2,500	1,100	+1,400	127
Crude birth rate	40	21	+19	90
Crude death rate	18	9	+9	100
Rate of reproductive change	22	12	+10	83
Annual growth rate	2·5	1·2	+1·3	108

* The nations of Europe, the U.S.S.R., North America, Oceania and including Japan and Israel from the developing regions.

Intercensal Increase in Population

Population dynamics are measured by comparing the results of two censuses, usually taken ten years apart. In addition, information is derived from registration of vital events in those countries where these statistics are available and reliable. It is obvious that the accuracy of the estimate will depend on accurate collection of the data, but most demographers accept that since errors are likely to occur in both censuses, they balance out, and the estimate has an accuracy of ±10 per cent.

For example, India took censuses in 1951, 1961 and 1971 as did many other nations, including the U.S.A. (1970) and Japan (1971). The figures in Table **9/2A** give an indication of the total amount of growth in the three populations studied, but they do not permit any comparison between the *growth rates* of the nations under consideration. However, this calculation is easy to make and is computed from the following ratios:

The *relative* change in the size of the population is measured by the ratio

$$\frac{P_t - P_0}{P_0}$$

or

$$\frac{P_t}{P_0} - 1$$

which is another way of expressing the same thing. In this formula, P_0 is the population at the initial census and P_t that at the next census. If this ratio is multiplied by 100, it is converted into a 'percentage change' between the two censuses.

INTERCENSAL PERCENTAGE CHANGE

As just noted, the intercensal percentage change can be calculated from the formula:

$$\left(\frac{P_t}{P_0} - 1\right) \times 100$$

Alternatively it can be computed by dividing the amount of change by the population at the time of the earlier census, and multiplying the result by 100 as

$$\left(\frac{P_t - P_0}{P_0}\right) \times 100$$

For example, between 1951 and 1961, India's population increased by 78,105,000. This means that the intercensal percentage change was

$$\frac{78{,}105{,}000}{361{,}130{,}000} \times 100 = 21{\cdot}7 \text{ per cent.}$$

Between 1961 and 1971, the intercensal percentage change, which also shows the growth rate, was 24·6 per cent, despite an intensive family planning campaign, which is calculated to have prevented 14 million births over the decade.

The calculation is obtained from the data:

$$\frac{108{,}132{,}000}{439{,}235{,}000} \times 100 = 24{\cdot}6 \text{ per cent.}$$

The reason for the increased growth rate is the greater number of children that are entering the reproductive era and are having children.

INTERCENSAL INCREASE IN POPULATION

In Table **9/2**, size of the population and the intercensal percentage changes are shown. It must be remembered, of course, that the components of population dynamics not only include reproductive change, that is births less deaths, but in the case of the U.S.A., particularly, also include net migration, that is immigrants less emigrants.

Table 9/2

The growth of the population and the intercensal change in the U.S.A., India and Japan since 1910

A. Population (in thousands)

Years	*U.S.A.*	*India*	*Japan*
1910–11	92,228	252,122*	50,297
1920–21	106,021	251,252*	55,391
1930–31	123,202	279,015*	63,872
1940–41	132,165	318,701*	72,540
1950–51	151,326	361,130	83,200
1960–61	179,323	439,235	93,419
1970–71	203,212	547,367	103,720

B. Intercensal change percent

1900–10	21·0	6·7	12·3
1910–20	15·0	−0·3	10·1
1920–30	16·2	11·0	15·3
1930–40	7·3	14·2	13·6
1940–50	14·5	13·3	14·7
1950–60	18·5	21·7	12·3
1960–70	13·3	24·6	11·2

* Relates only to areas of the Indian subcontinent now included in the Union of India.

The examples given in Table **9/2** are instructive. It can be seen that the intercensal change in population in the U.S.A. exceeded that of India until 1930. At this time, the U.S.A. was in an economic depression, the birth rate fell and immigration was curtailed; whilst in India increased health measures caused a reduction in the death rate with a higher intercensal percentage change. This has escalated since 1950. In the U.S.A.

meanwhile, the increased acceptance of birth control has reduced the rate of population growth. Japan is an example of a nation which has maintained a fairly steady intercensal percentage change. In the years 1900 to 1940 the mortality was high but was falling. From 1940 onwards, the mortality continued to fall, but birth rates also fell, initially due to war, and subsequently to Government action to control natality by permitting induced abortion and other birth control measures.

RATE OF POPULATION GROWTH

The rate of population growth is probably more informative than the actual growth of the population. It can be calculated with a reasonable degree of accuracy, if the crude birth rates and the crude death rates are known, and, when necessary, the net migration rate can be obtained. This produces the formula:

Rate of population growth = crude birth rate minus crude death rate + immigration rate minus emigration rate

= rate of reproductive change + net rate of migration

Reasons have been given in Chapter 8 why net voluntary migration today makes an unimportant impact on population dynamics, with the exception of a few nations, for example, Argentina, Australia, Brazil, Canada, Uruguay and the U.S.A. Even these nations are currently reviewing their immigration policies, and, if current political trends persist, may be expected to reduce their migrant intake in the next decade. Forced migration, because of fear, intolerance or hysteria will continue between contiguous nations in Asia and Africa, but the number will be small, apart from occasional exceptional migrations as, for example, the temporary flight of 10 million Hindus from Bangladesh in 1971, and the 'repatriation' of Chinese from Indonesia in 1960–66.

Population dynamics, therefore, is mainly a study of reproductive change leading to population increase, and this must be considered the major factor in the current accelerated rates of growth.

Annual rate of population growth

If one wishes to compare the rate of population growth between two countries, which have different intervals between censuses, the intercensal percentage change in population is meaningless. To make the information comparable, it is necessary to convert the data into annual rates of growth, or the percentage change per year. To do this the compound interest formula used in banking is adopted. If this formula is adapted to populations, it becomes:

$$P_t = P_0 (1 + r)^n$$

and

$$\frac{P_t}{P_0} = (1 + r)^n$$

where P_0 is the census count at the earlier census
P_t is the census count at the later census
r is the average annual rate of growth
and n is the time interval in years, or decimal fractions of a year, between the two censuses.

Without the use of logarithm tables the calculation to find the annual population growth rate (r) is complicated and tedious, but with them it becomes relatively simple, provided one recalls that by the rules governing logarithm calculations, $\log (1 + r)^n = n \log (1 + r)$. With this manipulation, the formula now reads

$$\log \left(\frac{P_t}{P_0}\right) = n \log (1 + r)$$

or

$$\log (1 + r) = \frac{\log \left(\frac{P_t}{P_0}\right)}{n}$$

To obtain the percentage growth rate, the result (which is a ratio) is multiplied by 100. This calculation implies a growth by regular increases, whereas of course, the growth is continuous. Once again compound interest mathematics using 'natural logarithms' tables (log *e* tables) enable this calculation to be made by the formula:

$$\frac{P_t}{P_0} = e^{rt}$$

The log *e* tables enable one to calculate *rt* by looking up the

e^x tables, where the values of rt can be found directly. From these tables not only the annual rate of growth (r) can be calculated, but the time (t) which the population will take to double can be readily calculated. Representative average annual rates of growth and population doubling times can be seen in Table **9/3**.

Table 9/3

The demographic data for the largest nations in each continent

Region	*Population* 1971 (*to nearest million*)	*Latest vital rates per* 1,000		*Annual population growth rate*	*Years to double population*
		Birth	*Death*		
World	3,634	34	15	2·0	37
Developing Nations	2,500	>30	—	2·5	28
China	700	34	11	1·4	50
India	541	43	21	2·5	28
Indonesia	120	45	20	2·9	25
Brazil	91	39	9	3·1	23
Bangladesh	74	45	12	3·3	22
Pakistan	59	45	10	3·5	20
Nigeria	64	50	24	2·6	27
Mexico	49	43	9	3·4	20
Developed Nations	1,100	<20	<15	<1·5	>50
U.S.S.R.	241	18	8	1·0	70
U.S.A.	204	18	9	1·1	63
Japan	103	18	7	1·1	63
Germany (West)	59	15	12	0·3	224
Britain	56	17	11	0·6	117
Italy	54	18	10	0·8	88
France	50	17	11	0·6	117
Australia	13	20	9	1·8*(1·1)	40(68)

* The higher figure is due to net immigration.

Demographic Transition

The study of various societies, both primitive and sophisticated, indicates that population growth has always been regulated to some extent and only recently has it escaped control. Since the population growth rate is merely a way of expressing the collective family size, it must be assumed that individual families made some decision about the number of children that they would like to have. The decisions are rarely arrived at by conscious rational discussion and, even today, seem to be made on the basis of conventional, cultural attitudes; imitation of respected or revered members of the society; or in deference to collective behavioural norms. Since these psychological attitudes are rarely verbalized, the social scientist is at a considerable disadvantage in analysing the population dynamics of past times. However, such evidence as there is seems to indicate that societies, as a whole, have sought to create populations in which births just exceeded deaths. When a disaster struck leading to a high mortality, it was followed 9 to 20 months later by a sudden spurt in the birth rate. This near balance of vital rates led to a slow growth in population over the centuries. The actual growth rate depended on the availability of food sources, the avoidance of famine, flood, war and infectious disease epidemics, and the cultural need for children as extra labour or for ritual purposes.

From the time, two and a half million years ago, when man first differentiated from the pre-hominids, population growth was very slow indeed, with a doubling time exceeding 100,000 years. Then about 10,000 years ago, perhaps following a sudden climatic change, primitive man began to domesticate wild animals and to cultivate the wild grains whose seeds he had previously merely picked when they were ripe. There is evidence that three centres of domestication and cultivation appeared at about the same time ($\pm$1,000 years). These were in West Asia, mainly in the Euphrates–Tigris river complex, in North China in the Yellow River area, and possibly in Central America (Figure **9/1**). From these centres agriculture spread to involve the Nile delta, the Indus river complex and the Amazon basin in South America respectively. With a better-balanced diet, the population growth rate increased and the doubling time shortened.

There were, of course, considerable fluctuations in the growth rate in each of the areas. When a succession of good seasons occurred, the population increased. When crops failed, or floods swept through, or drought cracked the land, deaths exceeded births, so that overall growth was slow. By the first year of the Christian era it is likely that the population of the world was 250 million. China had a population of 70 million, India of 100 million and the Mediterranean seaboard including the European, Asian and African shores, one of 50 million, the balance of 30 million being the population of Africa and America.

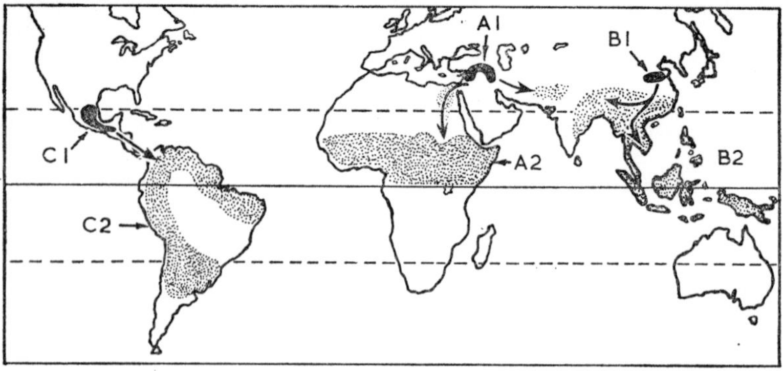

Figure **9/1** Centres of agricultural origins and probable secondary spread. A1. West Asian centre, B1. North China centre, C1. Central American centre.
Source: Harlan, J. R.

A review of the available evidence from incomplete historical records, and more accurate parish records in Europe in recent times, has led to the theory of demographic transition. This concept is particularly associated with the names of Professors W. S. Thompson and F. W. Notestein who separately developed the concept in the 1930s, when demographers were more concerned with population decline than with population growth. The dramatic changes in population growth since that time mar the theory to some extent, but if no time factor for change is postulated, the concept offers a theoretical basis for population dynamics.

In essence, this theory of population dynamics suggests that most societies seek to improve the welfare of their members, usually by the increased production of food and commonly used goods. Such an end is best achieved when there is a relative balance between deaths and births: only a slight excess of births being achieved, so that population growth is zero, or very low at most.

It is obvious that such an ideal state can be best obtained by low death rates and low birth rates; but it might equally be found in societies with high death rates and high birth rates. Between the two extremes are societies which have disparate rates of birth and death.

Viewed from an historical perspective, earlier societies had high death rates and high birth rates; and, as noted, population growth was slow. Most modern societies tend to have achieved

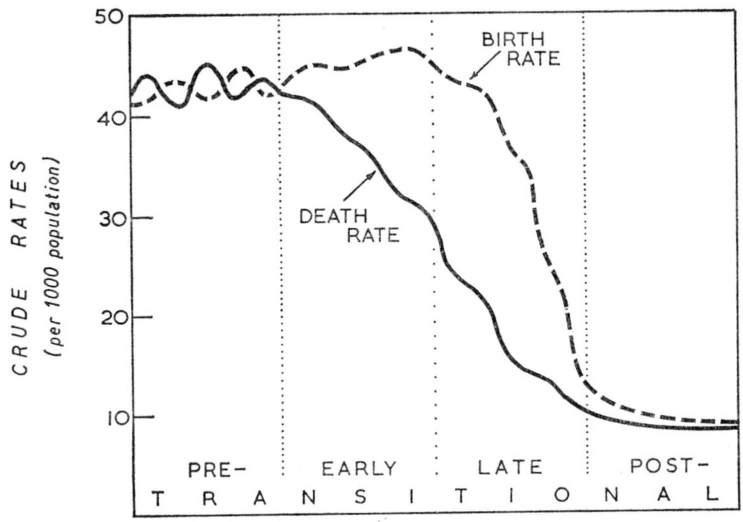

Figure **9/2** Stages of demographic transition.

some measure of death control so that death rates have dropped, but birth rates have not yet fallen, so that population growth is increasing at a high rate. A few modern societies have achieved birth control as well as death control, and are becoming in balance, demographically, once again, having gone through the demographic transitional process (Figure **9/2**).

These three types of society form a continuum (in the historical sense) in which change is occurring mainly in the direction of birth and death control. The process or change is termed *demographic transition.* Three stages are visualized: (1) pretransitional, (2) transitional, and (3) post-transitional.

In *pretransitional societies*, death rates are high and fluctuate widely as a result of epidemics, famine and war. No active death control exists. Birth rates are also high and, as with death rates, fluctuate widely. Few such societies exist today, apart from remote pockets in a few Asian, African and tropical American countries.

In *transitional societies*, the decline in the death rate has begun, or has advanced some way, with the reduction, particularly, of infant and childhood deaths. Because of this, the high birth rate may be increased, as more children live to reach the reproductive years. Population growth is occurring at an increasing rate, and causing concern, but considerable fluctuations continue to be seen, as control of the environment is inadequate or absent. In the later stages of this phase, the birth rate begins to fall because of birth control measures, whilst the death rate tends to fluctuate less and has fallen generally to a relatively low level. It may remain low or may rise as more people reach old age. The great majority of nations in the world today are in the transitional phase.

In *post-transitional societies*, both death and birth rates are low. Good preventive health care has reduced infant and childhood mortality to a minimum, although adult deaths still occur from the effect of over-eating, the misuse of drugs such as tobacco, alcohol and pharmaceuticals, and from environmental pollution. The birth rate is low and stable due to a wide knowledge of birth control and its general acceptance. Population growth is, therefore, almost zero.

It is possible to divide the nations of the world into their stage of demographic transition by making certain assumptions. These are that in the early transitional stage the annual population growth rate is more than 2·3; and in the late transitional stage it is between 2·2 and 0·5. In countries which have reached the post-transitional stage, the annual growth rate is 0·5 or less.

In Table **9/4** all nations whose population exceeds 5 million are graded into early transitional, late transitional and post-transitional stages. If this table is studied it will be observed that the more the nation has advanced through the transitional period, the more likely it is to be designated an economically 'developed' nation. It should be noted that the process of demographic transition is not a smooth, steady, onward

Table 9/4

The place in 'demographic transition' of nations with a population of 5 million or more (arranged in order of population size).

	Stage			
	Early transitional		*Late transitional*	*Post-transitional*
Annual growth rate	>2·3		2·2–0·6	<0·5
Years to double population	<30		30–140	>140
Population size (in millions) 100 or more	India Indonesia		China U.S.S.R. U.S.A. Japan	
20–99	Brazil Bangladesh Nigeria Pakistan Mexico Turkey Thailand Egypt South Korea Iran Burma Ethiopia Vietnam (North)		Britain Italy France Spain Poland Argentina Canada Romania Yugoslavia	West Germany
5–19	Vietnam (South) Colombia Congo (Zaire) Afghanistan Sudan Morocco Taiwan North Korea Algeria Peru Tanzania Ceylon (Sri Lanka) Malaysia Nepal Kenya Venezuela Chile Iraq	Ghana Uganda Malagasy Saudi Arabia Cuba Mozambique Volta Cameroon Syria Ecuador Rhodesia Angola Mali Haiti Bolivia Guatemala Tunisia Yemen	Netherlands Australia Portugal Greece Bulgaria Switzerland Denmark Finland	East Germany Czechoslovakia Hungary Belgium Sweden Austria

occurrence. Like all activities based on human behaviour, wide fluctuations occur. For example, in the 1930s much discussion was directed to the declining populations of Western industrialized countries, which were at that time considered to comprise the civilized world. It was felt that if the reproductive growth rate continued to decline the whole of Western civilization would collapse. Competent demographers (e.g. Whelpton) estimated that in 1970 the U.S.A., for example, would have a population of 154 million. The U.S.A. was, at that time, in the late transitional phase, information about contraception and simple contraceptives were available (see Chapter 12), the death rate was low (between 11 and 10 per 1,000), the reproductive growth rate was about 9·5 per 1,000, and the implied annual average growth rate was 0·79%. From 1940 on, for ill-understood reasons, young people decided to marry earlier and to have more children with the result that the birth rate rose; the average annual rate of population growth went up to 1·35% in 1940–49, and 1·82% in 1950–59. The demographers revised their estimates in 1959 and calculated that in 1970 the population of the U.S.A. would be 185 million. The actual census total for 1970 showed that the population was, in fact, 204 million. However, once again a change in reproductive behaviour may have begun. American women are having fewer children. In the 1970 census data are given showing that women under the age of 25 were opting to have no more than two children.

In Britain similar miscalculations were made. A paper in 1939 by Reddaway was accepted as authoritative. In this he estimated that by 1970 Britain would have about 44 million people of whom more than 15 per cent would be aged 65 or over, and less than 15 per cent would be 15 years old, or less. Eighteen years later a further estimate was made by Cole. He calculated that by 1970, Britain would have 55 million people, and twice as many would be under 15 years of age, as over 65 years of age. Evidence from the 1970 census indicates that Cole was more nearly correct. The population in 1970 was 56 million, and it is increasing at an annual rate of 300,000. The Royal Commission on Population predicted in 1959 that the population of Britain in the year 2000 would be about 54 million. This figure has already been exceeded, and present estimates are that by 2000 the population of Britain will be 66 million. These illustrations are given to show that demographic projections merely show trends; for the caprice of human reproductive behaviour may prove them false.

THE PROCESS OF DEMOGRAPHIC TRANSITION

Study of the process of demographic transition over a long period (which is the only valid approach) is impossible for most nations as the vital statistics needed are not available, or if available are highly inaccurate. Certain European nations, however, have information stretching back for two or more centuries and can be used as models to show the process. Two of these are Sweden and Britain. A study of the medical aspects of the process of demographic transition in Britain can be derived from the writings of McKeown and his colleagues, and it is from these that much of the following account is taken.

PRE-TRANSITIONAL PERIOD (1086–1770)

In 1086, the Norman overlords of England determined to make a census of the numbers of people, houses and resources of their occupied territory. The resulting Doomsday Book was the first census conducted in the country and showed that the population was about one and a half million. The pre-transitional period begins before 1086, but as no real information is available, for convenience this date is taken as a base line. Between 1086 and 1345 birth and death rates fluctuated considerably, but some population growth occurred so that by 1345 the estimated population of England and Wales was about 3·5 million. In 1348, the most severe epidemic of plague—the Black Death—reached England, and over the next twenty-two years deaths exceeded births, so that by 1370, the population had fallen to 2·5 million. As the epidemics waned, population growth was resumed and by 1670 England's population had doubled to 5 million, an implied annual growth rate of 0·2 per cent.

Over the next century, the growth rate accelerated because of the disappearance of the plague and the introduction of new agricultural practices, which greatly increased the food supply.

Between 1720 and 1770, the face of the English countryside changed as the Enclosure Acts enabled farmers to consolidate their holdings and to experiment with new agricultural techniques. Before, with much land held in common, and strips scattered everywhere, improvement had been nearly impossible. With consolidation of land and soil improvement, new strains of wheat were developed and food supplies increased. The introduction of marling the soil and of clover cropping (instead of having to let the land lie fallow) and the development of winter grasses enabled livestock to be kept alive all winter instead of being killed and salted in autumn. With this change,

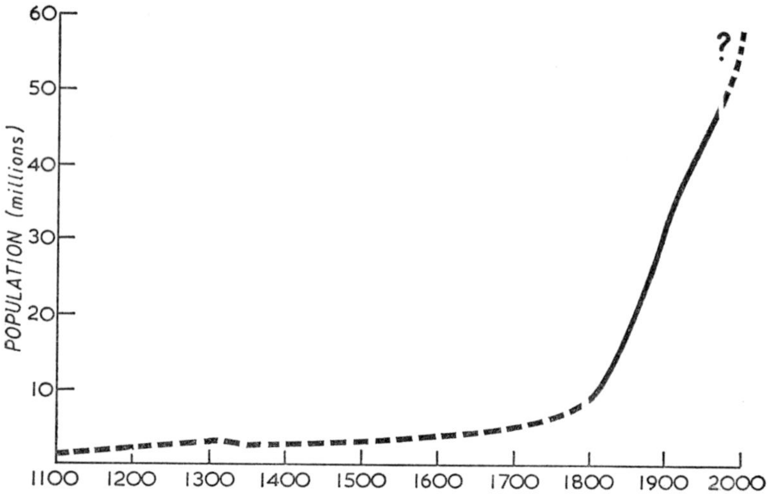

Figure **9/3** The growth of the population of England and Wales since 1066.

new breeds of sheep were developed which had a thicker fleece and a higher meat content. These changes led to an increase in the food supply and the cessation of gross food shortages, so that the population began to increase, although slowly at first, with a slight rise in the birth rate and a slight fall in the death rate after 1720. By 1770, the population had risen to 7 million, an increase of 5·5 million since 1086 (Figure **9/3**).

The effect of these changes, and the accelerated rate of population growth from about 1750, are shown in Figure **9/4**. Similar accelerated population growth rates were found in other North-West European nations.

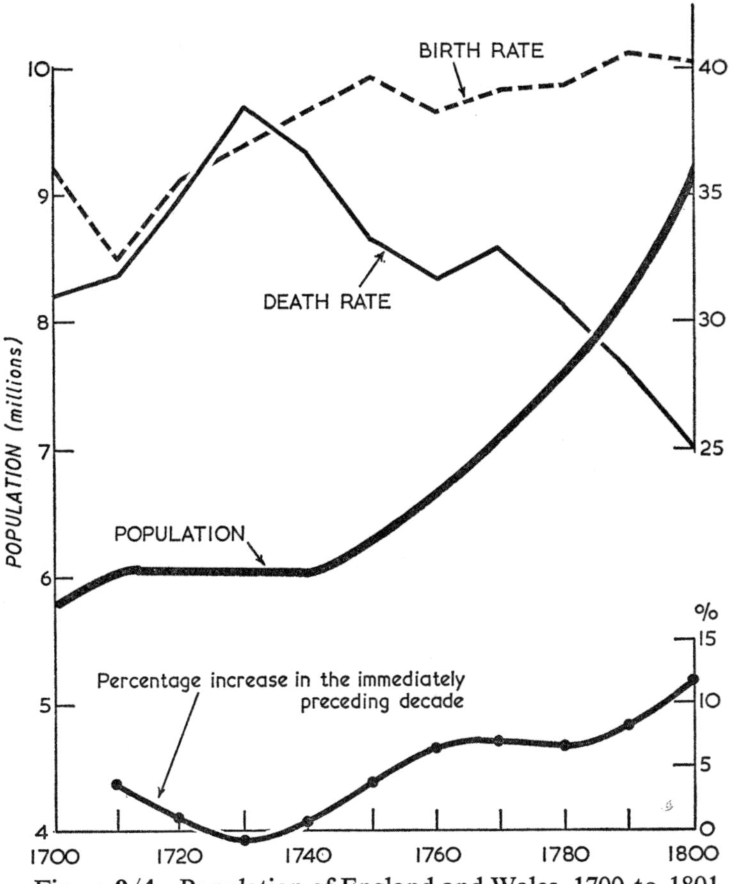

Figure **9/4** Population of England and Wales, 1700 to 1801.

EARLY TRANSITIONAL PERIOD (1770–1870)

From about 1770 the death rate began to drop, whilst the birth rate remained at its previous level, or for a short period (1770–1810) increased slightly (possibly, as Krause suggests, because more women married early owing to the changed economic conditions which followed the Agricultural and Industrial Revolutions). The fall in the death rate which continued throughout the period with a decline from 32 per 1,000 in 1770 to about 20 per 1,000 in 1870 (Figure **9/5**, p. 192), was not due to advances in curative medicine or to the provision of hospitals.

Curative medicine was still in the pre-scientific era: the number of drugs available was enormous, but the number which had more than a placebo effect was minimal. Of the total drugs available in 1870 only a few could be considered specific. These included laudanum and other opiates to relieve pain; digitalis for the treatment of 'dropsy'; purgatives; and, possibly, mercury for the treatment of syphilis. Physicians therefore relied on placebos, and supportive therapy, neither of which could have had much influence on the death rate. In surgery, the scene was just as uninspiring. Until the last few years of the period, anaesthesia was unavailable and the aetiology of infection unknown. Operative surgery consisted of amputations, transperineal lithotomy, incisions of abscesses, and the occasional removal of cataracts. The mortality of the first two operations was high; and even after inhalation anaesthesia enabled the surgeon to operate at leisure and to invade the peritoneal cavity, postoperative mortality remained high. McKeown quotes a London surgeon, Mr. Ericksen, who wrote in 1874 that 'skill in the performances has far outstripped the success in the result'.

The results in obstetrics were no better. Maternity hospitals had been established in Dublin in 1747 and in London in 1749, and were followed by others in many provincial cities. However, the majority of women were confined at home by midwives, usually untrained. Because of selection of patients and infection, the mortality in the hospitals was between five and ten times higher than that in domiciliary midwifery. No prenatal care was offered, and no preventive advice was given.

It is apparent that in all the main branches of medicine neither therapy, nor hospitals, could be causes of the declining death rate. It was even said, rather rudely, that most patients lived in spite of, not because of, the doctors.

McKeown's investigations showed that the causes of the decline of mortality in the years between 1770 and 1870 were due to three main factors. First, there was a marked improvement in the level of nutrition and hence of resistance to infection. This preceded by at least half a century the second factor, which was the improvement of environmental sanitation. The third factor, which operated interdependently with the other two, was a diminution in the virulence of infective organisms. McKeown's investigations have identified that most of the decline in mortality was due to a fall in the mortality from tuberculosis; typhoid, typhus and enteric fevers; scarlet fever and dysentery.

The relative importance of the three factors is under dispute, but all played a part in the process of demographic transition as well as in the general improvement of the health and welfare of the population.

Improvement of food supplies

There is much argument whether the diet improved after 1770, as more and more people left their homes in the conservative rural areas for the greater economic opportunities offered in the towns and factories. It has been suggested that in the rural areas a man could always keep hens or grow cabbages. The attractions of the rural areas were more apparent to middle-class travellers than to the inhabitants. Food consisted of bread and cheese washed down with beer or water, and meat was rarely eaten. Wages were minimal, often paid in kind, and working hours were long. Life in the towns was not much better, but there was a greater opportunity for employment and thus a larger income, and at that time the towns were small, the countryside was close.

In 1770, the only towns in England with a population of more than 50,000 were London (500,000), Bristol and Norwich (50,000 each). Forty years later there were eleven towns of more than 50,000 people, but apart from London (which now had one million inhabitants), Bristol and Plymouth, all were in the industrial north. Despite the increase in the urban population, for decades the Industrial Revolution was largely rural. This had profound results, the workers being dependent on the factory owner for housing, shops, food and drink. But despite the feudal control, wages were higher than in agriculture, and food more plentiful. Thus it is likely that, in fact, there was a rise in the standard of the diet from about 1770, and that the town dwellers did obtain a better diet than the country dwellers. The close connection between better infant nutrition and reduced infant mortality has been observed in the developing countries of the world today and it can be speculated that a similar event occurred in Britain 150 years ago.

Sanitary engineering

Despite the fact that the period 1770–1870 was that of the Industrial Revolution in Britain, with the rise of the manufactories, the expansion of the industrial towns, and the drift of the people from country to town, the factory owners, as much for profit as from humanitarian motives, soon realized that the efficiency of the labour force was reduced unless a certain amount of sanitation was provided in the festering slums which they had created. With the provision of piped water, protected wells, and with better personal and domestic cleanliness, the incidence of enteric disease fell, as did that of typhus, which was included in the enteric group in national statistics up to 1871. Dysentery and diarrhoea continued to be causes of death, particularly in infancy and childhood, but it would appear (from inadequate statistics) that these diseases were becoming less frequent towards the end of the period.

The reduction in virulence of infectious disease

The relative importance of this factor must remain speculative, for there are no objective data, but in the experimental situation various factors can influence bacterial growth and resistance. It is also known that the nature of bacterial virulence can change dramatically over a time period. There is evidence from many sources that scarlet fever was common in the eighteenth century and although the actual death rate from it is unknown, it is likely to have been high. At some time between 1830 and 1870, the death rate began to fall slightly and this persisted until the end of the period. Scarlet fever had a mortality rate of 700 to 800 per million in the period 1851–71, and the disease continued to be serious until about 1910, after which its incidence and virulence declined, so that today it is an uncommon disease. There is no evidence that the infectivity, or the virulence, of the organisms altered during the early transitional period, and in many ways their spread might be expected to have increased, as people moved to the towns into crowded slum dwellings.

Tuberculosis is spread by exposure to infection, caused mainly by overcrowding at home and at work. In the conditions of the English industrial towns in the period 1820–70, congestion of dwellings was increasing, hours and conditions of work in factories were deplorable, conditions which favoured the more rapid spread of the disease. On the other hand, evidence from World War II, and from concentration camps established by the Germans, indicates that increasing mortality from tuberculosis is related to deteriorating nutrition. McKeown notes that the mortality from tuberculosis began to fall from 1851, during a time when it is reasonably certain that the level of nutrition was rising. It must, therefore, be concluded that improved food supplies played a not inconsiderable part in the reduction of the mortality from tuberculosis between 1820 and 1870.

By 1870, Britain was in the middle of the period of demographic transition. The death rate was falling, the birth rate remained high, with a consequent high rate of reproductive growth, and a high annual population growth rate. These conditions apply to many developing nations in the world today.

LATE TRANSITIONAL PERIOD (1871–1971)

After 1870, the improvement in mortality from infectious disease control continued, and other measures began to play an important part. Advances in preventive and curative medicine occurred, particularly in the second half of the period, and medicine could now offer something more than mere reassurance and comfort. From about 1906, increasing attention was paid to maternity and child welfare, and to school health, and these, together with increasing advice about health and hygiene, have helped to reduce the death rate still further. Preventive inoculations against the common bacterial infectious diseases became increasingly available, and increasing numbers of children were protected. The introduction of chemotherapy in 1938 and of antibiotics ten years later further reduced the mortality from infectious disease. In the years from 1900, the main reduction has been in infant and childhood mortality, which in 1971 were 12 per cent and 3 per cent of the 1841–50 rates respectively. Infant mortality fell from about 175 per 1,000 in 1871 to about 18 per 1,000 in 1971. That this reduction is not unique is shown by reliable statistics from Sweden, where in 1751 the infant mortality was 210 per 1,000 live births but by 1951–60 it had fallen to 17 per 1,000, and by 1970–71 to 13 per 1,000 (Table **9/5**).

The period 1871–1971 also saw a marked reduction in the

Table 9/5

Infant and childhood mortality in Sweden since 1751

	1751–70	1951–60	1968–70
Infant	210	17	13
Childhood 1–4	35	0·8	0·6
5–9	13	0·4	0·3

Source: Central Bureau of Statistics, Sweden.

birth rate in Britain. The start of this decline coincided with widespread publicity about contraceptives following the Bradlaugh-Besant trial (see Chapter 10) and has continued. In 1971, the birth rate was 17 per 1,000, the death rate 12 per 1,000, and the reproductive growth rate 0·5 per cent. Britain was therefore about to leave the late stage of demographic transition and enter the post-transitional stage (Figure **9/5**).

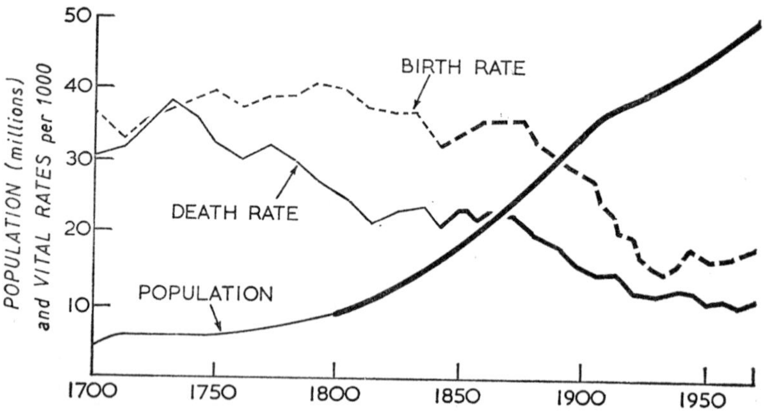

Figure **9/5** Population growth, England and Wales 1700 to 1970.

Cultural Influences on Demographic Transition

The model of England and Wales as a nation which has almost completed demographic transition has been given to show how the process may occur, and be analysed by a study of vital rates. The effects of social and economic change have also been demonstrated. The effects of the less readily observable cultural traditions have not been considered. Yet they are most important. The demographic transition undergone by England and Wales was also followed by the majority of North-West European nations. But there were two exceptions—France and Ireland.

During the period between 1770 and 1870, France's population growth rate was half that of the growth rate of 1·0 to 1·5 per cent of other European nations, and in the latter year was almost stationary. The reasons for this slow growth appear to have been cultural. Not only did the French peasant attitudes encourage small families, but Napoleon's Civil Code had introduced an economic basis for the tradition. This was that parents had to bequeath a determined portion of their property to each child. Being intensely conservative and realist, the French peasant and small landowner saw that his hard-won property would be dispersed and disintegrated if he had too many children. It was, therefore, necessary to limit the size of the family.

Examination of population growth in Ireland also shows how cultural influences as well as natural phenomena affect population dynamics. In common with England and Wales, and with the Scandinavian nations, a surge of population growth occurred in Ireland between 1770 and 1841. The increase has been estimated by Griffeth to be about 175 per cent, although his estimate may have been high. As in England and Wales, this increase coincided with an increased supply of very cheap food, particularly potatoes and milk. At the same time the age of marriage fell. Young, after touring the country, claimed that 'marriages are daily contracted with the most reckless improvidence. Boys and girls marry literally without habitation or means of support, trusting, as they say, to Providence as others have done before them.' Indeed the quality of life was so low, that it seemed, as the Roman Catholic Bishop of Raphoe told the Poor Law Enquiry in 1835, that the people married young 'as they cannot be worse off than they are . . . and they may help each other'.

By 1841, the population was over 8 million, making Ireland one of the most densely populated nations in Europe, and it appeared to be increasing at over 3 per cent per annum.

This exploding population led to increasing subdivision of land, as peasants struggled to obtain sufficient to grow the staple potato. By 1835, holdings were being divided and divided again, rents were rising and families of six and more were attempting to live on 0·25 to 0·5 hectares. At the same time a large number of the peasants had no employment except during planting and harvesting the potato crop. A situation of overpopulation, under-employment and high natality threatened. Then in 1845, potato blight, which had been introduced from North America, struck the crop, and over the next four years the crop repeatedly failed. By mid-1846, famine was everywhere; there was, declared a leader-writer in the London newspaper, *The Times*, 'total annihilation'.

In the six years between the onset of the potato blight and 1851, the population of Ireland dropped by 2 million. Of these people about 1 million perished from starvation or from disease, and 1 million emigrated. The traumatic experience of seeing a devastated countryside and the realization that the disaster had been due to the combined effects of an unexpected natural disaster and uncontrolled population growth had a profound effect on the cultural outlook of the people. Land hunger remained intense, but the small peasant land-holders resisted subdivision by deciding that the tenancy of their small-holding would be given to the eldest son; the others would have to make their own way elsewhere. It also became a cultural tradition that marriage should be postponed until the man's father was too old to work the farm. Uniquely, amongst the nations of Europe, the Irish adopted Malthus' suggestion of sexual abstinence as a method of population control. This led to a low birth rate and a slow population growth. At the same time, the younger sons who saw no hope of ever having land, and many of the women who saw no hope of marriage, emigrated from Ireland in increasing numbers between 1825 and 1925, both to the U.S.A. and to England. However, once marriage occurred, natality rates were high, and the census of 1911 showed the average number of children born to a woman aged 45, whose marriage had lasted 13 years, to be 6·77.

The combined effects of these cultural patterns reduced the growth rate of the Irish population, despite a religious environment in which all forms of contraception were prohibited.

Between 1860 and 1960, the birth rate fell from 25 per 1,000 to 21 per 1,000, the death rate declined from 18 per 1,000 to 11 per 1,000 and emigration continued. Throughout the period the population had a negative growth rate, declining by about 150,000 each decade until 1940, after which a slow increase in population has occurred.

Demographic Transition and Economic Development

Economists have divided the nations of the world into developed nations, and the developing nations. A demographic study of the population structure of the two types of nation was made by the United Nations and the results are shown in Table **9/6**. In the developing nations 42 per cent of the population are under the age of 15, and the proportion is rising, compared with

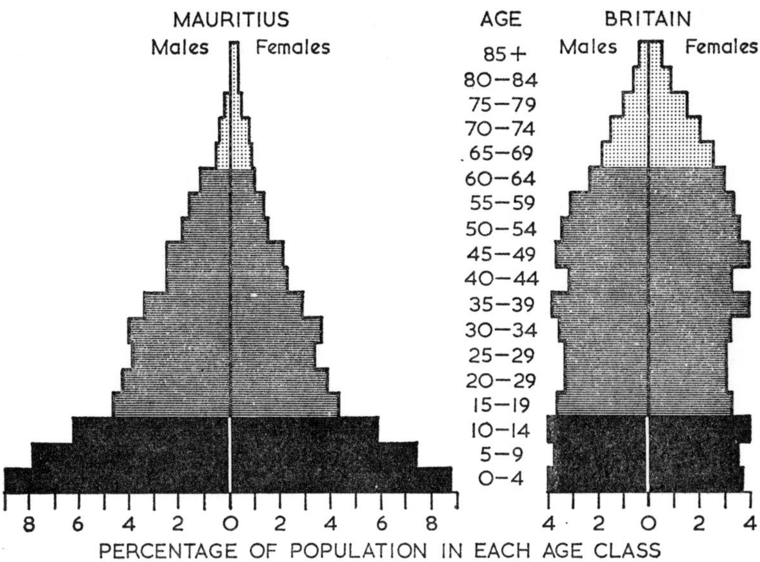

Figure **9/6** The population profiles of Mauritius and Britain for the year 1960. The contrast between the population structures is clearly shown. In the developing nations, young people predominate. In the developed nation the population is more evenly distributed. Source: *Pop. Bulletin*, **18,** 5.

Table 9/6

The demographic and socio-economic characteristics of the developing and the developed nations (1971)

	Developing nations Early transitional	*Developed nations Late transitional*
STATISTICS		
Total population	2,510 million	1,082 million
Average birth rate	30–50	15–25
Average death rate	10–25	5–15
Rate of reproductive change	35–5	20–0
Dependency (%)		
Youth (0–14)	42·1	26·4
Age (65 or more)	2·9	8·6
Total	45·0	35·0
CHARACTERISTICS		
Economic	Generally poor Low per capita income Low industrialization Low consumption of energy Poor communications Poor transportation facilities High un- and under-employment	Generally affluent High per capita income High industrialization High consumption of energy Good communications Good transportation facilities Low unemployment
Environmental	Low environmental pollution Low mobility of people Predominantly rural	High environmental pollution High mobility of people Predominantly urban
Most usual occupation	Farming Unskilled labour	White collar Skilled labour
Social and Medical	Low literacy Low educational standards Low health-worker to population ratio Low calorie and protein intake Falling death rate	High literacy High educational standards High health-worker to population ratio High calorie and protein intake Low death rate

26 per cent of the population in the developed countries. In the developed nations 9 per cent of the population is aged 65 or more, compared with only 3 per cent in the developing nations. In the developing nations about 50 per cent of the population is in the reproductive age group, which is also the age group of maximal economic activity, and in the developed nations, the proportion is 55 per cent. The greatest burden has been placed on those nations with the least financial resources.

In the developing nations, the high proportion of young people imposes a need to finance health-care and education of an economically dependent group, and this limits the accumulation of capital for agricultural and industrial development. The population profile also indicates that increasing numbers of children are living to reach the reproductive years, with the result that more children will be born to increase the 0 to 4 cohort (Figure **9/6**).

This is typically the pattern found in nations in the early transitional stage of demographic development, whilst the developed nations are either in the late transitional stage or are about to enter the post-transitional stage.

Trends in the Growth of the World's Population

A nation cannot plan ahead unless there is reasonably reliable information about the probable population, its age structure and its distribution at any given time in the future. One of the main objectives of demographers is to provide this information. But since any projection must be based on the trends of current mortality and natality rates, the population forecasts are not what *will* happen, but what *would* happen if existing natality and mortality rates continued, or the observed trends in the rates persisted. In this regard it is easier to forecast the future trends in mortality rates than in natality rates, for the latter are so much more subject to the vagaries in human behaviour, to the influence of fashion and to the multiple factors which lead to decision making. The vagaries of human behaviour are nowhere more marked than in the movement of people within a nation, but luckily this can be disregarded when the growth of the population of the world is under study, and in view of current trends, migration between nations may be disregarded, as was discussed in Chapter 8.

For these reasons, demographers normally try to make as much allowance as possible for unexpected changes in natality and mortality rates by making three estimates of population. These are a high estimate, an intermediate (or medium) estimate and a low estimate. The assumption is made that the population projection for a given date will fall somewhere within these estimates, and that it is unlikely to be greater than the high estimate, or less than the low estimate. The U.S. Bureau of the Census makes four estimates in its projections of the population of the United States. In the introduction to the 1967 report, it is stated specifically and explicitly: 'In view of the many uncertainties in predicting future fertility, the Bureau of the Census does not recommend any one series as the "best" series. Long-term projections, such as those for 1995 to 2015, are necessarily subject to the possibility of considerable error, in as much as they require the projection of births, deaths and net migration up to half a century ahead.'

If the highly efficient Bureau of the Census of one of the most affluent nations in the world has to make this disclaimer, the chances of error in the projected populations of other less fortunate nations are correspondingly greater.

Although population projections are subject to error, they form essential data for the study of the future of man on this earth. The importance of this information is clear to the United Nations, and its Population Division has been engaged in the study of this since 1950. At that time the components of population dynamics were unknown for most of the nations of the world. Accurate data about birth rates were lacking, as many births were not reported, and death rates were equally inaccurate. Despite the inadequate data, the Population Division devised procedures for estimating the components of growth, and in 1952 published its first report: *The Past and Future Growth of World Population—A Long View*. The findings were startling. It appeared that in most of the world, and in the developing nations particularly, population growth was occurring at an alarming rate, mainly because death control was being achieved increasingly, whilst there was no birth control. In 1954, a conference was called to consider the report and to speculate on its consequences. In 1958, it published its findings as a book, *The Future Growth of World Population.* This report was even more startling for it showed that the estimates of 1953 were underestimates, and that population growth was proceeding even more quickly than had been believed.

In 1963 the Population Division of the United Nations prepared projections for each country and region for the years 1965 to 2000. These estimates were considerably higher than

Table 9/7

World population projections to the year 2000. The 'medium' variant of the U.N., and the 'constant natality, diminishing mortality' variants are shown

U.N. ESTIMATE: MEDIUM VARIANT

	Year			
Type of nation	1970	1980	1990	2000
Developing	2,500	3,200	3,900	4,700
Developed	1,100	1,200	1,300	1,400
World Total	3,600	4,400	5,200	6,100

U.N. ESTIMATE: CONSTANT NATALITY VARIANT

	Year			
Type of nation	1970	1980	1990	2000
Developing	2,500	3,300	4,400	5,900
Developed	1,100	1,200	1,400	1,600
World Total	3,600	4,500	5,800	7,500

those of 1958 which had so startled the world leaders, and further projections in 1968 showed that the new population estimate for the year 2000 was 6 per cent higher than that made five years earlier.

The medium estimate made by the United Nations in 1968 is shown in Table **9/7** and in Figure **9/7**. This estimate, and the other two, all anticipate some degree of family planning in most nations. If no family planning programmes are undertaken, an estimate assuming a continuation of current natality rates can be made. This estimate is also shown.

The accuracy of these estimates has been subjected to much analysis and study, by demographers, who appear to fall into two main classes; the optimistic, who consider that even the

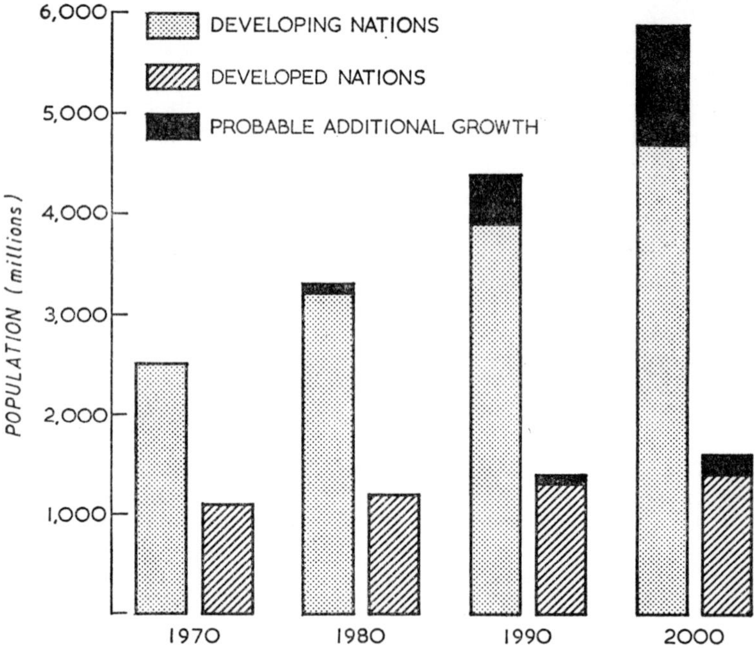

Figure **9/7** The projected population increase in the developed and developing nations (U.N. medium variant) 1970–2000, with the probable additional growth if natality rates remain constant.

low population estimate is too high, and the pessimistic who await the results of the 1970–71 censuses to confirm that the highest U.N. estimate is too low.

The optimists (e.g. Bogue) point out that although death rates are falling in most developing nations, mainly due to reduction in infant mortality, the rate of this reduction may become slower in the next thirty years. This is because the effect of better sanitation and environmental health is now probably nearing its maximum; and preventive inoculations against infectious disease are now readily available. These two measures can effectively reduce the crude death rate to between 15 and 20. But any reduction beyond this is expensive, it demands an educated and motivated population, it is difficult to mount and requires considerable numbers of health workers. In addition, since good infant nutrition is a factor in reducing mortality, the possibility of recurring food shortages may hinder any further reduction of infant deaths. The optimists also point out that the United Nations projections may have underestimated the rapidity with which family planning programmes progress. In other words, they fail to make allowances for acceleration in natality control, and hence in natality decline as family planning measures are more readily accepted. These, they argue, should have a cumulative effect on birth rates by the year 2000.

The pessimists take the opposite view. The expectations of the leaders, and the people, of the developing nations will not be met if the death rate does not continue to be reduced, so that levels approaching those of the developed nations are achieved by 1990. They hold that all the evidence so far indicates that, except in Singapore, Hong Kong, Taiwan and perhaps South Korea, family planning programmes have had a low cost benefit and that neither the leaders (particularly if military), nor the people, have really accepted the need for limitation of natality.

There is not enough reliable information to support either the optimistic or the pessimistic position, and the only rational course is to accept the medium estimate of the United Nations as being likely, and to determine if any solutions exist to the problem that the current annual growth rates in too many nations exceeds 2·0 per cent, and that by the year 2000, the population of the world will be about 6,100 million people, who will require food, housing, education, health-care and jobs. Failure to provide these necessities will lead to an increased death rate, turbulence and possibly to the Malthusian correctives of famine, pestilence and war.

Possible Solutions to the Problem of Population Growth

Many authorities hold that there are two approaches to the main problem, which is the relationship between population growth and food supplies. The first is to increase the food available, and the second is to restrict population growth by controlling natality. If the first approach is adopted, it is nevertheless a simplistic solution for it fails to allow for the economic and social consequences of unrestricted population growth. These are the high dependency ratio, the need for a large expenditure on health and education, and the necessity to create jobs, all of which constrain the socio-economic development of a nation. It is largely propagated by the pro-natalists, who believe that technology can solve all our problems, and that consequently population growth restriction is unnecessary, and somehow immoral.

The anti-natalists point out that even after large inputs of technology, fertilizer, water and machinery, food production is barely keeping ahead of population growth, and the exponential surge of the latter will cause food production per capita to fall in the next decades.

The conflict between the two view-points is, of course, a false one. They are not antithetical. Indeed any rational approach, in this unique period of the world's history, must seek simultaneously to reduce the population growth rate and to increase the rate of food production.

Since 1950 the increased application of agricultural technology has enabled food production in the world to increase at about 3 per cent per annum, with the result that the total food produced has doubled in the 20 years to 1970. This increase has only been achieved by very considerable increases in the use of fertilizer, in the use of pesticides and by the purchase of agricultural machinery, especially tractors. Between 1950–51 and 1970–71, the quantity of fertilizer used has risen from 15,227,000 metric tons per year to 67,916,000 metric tons per year, an increase of 350 per cent. In the same period the quantity of pesticides used has also increased by 350 per cent, and the number of tractors in use has risen from 6,038,000 in 1950–51 to 15,558,000 in 1970–71 (FAO).

These massive inputs have been predominantly in the developed world, where the food production per head has risen by 32 per cent. In the hungry, developing world, total food output per person has risen by only 6 per cent in the 20-year period, and current indications are that since 1971 it is actually declining because of the more rapid rate of population growth (see Figure **9/8**).

Today, despite the large inputs of the past 20 years, between 20 and 30 per cent of people in the developing nations still receive insufficient calories per day, even taking a modest mean

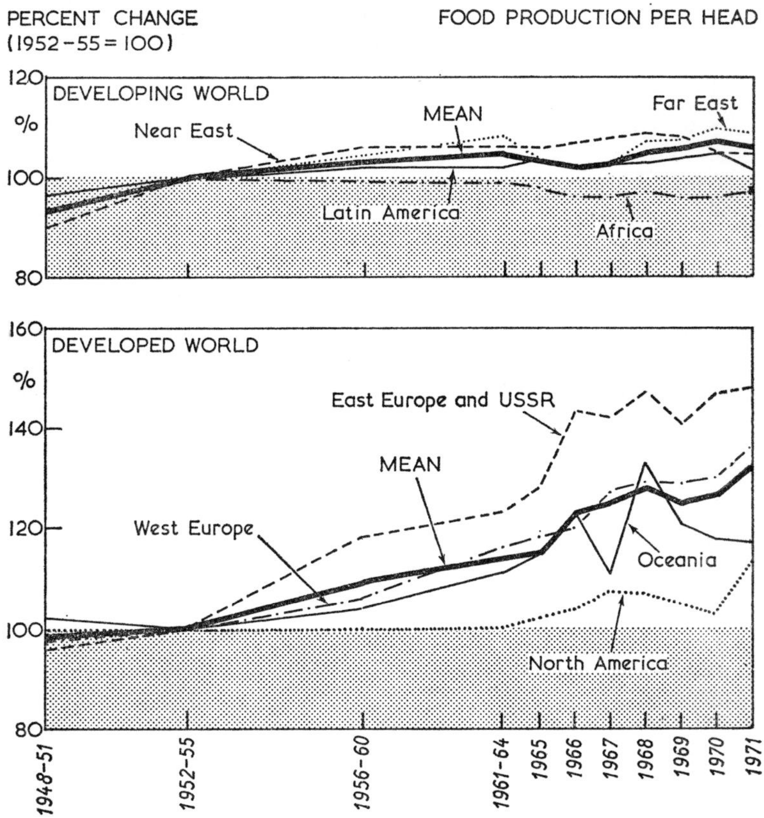

Figure **9/8** Food production in the developing and developed regions of the world, 1948–71.
Source: *FAO Monthly Bulletin*, January, 1972.

daily requirement of 2,100 K-cals per head (Table **9/8**), and are undernourished. Between 15 and 25 per cent of the people receive insufficient protein, vitamins or minerals (especially thiamine and iron) and so are malnourished. To meet the requirements of the projected population of the world in AD

Table 9/8

Minimal K-calorie requirements for the 'average' person in the developing and in the developed nations

DEVELOPING NATIONS

Age group	*Proportional percentage in age group*	*K-cals required for maintenance and growth*
0–4	16	1,000
5–9	13	1,200
10–14	12	1,500
15–64	54	1,950
65+	5	1,750

Mean K-calories required for maintenance and growth	1,600 K-cals/day
Mean K-calories required for activity	300–700 K-cals/day
MINIMAL REQUIREMENT per head per day	1,900–2,300 K-cals

DEVELOPED NATIONS

Age group	*Proportional percentage in age group*	*K-cals required for maintenance and growth*
0–4	9	1,000
5–9	9	1,200
10–14	9	1,500
15–64	63	2,400
65+	10	2,000

Mean K-calories required for maintenance and growth	2,045 K-cals/day
Mean K-calories required for activity	300–800 K-cals/day
MINIMAL REQUIREMENT per head per day	2,345–2,845 K-cals

The population structure was obtained from *The World Population Situation in 1970*, U.N., New York, 1971. The K-cals required for maintenance and growth from Payne, P. R. and Waterlow, J. C., *Lancet*, **2**, 210, 1972. The calorie requirement for activity was derived from Brockett, J. H. et al., *Report 212*, U.S. Army Medical Nutrition Laboratory.

2001 demands an increased use of potentially arable land; the continued development of new strains, particularly of cereals; the improvement of harvest yields by increased irrigation and the heavy use of nitrogenous fertilizer; the reduction of food losses by controlling rats, birds and plant disease; and the possible development of alternative food supplies, for example fish or plankton, by harvesting the sea. These inputs all have ecological significance.

INCREASED USE OF POTENTIALLY CULTIVABLE LAND

About one quarter of the world's 14,500 million hectares is suitable for growing crops, and another quarter is suitable for grazing. The remaining half, which includes desert, tundra, mountains and forests, is of little or no use for producing food. Of the 3,600 million hectares suitable for growing crops, just under half is now cultivated, and the rest is potentially cultivable. Calculations show that in Asia 17 per cent, in Africa 78 per cent and in Latin America 89 per cent of potentially cultivable land is not being cultivated. All that needs to be done, say the optimists, is to cultivate it, and a much larger population than that existing today can be fed. Unfortunately this optimistic viewpoint is not valid. At least half of the land in Africa is in the tropical zone and of limited potential, whilst a further proportion is in the desert zone. In Latin America most of the potentially cultivable land is in the tropical zone.

The cost of clearing land, particularly in the tropics, is high. The estimated cost per hectare cleared is about $1,000, and one hectare will barely support a married couple in the tropics. The soil is thin, and if incorrectly farmed will leach away, leaving a raw, eroded, useless desert.

Because of its poor nature, most of this potentially arable land will not support the regular growth of crops without heavy fertilization and controlled irrigation, so that it is not a practical proposition to develop it, except slowly and after a careful analysis of the ecological problems involved.

IMPROVED STRAINS OF CEREALS

The great success of the new strains of wheat and rice have heralded what has been called the 'Green Revolution', and research for better strains continues. However, the evidence so far suggests that although greatly improved yields are being obtained, the crops need a high fertilizer spread, abundant water, a heavy spread of pesticides and a precise knowledge of when to apply each of these additives. In addition, considerable expenditure is needed to build rat-proof stores to hold the harvested grain. These constraints suggest that the only methods of efficient farming are increased landlordism with more landless peasant workers, or the alternative of farming on a communal basis with increased mechanization. As a solution to existing food shortages, the Green Revolution is making an impressive, if limited, contribution; but to meet the needs of the projected population it is likely to be inadequate. Even Borlaug, who developed the new strains, states that the success in increasing the world supply of food is 'only a stop-gap, not a solution'. There is evidence that the initial successes of the first two or three years are followed by lower yields, even if great care is taken to continue fertilization, irrigation and the use of pesticides. Even more serious is the evidence that the new strains are becoming susceptible to viral diseases and the ecological balance is threatened. There is also concern that the farmers may reject the new strains, which require much greater care during the growing period than the older ones, as they find that the glut induced by the higher yield leads to a fall in the price of the cereal, and a lower return for their labour.

LARGER YIELDS

Larger yields of food grains per hectare, diversification of crops to grow those high in protein, the improved care of livestock, the use of new fertilizers and better irrigation are obviously desirable. Ultimately, the key to higher yields is not agricultural science alone, but the flexibility of the farmers to adapt to new practices. Rural people are traditionally conservative and suspicious of new ideas, especially if introduced by strangers. If the new ideas demand that the farmer make changes from traditional farming practices, the difficulties are compounded. Advances are being made, especially in India, to alter farmers' attitudes, but the key is education and the reduction of illiteracy. And this costs a great deal, particularly in those nations with a high rural population and a large youth dependency-ratio.

REDUCTION OF FOOD LOSSES

Once cereals have been grown they require to be stored until they are required for consumption. Experience in India, as an example of a developing country, indicates that a very large proportion of the crop is eaten either by birds when growing, or by rats when in store. For example, in 1968 the Ministry of Food and Agriculture of India estimated that rats ate 10 per cent of India's grain crops, and it is likely that a similar or greater proportion of cereal crops is lost in other developing nations. In addition, birds are estimated to eat between 2 and 5 per cent of cereal crops.

The only solution to the problems of food losses is expensive. It is to build and maintain central communal storage silos, a method which is against all rural tradition, in which the farmer stores his own requirements of grain in the family house and sells the rest at the best price he can get.

HARVESTING THE SEA

In view of the uncertainty of food production and the relatively high cost of producing protein on land (except by the cultivation of soya bean), the novel method of harvesting the sea has been suggested. Fish are an excellent source of protein, either as the whole fish or as dried fish protein, which can be added to traditional diets. If fishing were encouraged there would be lavish supplies of protein for the malnourished people of the world. Unfortunately the ecological balance and the life cycle in the sea cannot be disturbed too much, or catches fall off greatly and the cost of fishing rises to render the return uneconomic. One expert, Dr. Ryther, has calculated that even with controlled but intensive fishing, only an additional 40 million (metric) tons could be annually harvested in the first 10-year period, and the harvest would decrease over subsequent 10-year periods, as the ecological balance in the oceans was disturbed. And even if his estimate is 100 per cent too low, as has been suggested, the additional 80 million metric tons annual harvest will be insufficient to meet the increased needs of the population unless natality is controlled concurrently.

IS INCREASED FOOD SUPPLY THE ANSWER?

The opinion of most experts in the field indicates that whilst food production can be increased considerably, the cost is great. In fact, food production is increasing by between 1 and 2 per cent per capita per annum, but simultaneously population growth is increasing at a rate of over 2 per cent per annum, so that even with expanded programmes, food production will tend to lag behind population growth.

One is drawn uncomfortably to the conclusion that increased food production alone cannot meet food requirements at the end of the century. Malthus' statement, in the first edition of his Essay, remains valid. He postulated: 'First, that food is necessary to the existence of man. Second, that the passion between the sexes is necessary, and will remain nearly in its present state. . . . Assuming then, my postulata as granted, I say that the power of population is infinitely greater than the power on the earth to produce subsistence for man.' Luckily today there is no need to take for granted the result of the 'passion between the sexes'. Birth control is not only possible but necessary.

THE LIMITS TO EXPONENTIAL ECONOMIC GROWTH

In the first pages of this book, it was argued that two main problems posed grave dangers to the survival of man. The first was exponential population growth and the need for food supplies to keep up with it. The second, and interlinked problem, was that of exponential economic growth. Estimates of the remaining supplies of many mineral resources, even allowing for the discovery of unexpected, hidden wealth, shows that the current rate of economic growth cannot be supported for much longer. The current rapid depletion of unrenewable mineral resources, by consumption and wastage, could be limited by improved technology which would involve the search for less scarce substitutes, and by improving recycling processes. But this will only buy time, and will add considerably to the increasing pollution of land, water and air, which in turn threatens to reduce food supplies and to increase disease. This has led to the belief that industrialization and economic growth must be rapidly reduced. It is noticeable that the majority of people supporting this thesis are members of the affluent third of humanity. To the people of the developing nations, this reversal of a long-held opinion of the primacy of continued economic growth seems cynical. For nearly two centuries the developing nations have been the quarry, the farm, the plantation and the fibre shed of the industrialized nations. The latter bought their agricultural products and their minerals cheaply, turned them into manufactured goods and sold them back expensively. The third world has seen this process continue until today, and now when the potential for industrialization is theirs, the United Nations, and informed opinion, have suggested that economic growth must cease. It is little wonder that cynicism and suspicion of the motives of the developed nations are voiced. Yet the evidence is so strong, so persuasive and so urgent that economic growth must decline, and that accumulated capital must be diverted from consumer goods to social ends, it would be unwise to ignore it.

To many leaders in the developing world, a larger population means a larger market, a stronger nation and cheaper industrialization. That this is a mirage is difficult to explain, and hard to make convincing. Yet it is so.

One way in which developing nations might accept the honesty of the affluent world is if the rich nations at once reduced considerably their own economic development, instituted favourable terms of trade for developing nations, gave them massive aid, encouraged specific social and industrial progress in the developing world (ensuring bilaterally that *total* economic growth was reduced) and instituted a world food bank. Simultaneously, all nations would agree to reduce the rate of their population growth, for this is the greatest of our problems.

Reduction in the Rate of Population Growth

The first part of this book has sought to present objective evidence from which the reader could reach a decision about population dynamics. The evidence indicates that the annual increase in population is now so great that unless food production is increased, environmental pollution controlled, and population growth reduced considerably, preferably to zero growth, the prospects for all the human race by the year 2000 are serious. Evidence has been advanced that an increase in food production is inadequate to solve the problem, and that concurrently there must be a restriction of population growth. The environmental pollution issue is linked with these other problems, and must be tackled simultaneously but separately. Since this book is concerned with human reproduction, the threat to the environment will not be discussed, but interested readers should obtain Paul Ehrlich's book, *Population, Resources and Environment*; or my book, *People Populating*. Conception control does require consideration, however, as the opponents of family planning continue to give reasons why it is unnecessary or counter-productive.

The first argument is that every increase in the population is beneficial, as the country becomes a larger consumer group, is better able to defend itself and better able to diversify its activities. The fallacy is that it is not an increase in the total population that adds to a nation's wealth, but the increase in the proportion of healthy, educated, thrifty people. Even if one accepts that demographic growth is beneficial, the rate of growth is crucial: too fast a growth rate is the opposite of beneficial.

The second argument is that increases in population can be matched by increases in agriculture and industry. This has been shown to be doubtful and can only occur at the cost of increased usage of finite resources, and with increasing pollution. The question which should be asked is not 'How many human beings can be kept alive on a minimal diet?', but 'How many human beings can be given a life which is not entirely taken up by the effort of mere survival?'

The third argument is that urbanization and industrialization in themselves automatically reduce the birth rate. Historically there appears merit in this argument. In the nineteenth century, urbanization and industrialization of Western nations were associated, after a time lag, with a reduction in the birth rate, but there is evidence that much of this was due to voluntary contraceptive measures. As well as this, emigration to the U.S.A., to Canada and to Australia reduced the total populations of many European nations. There is no direct relationship between the curves of a falling birth rate and economic growth.

Urbanization without marked industrialization merely compounds problems. Industrialization and urbanization together increase environmental pollution. To be economic, industrialization increasingly demands an educated work force, and education is expensive and slow. Time is not available at the current rate of population growth for this solution to be effective, although with better communication techniques the process of demographic transition is likely to be faster in the next three decades.

The fourth argument is that limitation of births will lead to a disproportionate number of old people in the population. Temporarily this argument is valid, but in time the population profile becomes the normal one for a slow, or zero, growth population. Meanwhile, the resources which would have been given to the health-care and education of the additional children can be transferred to the care of the aged. Since the aged often have made some savings, the cost to the community would, in fact, be less than that required for the care of the young.

The fifth argument is that if the growth of the population is regulated, economic growth stagnates. There is no real evidence that this is so. In the World Bank's view, 'the most immediate and measurable effect of slow population growth is the increase in per capita income'. In a thrifty nation this permits higher savings and the accumulation of capital, which in turn can be used for investment in human resources, such as improving the quality of education, enhancing social services or for financing technological research. In the long term, this investment, used wisely, will increase economic growth. However, increasing opinion questions if unlimited economic growth is not perhaps a dangerous illusion leading to immense environmental problems. Economic growth is needed, especially in the hungry developing world, but the technology involved must be one which does not distort ecosystems, and lead to environmental deterioration.

The consensus of informed opinion is that unless the rate of population growth is controlled, and eventually is reduced to no more than replacement level, which means a stable population, the outlook for mankind is very bleak indeed.

What Hope is there of Reaching a Stable Population?

The attempt to change a pronatalist attitude to an antinatalist one is unlikely to be quick, unless coercion is used. To most people in most nations, the idea of coercion in natality is unacceptable at present, and it is likely that only persuasion will be used to effect birth control, at least for the next twenty-five years. The question is: Have we time, is this sufficient?

Even if natality is reduced, so that zero population growth (a net reproduction rate of 1·00) is obtained by 1995, the momentum of the world's population growth rate is such that it would take between 35 and 60 years before the population of a nation stopped growing and became stationary, or stable. This is because population growth in any country depends on its age-structure. The greater the proportion of young people, the greater is the potential for growth even after the two-child family (actually between 2·1 and 2·3 children are required for replacement) has been accepted by a great majority of the population.

The fear of some national leaders that zero population growth will lead to a weak, defenceless nation is unfounded. Calculations made by Nathan Keyfitz and by the Bureau of the Census in the U.S.A. confirm this view. Keyfitz has proved mathematically that in the hungry developing nations the reduction of the birth rate to replacement level (i.e. zero population growth) by 1990–95, will still mean that the final stable population of each nation will be an average 2·5 (range 1·8–2·9) times as large as it was in 1970. The momentum of population growth in the developed nations is less, as they have practised birth control for some years on an increasing scale. But even in the affluent nations, the stable, stationary population will be about 1·2 times as large as that counted in 1970.

Table **9/9**, which has been derived from calculations by the U.S. Bureau of the Census, indicates this. A rapid calculation shows that even if the world urgently realizes the magnitude of the dangers of the current population growth rates and all nations have a zero population growth rate by 1995 (which is unlikely), the world's population will finally stabilize at over 7,400 million people in 2060. Of these people, 6,000 million will live in the hungry developing nations, and 1,400 million in the affluent nations.

The question which national leaders should be asking today, and should be asked by concerned citizens, is: 'Can my nation feed, house, keep healthy, educate and find employment for the inevitable increase in the population, or will the only redress be the Malthusian correctives of famine, pestilence and war?'

If the question is difficult to answer, assuming that the two-child family is the norm by the year 1995, how much more impossible will it be to answer if the current natality patterns persist, and the world's population reaches 7,400 million in 2010 and by 2060 may exceed 60,000 million, seventeen times today's world population?

Logic would suggest that all nations should urgently, efficiently and effectively induce their citizens to adopt zero population growth with the least delay. However, in politics emotion all too often replaces logic.

At this time the main effort is being put into informing people of birth control facilities, in providing contraceptives readily and easily for all interested couples, in encouraging voluntary participation in the family planning programmes, and in offering inducements for participants. It is questionable what impact this approach is making. Nortman has examined the progress of birth control programmes in 24 nations. In eight: Barbados, Jamaica, Korea (South), Malaysia (West), Mauritius, Singapore, Taiwan and Tunisia, the target has been achieved. She notes that 'the successful list consists exclusively of small, rapidly modernizing countries which are either islands or peninsulas'. In six nations: Dominican Republic, Ghana, Indonesia, Philippines, Thailand, Trinidad and Tobago, the programme has been in operation for too short a time for evaluation. Three nations cannot be evaluated because of lack of vital data. These are Kenya, Nepal and Turkey. In seven nations, which together contain 780 million people, 'progress has been poor at least in relation to targets'. These are Bangladesh, India, Iran, Morocco, Pakistan and Egypt. Nortman wonders whether voluntary family planning programmes can have a significant impact on demographic change, or whether social and economic change must not come first. The evidence of the consequences of the current exponential population growth

Table 9/9

The estimated stable (or stationary) population of selected nations if zero population growth achieved by 1995, and the year in which the stable population will be reached

(*Population in millions*)

Nation	*Population* 1970	*Stable population if two-child family the norm by* 1995	*Factor of increase over* 1970	*Year stationary population achieved*	*Population in same year if constant natality persists*
Latin America					
Argentina	24·0	34·8	1·4	2050	60
Brazil	93·5	237·8	2·4	2050	1,677
Chile	9·5	18·9	1·9	2055	62
Colombia	20·8	56·6	2·7	2050	443
Cuba	8·3	15·1	1·8	2050	55
Ecuador	6·0	16·5	2·7	2050	146
Guatemala	5·2	13·4	2·6	2055	110
Haiti	5·2	12·4	2·4	2055	98
Mexico	50·1	134·8	2·7	2050	1,035
Peru	13·2	33·5	2·5	2050	235
Venezuela	10·4	27·3	2·6	2050	199
North America					
Canada	21·4	30·4	1·4	2035	36
U.S.A.	204·3	278·7	1·3	2035	341
Europe					
France	50·0	64·1	1·2	2045	103
U.K.	55·6	67·5	1·2	2045	102
Oceania					
Australia	12·4	17·7	1·4	[illegible]	[illegible]

Africa					
Egypt	32·8	80·8	2·5	2050	583
Ghana	8·7	21·5	2·5	2060	270
Morocco	15·6	44·7	2·2	2055	735
Nigeria	63·4	145·0	2·3	2065	1,475
Tunisia	5·2	12·8	2·5	2060	138
Uganda	9·6	22·5	2·3	2055	213
West Asia					
Afghanistan	17·0	38·7	2·3	2060	399
Bangladesh	73·7	191·9	2·6	2055	2,044
India	576·0	1,450·9	2·5	2055	13,905
Iran	28·2	80·5	2·9	2050	985
Nepal	11·3	22·5	2·0	2065	172
Pakistan	59·0	153·2	2·6	2050	1,284
Sri Lanka	12·4	27·1	2·2	2050	96
Turkey	34·9	82·8	2·4	2050	569
East Asia					
Burma	22·7	60·3	2·2	2060	541
Cambodia	6·8	16·5	2·4	2060	164
China	750·0	1,661·0	2·2	2060	14,541
Indonesia	120·0	275·0	2·3	2060	3,019
Japan	103·7	132·2	1·3	2025	133
S. Korea	31·4	69·9	2·2	2050	333
Malaysia	10·9	28·4	2·6	2060	260
Philippines	38·2	103·4	2·7	2050	879
Thailand	36·4	93·4	2·6	2045	567
S. Vietnam	18·2	44·4	2·4	2050	339

Source: U.S. Department of Commerce, Bureau of the Census. *The Two-Child Family*, Washington 1971.

rate, just given, indicates that there is not enough time to achieve demographic transition through economic change. This is not to say that social and economic changes should not be encouraged: they should, but simultaneously, a reduction in the population growth rate is essential. Indeed the two are interlinked.

It is depressing, nevertheless, that despite a considerable effort in the past decade, the total effect of birth control programmes in developing nations, in 1970, reduced the birth rate by only 3·3 per cent: and an excess of 73 million births over deaths occurred in that year.

This very limited success raises the question of whether voluntary measures are sufficient or whether compulsion, or at least heavily motivated persuasion, should not be used. The example of China should be considered.

By official encouragement to delay marriage, through the widespread dissemination of information about contraceptives, through the ready availability of all birth control measures, including abortion, China appears to have made a significant impact on her birth rate. The experience of China needs to be studied, now that the People's Republic is a member of the United Nations.

At present the answers are obscure, but of all the problems facing man—unbridled economic growth, increasing use of non-renewable minerals, increasing pollution—that of exponential population growth is the most serious.

Population Control and Family Planning

If the evidence presented is accepted, there can be no doubt that control of the growth of population is essential, and measures to decrease the rate of population growth must be applied to all nations.

There has been considerable confusion in recent years as to what this means, but many Governments have accepted the belief that family planning should be the key in any campaign to reduce the population growth rate. However, most have confused population control and family planning.

Family planning implies that individual married women, with or without their husbands, unmarried men, and women who are at risk of becoming pregnant, are offered contraceptive advice and appliances. The slogan adopted has been that 'every child should be a wanted child'. In an increasing number of countries, such contraceptive help includes the offer of legally induced abortion provided that the gestation period (calculated from the first day of the last menstrual period) has not exceeded 12 weeks. In family planning the decision whether or not to have another child, when to have that child, and whether to continue with, or abandon, birth control, is individual. Governments may help by making contraceptive services available through Maternity and Child Health centres, or through physicians, but the decision whether or not to seek the services is a personal one. The technology of birth control is discussed in Part II of this book.

Family planning is only one aspect of population control. It has the possible disadvantage that it stresses the medico-technical aspects of population control whilst minimizing the crucial fact that decisions about procreation and child rearing are social and cultural ones. It may also hinder population control as it places reliance on a single method. This may lead to the postponement of other necessary methods of curtailing population growth, as Davis has pointed out. If the crucial decision about population control is a psychological one, it must, if it is deemed socially and economically necessary, involve Governments in social manipulation. Such manipulation may range from the prohibition of all pregnancies beyond a certain number by compulsory abortion, and the prevention of all extramarital conceptions by threat of punishment or by compulsory abortion, to the milder, more humane approach of discouraging conception.

Even in advanced countries where the birth rate is relatively low, the decision by women to have three rather than two children, makes the difference between a stable population and one which doubles about every 43 years. In view of the current concern amongst biologists that the rate of growth of population is a major factor in the current environmental threat to the well-being of all mankind, the impact of uncontrolled population growth in the developing countries, particularly, is even more serious, as their resources to cope with the problem are limited. Admittedly, the reproductive growth rate in the developed nations is not excessive (0·5–1·0 per cent per annum) but it could beneficially be reduced further, not for urgent demographic reasons, but for social reasons. Currently in many developed nations, between 10 and 15 per cent of births occur extranuptially. Half of the mothers remain single, the other half undergo hasty marriages which are rather unstable (see Chapter 15). If these unwanted births were eliminated, the reproductive growth rate would fall still further, enabling the nation to develop the new technological techniques necessary for control of environmental pollution. This is a matter of some importance as current calculations suggest that one child born in a developed nation, in his lifetime will consume and pollute between 10 and 40 times as much as a child born in an underdeveloped nation. It would be unrealistic and insulting, moreover, for members of affluent nations to tell the people of the developing, underprivileged world to limit their families, if they themselves are not prepared to do so as well. The psychological affront implied by such a suggestion might be sufficient to cause the leaders of the developing nations to induce their people to do just the opposite.

There need not be concern that world-wide limitation of population growth is unacceptable to reasonable people. If the rate of population growth poses as marked a threat to human well-being as it appears to do, society can be induced to accept controls. In most societies sanctions are placed on criminals who threaten society, on the mentally disturbed, on dangerous drivers, and on those who take certain drugs. Such activities are considered anti-social. There is no intrinsic reason why uncontrolled natality should not also be considered anti-social.

In this period of the twentieth century, population control is necessary for all nations. In certain nations religious prohibitions, such as those which put a high value on premarital chastity, if accompanied by insistence on delayed marriage and by abstinence from coitus within marriage, might be sufficient. Indeed these were Malthus' recommendations. They were shown not to be practicable 150 years ago (except in Ireland) and it is very doubtful if they would be effective today. Nor is infanticide a solution currently acceptable, although legal abortion as a method of conception control is currently spreading.

There are two ways to reduce population growth; one can

either increase mortality or reduce natality. The former is clearly unacceptable to reasonable men. For the latter to succeed the restraints of uncontrolled fertility must be such that they can be introduced with minimal administrative disturbance and at the minimum possible human cost. The type of approach adopted will depend on the situation in a particular nation, but since it is desired to manipulate socio-cultural factors, certain general methods can be outlined.

The approach would be to use rewards and sanctions to achieve the desired stable population. In applying these rewards and sanctions a principle should be that they would not penalize any child which is born, as it is innocent of the act of conception and should be given the full opportunity to develop its potential. For this reason any sanction penalizing existing children is unjustifiable. Sanctions are only effective if the reason for them is understood, if they are equitable, and if the individual can easily avoid being put in danger of their application. Since the objective is to reduce natality, and the sanctions are applied to those who fail to reduce natality, strategies can be developed after analysis of the data applicable to a particular nation.

Such strategies might include a mix of some of the following suggestions, but these are only given as examples, and the reader may wish to devise his own. In this he might read, with profit, the articles by Berelson, Davis and Spengler listed in the bibliography.

The suggestions include:

1. The institution of campaigns to make all the people, of all ages and at all levels of intelligence and perception, constantly aware of the danger of uncontrolled natality. If such campaigns are supported by the example of the nations' leaders and cultural heroes, who themselves are seen to practise birth control, and who encourage others to do the same, such campaigns will have more chance of success. The objective would be to establish within the society a new cultural norm that two children are the maximum required for satisfying social status needs, and that barrenness of some couples is not only desirable but to be encouraged. There is little likelihood that this concept would be achieved immediately, particularly in the developing nations, where high natality has a high status value, but the acceptance of the concept should be encouraged.

2. The provision of sex education in all schools from before the age of puberty, in which sexual responsibility is stressed, anatomy and physiology are explained, and contraceptive measures are discussed.

3. The alteration of the prevalent cultural view that women's only real destiny is to bear and rear children, and that the single woman, the infertile woman, the career woman is to be mocked and despised.

There should be encouragement for women, by education and by offering employment, to take up roles alternative to, or supplementary to marriage, so that excessive natality has competition. It has been observed in the developed nations particularly, that natality rates fall when women have opportunities to obtain employment outside the home. For this reason, employment opportunities for women, with the provision of day crèches for existing children (up to an agreed limit) might discourage child-bearing and encourage economic development.

4. The provision of the best possible health-care, education and job opportunities for all children, up to the limit of two in each family, at minimal cost so that parents can be secure that their children will have every opportunity to achieve success, and will survive to be a comfort to them in old age.

The aim of all these restraints is to induce men and women to *desire* fewer children, preferably no more than two in any family, and to offer them measures, easily and conveniently, which will help them achieve their desires.

In many societies a reason for reproduction is the expectation by the parents that their social and economic support in old age will be provided by their children, and the urge to have many children is strong. If a nation introduced a social security system which provided adequate support for the old, for the invalid and for the sick, the cultural need for high natality would diminish, although children, in fewer numbers, would be welcomed for the social support they provide for ageing parents. The introduction of such a scheme could be linked to population control. Parents who at the start of the scheme had more than two children would be eligible for a full pension, but future parents who chose to have more than two children would receive a reduced pension. The equity of this proposal is that as the community largely bears the cost of educating and providing health care for children, it should not be doubly burdened by having to provide a full pension for a socially selfish person.

Economists have calculated that the cost of the scheme would be less than the cost of rearing the children who would be born (i.e. the cost of the youth dependency) if the scheme did not exist.

5. To further reward those couples choosing to have only two children, Spengler suggests that an interest-bearing insurance fund is established. If one of the couple died, this fund would provide support for the surviving spouse and any children, up to a determined age. Should the couple remain childless, or have no more than the target number of children, the insurance (with interest) would mature when the wife reached the age of 45. For each additional child above the target, the sum payable would be reduced by 50 per cent or some such figure. If during the time the policy was operative either parent decided to have a tubal ligation or a vasectomy, the policy would be payable, with perhaps an enhanced bonus, after the operation.

Since the sanctions must be equitable and avoidable, it implies that contraceptive advice and materials would have to be easily and freely accessible to all couples, at a minimal, or no cost. It also implies that legally induced abortion should be available as a 'back-up' for failed contraception.

There are, of course, other measures. For example, Berelson lists 29 in his article, and concludes that currently the provision of birth control information and appliances offers the best hope. This is disputed by Spengler who feels economic measures will produce the most rapid results, whilst Davis believes that 'the emphasis on family planning (is) a major obstacle to population control. The creed is not to abandon family planning but to put equal or greater resources into other approaches.'

It is obvious that the experts disagree; and unfortunately too few national and community leaders have analysed the problems of the rate of population growth in their own countries to enable them to ask the right questions and seek the answers. It must be stressed that birth control is not an end in itself. A reduction of the rate of population growth does not absolve national leaders from tackling the social problems of the increasing gap between the developed and the developing nations; the existing inequalities, in many nations, of the distribution of land and of wealth; the inadequate educational and health services; the exploitation of a nation's natural resources, and world problems of ecologically uncontrolled economic growth, environmental pollution and excessive use of non-renewable materials. Yet the problem of the rate of population growth is paramount and it is to be hoped that key people in all nations, such as physicians and other health workers, social scientists and social workers, and informed people at all levels, will begin to exert pressure on their political leaders. It is not too late, but time is short.

PART II

The Technology of Birth Control

The fact itself of causing the existence of a human being, is one of the most responsible actions in the range of human life. To understand this responsibility—to bestow life which may either be a curse or a blessing—unless the being on whom it is to be bestowed will have at least the ordinary chances of desirable existence, is a crime against that being.

On Liberty
JOHN STUART MILL

TEN

A History of Contraception

Throughout history there has been a desire to control conception, at least to the level accepted by a particular society in which the woman lived. This applied to all societies, even to those which disapproved of sterility, and those which encouraged the birth of at least one son. The degree of control varied, and in each society seems to have been determined by the then current needs of the society as a whole. In general the aim appears to have been to replace the deaths by a slight excess of births. This enabled the society to meet its needs for food gathering and production, for specialized occupations, for ritual and for defence against human and animal predators. The desire to control natality was supplemented by some knowledge of contraceptive practices, although much of it was based on magical or inadequate preventive measures. In a few societies, conception control was supplemented by abortion and infanticide until the desired size of family, or at least that most acceptable to prevailing cultural norms, had been obtained. The reason for the reliance on the positive checks (to quote Malthus) of abortion and infanticide was that until the past twenty years no really effective method of conception control was available.

Throughout history, too, runs a thread binding contraceptive practices from one era to the next. What probably happened in primitive tribal societies is reflected in today's few remaining ones (such as the Australian aboriginal) where these practices persist. Such societies are a model of the pre-literate societies of the past. The main methods amongst such groups were sexual constraints, coitus interruptus and the use of magic, whether in the form of amulets or as potions containing pounded seeds, herbs and pulses. A few of these primitive groups were rather more sophisticated and realized that in some way the male ejaculate in the vagina led to conception. To prevent this event they placed a barrier in the vagina. In Indonesia, for example, the Batak people in the Lake Toba area of Central Sumatra and the Achenese of North Sumatra, used a vaginal plug impregnated with tannic acid which is an excellent spermicide. Despite these preventive methods, it is likely that abortion and infanticide were also practised, particularly in times of famine.

The first mention of contraception by the Egyptians is in the Petrie papyrus of 1850 BC in which a variety of magical potions are mentioned, but which also suggests the use of a vaginal plug formed from crocodile dung and honey, which was to be inserted into the vagina prior to coitus. The Ebers papyrus, written 300 years later, also mentions a vaginal pessary of lint soaked in the juice from the tips of acacia shrubs, mixed with honey. The honey would form a film penetrated with difficulty by the spermatozoa, and the acacia tips contain gum arabic which releases lactic acid, a fairly efficient spermicide.

Although the Jews appeared to condemn birth control, recent scholars suggest that the prohibition was directed more to abortion and infanticide rather than contraception. Certainly there is evidence that a vaginal sponge made of wadding and called 'mokh' was used; and coitus interruptus was not disapproved in certain circumstances, provided the couple had had at least two children to obey the injunction to replenish the race.

There is unfortunately little information about contraceptive practices in China, India and Japan, but such evidence as there is suggests that sexual restraint and coitus interruptus were practised. And, as in other cultures, many magical potions were available.

Both the Greeks and the Romans subsequently made use of magical incantations and potions, but Aristotle mentions the use of cedar oil prior to coitus, whilst Soranus, 500 years later, gave a specific method of compounding a contraceptive ointment of olive oil, honey and cedar gum which was mixed with white lead and smeared on soft wool. This was then introduced high into the vagina.

During the Islamic cultural period from AD 800 to 1500, Muslim scholars held that as the embryo and early fetus had no human identity, abortion was permitted. As an alternative, coitus interruptus was practised, and some medical authors recommended vaginal plugs of the rennet of a rabbit or the leaves of the weeping willow.

In Europe up to 1650, there was an ecclesiastical prohibition against conception control based on Aquinas' view that 'in so far as the generation of offspring is impeded, it is a vice against nature which happens in every carnal act from which generation cannot follow'. Because of this, it is likely that the only contraceptive measures used were the ineffective ones based on folk remedies, although to some extent coitus interruptus was practised, particularly amongst the nobility and richer merchants. This is a possible explanation for the smaller size of the families of the wealthy and powerful who, being better fed and housed, might be expected to conceive, deliver and rear more children to adulthood. In North America the puritan ethic and the emptiness of the land inhibited contraception, as large families seemed desirable; whilst in Latin America the power of the Roman Catholic Church was supreme.

Mechanical methods of contraception were unknown in Europe, although in 1564 Fallopius had recommended a linen covering of the glans penis as a protective against syphilis, which was then epidemic throughout Europe; but its usage was limited, except in brothels, until about 1720. At that time, the condom (as it was now called) was made from the caecum of sheep and was drawn onto the erect penis to cover both glans and shaft. The condom was advertised widely in London between 1750 and 1820 and again was mainly used as a protection against syphilis rather than as a contraceptive.

By the last decade of the eighteenth century, the cultural climate was much more enquiring; urbanization and industrialization were proceeding, and the benefits of the earlier agricultural revolution, which had led to enclosures and crop rotation, were apparent. At the same time ecclesiastical dominance in sexual matters was diminishing, with the resulting increasing interest in conception control. With the better food available, infant and childhood mortality fell, and rural families reared more children to adolescence, so that the urge to reproduce diminished. As more parents moved to the towns and the manufactories, young children began to become a liability requiring food, rather than an asset for exploitation as a cheap source of labour. This changed attitude was accelerated after the legislation restricting child labour in 1832. In this more permissive atmosphere the use of coitus interruptus as a contraceptive method appears to have increased amongst all socio-economic groups. With the publication of Place's *Illustrations and Proofs of the Principle of Population* in 1822, and his handbills, the knowledge that contraception was available also spread widely, particularly amongst the wealthy and educated. Francis Place (1771–1854) can be called the founder of the birth control movement, and his influence in informing the people about contraceptive methods was considerable. It is significant that by 1822 he had rejected Malthus' solution of 'moral restraint' by delaying marriage, as he believed that this would lead to vice and prostitution. In place of moral restraint he favoured the more realistic approach of contraceptive measures. His book reached the affluent, his single sheet handbills were distributed widely amongst the workers in London and in the industrial towns of Northern England. The handbills of 1823 were addressed to 'The Married of Both Sexes of the Working People', as well as to other groups. Although Place took a moral tone against vice and debauchery, he suggested that by limiting the size of their families, the 'misery of the poor children' and the parents' 'own sickness' might be mitigated. Place recommended that the women use a 'piece of soft sponge tied by a bobbin or penny ribbon, and inserted (. . . into the vagina . . .) just before sexual intercourse takes place'. The sponge was to be the size of a green walnut or small apple and would not 'diminish the pleasures of married life'. Only when the sponge was not available did Place recommend coitus interruptus. In addition to the medico-social advantages of contraception outlined in his handbills, Place also stressed the economic advantages of small families which would prevent poverty, reduce the need for child labour and raise the standard of living—attitudes echoed today in the stress in many nations on family welfare in contraception programmes.

The main effect of Place and his followers, Carlisle, Hassell and Campion, was not that a substantial reduction of the birth rate followed the spread of the pamphlets, but that attitudes were altered, and a cultural change which recognized the need for family planning began.

At the same time in the United States of America, Robert

Dale Owen, the son of the Scottish philanthropist and social reformer, published a book *Moral Restraint* (1830) in which coitus interruptus was recommended in preference to the vaginal sponge and the condom. He claimed that the former was of doubtful efficacy and 'physically disagreeable', whilst the condom was 'inconvenient'. Although Owen's book had sold 75,000 copies by the time of his death in 1877, it did not have the impact of Dr. Charles Knowlton's *The Fruits of Philosophy: or a private Companion of Young Married People* which was first published in 1832. Knowlton's book had gone through 10 editions by 1877, and was reprinted in Britain in that year, an incident which led to the trial of Bradlaugh and Besant, with resulting widespread publicity about 'birth control'. Knowlton's recommended method was douching, using an 'astringent vegetable' infusion, or soda bicarbonate, but he was 'quite confident that the liberal use of pretty cold water would be a never failing preventative'. He did not think coitus interruptus safe, and apparently rejected the vaginal sponge as unaesthetic.

By 1860 in England, it was considered safe to write about contraception, and Charles Bradlaugh published articles recommending consideration of 'Neo-Malthusian principles' (which was a euphemism for contraception) in his journal *The National Reformer*. Early in 1877, a Bristol publisher, Henry Cook, had printed and distributed an edition of Knowlton's *The Fruits of Philosophy* in which it was alleged he had interleaved obscene pictures. For this he was sentenced to two years' imprisonment with hard labour. As the book had been circulating for over twenty years, Bradlaugh, together with his fellow reformer Annie Besant, objected to this and invited prosecution by publishing another edition (without the pictures). They were duly prosecuted and after two trials, which were attended by much publicity, were acquitted, and the right to publish contraceptive information was established. At the same time another reformer, Edward Truelove, then nearly seventy years old, published a new edition of Owen's booklet and was prosecuted as the booklet 'would have an injurious effect on the minds of the young'. Again two trials were needed before Truelove was convicted and sentenced to four months' imprisonment.

The effect of these two trials scandalized intellectual society, many of whom were already using birth control (Figure **10/1**), and radical journals printed denunciations of the prosecutions. Not only was intellectual opinion incensed, but the general public began to be interested, as they read that contraceptive methods were available, and knowledge of them might be obtained legally and without hazard. By this time, too, the condom had come into general use. In 1843, vulcanization of rubber had been discovered which lowered the cost of making

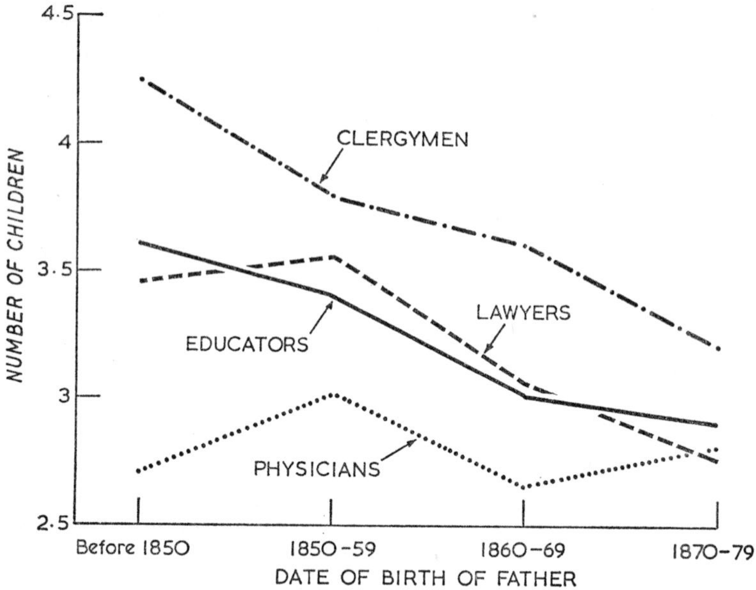

Figure **10/1** The reduction in family size, selected professions, U.S.A. 1850–80.

thinner, stronger sheets of crêpe rubber. Between 1844 and 1875, rubber condoms largely replaced gut condoms. Costs of production were lowered, the new condom was aesthetically better, and its popularity and use rose rapidly.

Following the Bradlaugh–Besant trial, public interest in contraception increased and sales of books dealing with birth control rose dramatically. For example, the edition of Knowlton's *The Fruits of Philosophy* published by Bradlaugh and Besant, sold 185,000 copies in the next four years, and other editions were published in industrial towns in the North of

England. In 1879, Anne Besant wrote and published a book which replaced Knowlton's dated work, and had the effect of further spreading knowledge of contraception. This book, *The Law of Population: Its Consequences, and the bearing on Conduct and Morals*, was dedicated 'To the poor in the great cities and agricultural districts, dwellers in stifling courts or crowded hovels, in the hope that it may point out a path from poverty and may make easier the life of British mothers, to them I dedicate this essay.' The sales were large, 175,000 copies having been sold at sixpence (7c) a copy by 1890. Mrs. Besant condemned abortion and felt the 'safe period' (which had incorrectly been assumed to be from the 5th to the 15th day of the menstrual cycle!) was uncertain. She accepted coitus interruptus as 'absolutely certain' and without injurious side-effects, but considered the vaginal douche and the use of the condom to have obvious aesthetic disadvantages 'as a matter of taste and feeling'. She felt that the vaginal sponge was the preferred method, and in later editions also approved soluble vaginal pessaries. By 1885, she added that the sponge should be soaked in a dilute quinine solution, and that the following morning the wife might douche using a quinine solution. She also recommended a rubber cervical cap in place of the vaginal sponge as it was 'absolutely unobtrusive'. In 1885, a Leeds physician, Dr. Allbutt, wrote *The Wife's Handbook* in which one chapter deals with 'How to Prevent Conception when Advised by the Doctor'. Allbutt described in careful, non-sensational detail the methods then available for birth control, including the use of the vaginal diaphragm, which had recently been introduced in Germany. Two years later he was indicted for unprofessional conduct and was examined by the General Medical Council. They found him guilty of the 'offence' charged against him; 'that is to say, of having published and publically caused to be sold, a work entitled *The Wife's Handbook* in London and elsewhere, at so low a price as to bring the work within the reach of the youth of both sexes, to the detriment of public morals'. This act, the Council decided, was 'infamous in a professional respect', and Allbutt's name was removed from the Medical Register, his licence to practise medicine thus being revoked. This action again led to widespread publicity, and according to a weekly journal, *The Pall Mall Gazette*, was 'one of the most glaring illustrations of professional prejudice and human folly'. It also led to a large sale of *The Wife's Handbook*.

The effect of all this publicity from 1877 onwards was to induce people to question whether they had all the children they desired, and if they reached the decision that they had, to use one or other of the contraceptive methods available. It also led to anticontraceptive legislation initiated by Anthony Comstock, the secretary of the 'New York Society for the Suppression of Vice'. Comstock was a puritanical fanatic whose slogan was 'Morals, not Art or Literature'. Legislation inspired by him led to the passage of the Comstock Act of 1873. This Act was a broad-based anti-obscenity law which prohibited the importation, transportation between States, or the mailing of 'any article whatever for the prevention of conception'. Under the Act authors of articles on contraceptive advice were regularly prosecuted. Although this effectively hindered the dissemination of birth control information, the use of contraceptive measures increased in the forty years from 1880 to 1920, particularly amongst the upper and middle classes.

In Scandinavia contraceptives were freely available from about 1880; and in Britain, contraceptive advice and devices were freely disseminated following the decision in the Bradlaugh–Besant trial. That this had some influence on the birth rate, which began to fall from 1877, is evident in Figure **10/2**. In the U.S.A., because of the Comstock Act, the dissemination through the mails of birth control advice was prohibited and appliances could only be prescribed by physicians for medical reasons and then at risk of prosecution. After working with the urban poor in New York, Margaret Sanger became convinced that many women who needed contraceptive advice for social or economic reasons were being refused such advice by physicians. Accordingly she began a campaign, culminating with her 'Contraceptive Advice Station' opened in Brooklyn in 1916 and rapidly closed by police action. However, the experience she obtained was influential in securing a decision by the Court of Appeals that it was legal for physicians to give contraceptive advice 'for the cure and prevention of disease', which could be widely interpreted.

This movement was encouraged by the formation in the 1920s of the National Committee on Maternal Health Inc. But it will be noted that all the efforts mentioned were made by voluntary organizations, usually in the face of official indifference.

Despite the obvious need for birth control information, the situation in the U.S.A. was hindered by government and institutional policies which made it difficult for health workers to dispense, and for couples to practise, birth control. From 1936 several court decisions moderated the impact of the anti-contraceptive Comstock laws, but twenty-two years elapsed before the ban on prescribing contraceptives in public hospitals in New York was lifted. This started the trend to publicly

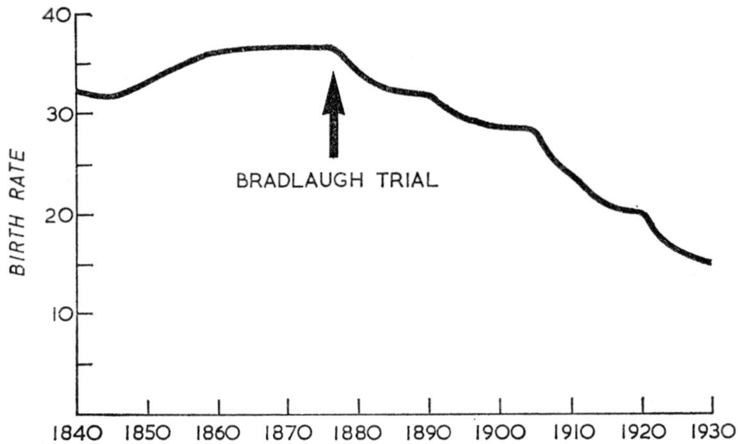

Figure **10/2** The effect of the Bradlaugh trial on the birth rate.

financed family planning services, but it was not until 1967 that the U.S. Congress adopted any specific legislation on family planning.

Since 1967, the changes have been rapid. Federal and State agencies have initiated policies favouring family planning; and increasing numbers of States have liberalized their abortion laws. At the apex of the changes is the federal family planning agency which was set up after the passage of the Family Planning Services and Population Research Act of 1970. It is now public policy to help American women avoid unwanted, unwelcome pregnancy, and this measure should play a significant part in helping the U.S.A. to achieve population stability.

In Britain the situation was similar. Birth control information and advice was left to voluntary organizations, and was opposed by legislators. However, changes were occurring. The effect of World War I, the Suffragette movement and the general emancipation of women led, in the early 1920s, to the formation of The Birth Control League; and Marie Stopes and Norman Haire popularized birth control. More important, birth control clinics were established by interested private organizations to give advice and to provide devices for those too poor, or too shy, to visit their family doctor. However, no support was received from the Government, although a resolution in 1926 by the House of Lords had called for the removal of 'all obstacles to the introduction of birth control advice in Maternity and Child Welfare Centres'. This was not implemented. But six years later the Minister of Health issued a circular permitting the M. and C.W. Centres to give contraceptive advice in cases 'where a further pregnancy would be detrimental to health', but in no other cases. The Government was not anxious to be involved politically with birth control. By 1930, it appeared that over 70 per cent of married women of the upper socio-economic groups used contraceptive methods, whilst in the lower socio-economic groups about half of those who were sufficiently motivated to attend a birth control clinic said they had used some form of contraception prior to the visit. Kopp (1934) studied this in New York and found that the methods used had been various, and the failure rate high, which indicated that the knowledge of contraceptives and the application of that knowledge was defective (Table **10/1**). It is also clear from other studies that the higher the socio-economic level of the women, the lower was the failure rate, which stresses the importance of education in family planning programmes.

Between 1935 and 1955, contraceptive advice continued to be given and contraceptives to be obtained either from birth control clinics, pharmacists' shops or other sources on an increasing scale. During this period, neither political party in the United Kingdom had any policy about population dynamics. This was understandable in the 1930s, when demographers foretold a decline of population; but after World War II the policy continued, despite the recommendation in 1949 by the Royal Commission on Population that the population needed

Table 10/1

Contraceptive use and 'failure' rates (three collected series involving 16,835 U.S. women), 1933–34. (The number 27,601 indicates the total number of women reporting the methods they used; as some used more than one method the total exceeds the 16,835 women investigated.)

Method	*Total instances*	*Usage (per cent)*	*Failure rate (per cent)*
Coitus interruptus	7,773	28·2	60
Douche	6,922	25·1	55
Condom	6,528	23·6	42
Suppositories or jellies	2,230	8·1	40
Diaphragm or cervical cap	921	3·3	25
Other methods, or combinations of methods	3,227	11·7	—
	27,601	100·0	

Sources:
Kopp, M. E. *Birth control in practice*, McBride, New York, 1934.
Pearl, R. 'Contraception and Fertility in 4945 Married Women'. *Human Biology* **6**, 355, 1934.
Stone, H. M. *Medical Journal and Record*, **137**, 7, 1933.

to be stabilized and 'control of men and women over the numbers of their children is one of the first conditions of their own and the community's welfare'. Religious and other pressure groups echoed Sir Norman Birkett's 1939 remark that birth control ought not to be made generally available as it would 'tend to lower the traditional and accepted standard of morality' and might often be 'a source of temptation'. Their influence delayed any implementation of a population policy, although the world's rate of population growth was now a matter of grave concern to many.

It was not until 1967 that the Family Planning Act was placed on the statute book. This Act gave the Minister of Health the power to order any local authority to provide family planning services as a statutory duty. But between 1967 and 1970, few local authorities had taken much action, pleading shortage of funds. The introduction in 1968 of the Abortion Act widened the indications for legal abortion, and in the first three years the rate rose to 120,000 abortions annually. Belatedly the Government realized that many of the abortions were being performed because pregnancy had resulted from the unavailability, inconvenience or cost of obtaining contraceptive advice. It was estimated by the Select Committee on Science and Technology that between 200,000 and 300,000 unwelcome, often unwanted children, were born each year in England and Wales alone. The rising rate of legal abortions, together with the evidence of the large number of unwanted pregnancies, has led to a realization that the Abortion Act was introduced prematurely, and was not preceded by a vigorous campaign to provide birth control measures to those most vulnerable—unmarried girls under the age of 25, and married women, largely urban dwellers, whose income was low, and whose social environment was depressed. A further factor was that under the Abortion Act, abortions were provided free in National Health Service Hospitals, but contraceptive advice had to be sought privately, and the contraceptive equipment had to be purchased.

These defects aggravated the situation and increased the requests for abortion as a birth control measure. Middle-class women were able to obtain contraceptive advice from their family doctors or from the Family Planning Association clinics. Lower-class women, and particularly unmarried girls, not only found it difficult to seek advice from predominantly middle-class, usually male, family doctors, or the mainly middle-class workers in the F.P.A., but tended to be deterred by the complex administrative arrangements, in particular the need to walk into a building which existed solely to give contraceptive advice. This constraint is due to the sexual prudery of many women, and to the lack of adequate sex education in childhood and adolescence. It has had the effect that contraceptive measures have not been sought by many women at risk of becoming pregnant. It has been calculated that failure to use contraceptives was the cause of 70 per cent of 120,000 pregnancies terminated in 1971.

Despite this evidence, the British Minister of Health declared in 1971 that free contraceptives would be a gratuitous waste of the taxpayers' money, as the vast majority of people in Britain were capable of seeking and paying for contraception. More significantly he rejected the suggestion that maternity hospitals and M. and C.W. clinics were suitable places to give contraceptive advice, although most experts, including the World Health Organization, consider that family planning is most suitably linked with maternity and child welfare. Linking family welfare and family planning enables easy referral to take place when gynaecological problems are discovered, enhances the service of each, and reduces costs considerably.

Opposition to the dissemination of contraceptive advice by community leaders has had the effect that although local authorities have had the power to provide birth control facilities since 1967 (and have had funds made available by the State for the purpose), by 1972 only one-third offered such a service, and then not all offered a 'consumer oriented' service.

The lack of enthusiasm and co-operation by local municipal and county authorities was, in part, due to the fear that increased contraceptive availability, particularly amongst unmarried women, would lead to increased promiscuity. Unmarried men had always been able to purchase condoms from pharmacists' shops, or more usually from men's hairdressing shops, but the double standard of sexual morality inhibited the thought of many community leaders.

There is no evidence that contraceptive availability increases promiscuity. Both have increased in an increasingly sexually permissive atmosphere. Two careful studies, one in Birmingham by Jordan and Studd, the other in London by Newton, confirmed that 96 per cent of the 1,500 unmarried girls studied were sexually active when they sought contraceptive advice; that only 7 per cent had changed their sexual partners in a follow-up survey made 18 to 24 months after their first visit to the clinic; that the girls attended of their own free will; that 25 per cent had informed their parents, and that using a personality questionnaire the girls were indistinguishable from the population at large.

Sociological studies suggest that a consumer demand exists in Britain. Surveys seeking information about birth control get a higher response than those seeking information about income and expenditures. Newspapers and magazines emphasizing sexual exploits have a large circulation. The constraint to accepting birth control seems to be fear of being snubbed by the health worker and the cost, not a lack of desire.

In 1973, the British Minister of Health had second thoughts about his 1971 statement, and in introducing changes in the National Health Service, to operate from mid-1974, he announced that he would include contraceptives in the Health Service. The pill, and contraceptive appliances, would not be free but would carry a prescription charge. He came to this decision despite the obvious concept that prevention of unwanted pregnancies is as much a part of preventive medicine as are immunizations, cancer smear tests, routine chest X-rays, and the provision of pure water—and in England preventive health measures are provided free. He also ignored the remarkably successful experience of those few local authorities who have provided a free contraceptive service to the poor in their area. The Minister's change of mind is hardly a giant stride in social reform, but is a first small step to making all pregnancies wanted.

Any nation concerned with the rate of population growth, the number of illegal abortions, and the number of births to unmarried mothers, should first institute a well-organized information campaign about family planning; should institute sex education (including information about birth control) in primary and secondary schools and should offer contraceptives which can be obtained easily and at little or no cost. If this sequence is adopted, legal induced abortion should only be needed as a 'backstop' when contraception fails, and to help the ignorant, the unlucky and the unfortunate woman who becomes pregnant.

Although political hostility, or at least indifference, has hindered the dissemination of contraceptive knowledge and the use of contraceptives, the advances in contraceptive technology since 1935 have led to a move away from the less effective methods of conception control (the douche and coitus interruptus) to the use of the vaginal diaphragm, whilst the condom continued to be used at the same proportional rate (Table **10/2**). It will be noted, too, that the 'Safe Period' which was acceptable to Roman Catholics, was used increasingly up to 1955 but became less popular after that date. This coincided with the development of oral contraceptives.

In 1935 a technological change in the manufacture of condoms occurred, liquid latex replacing masticated crêpe rubber

Table 10/2

The changing pattern of choice of contraception in the U.S.A. between 1935 and 1970

Method	*Per cent in* 1935	*Per cent in* 1955	*Per cent in* 1965	*Per cent in* 1970
Coitus interruptus	29	7	7	2
Douche	26	10	4	4
Condom	24	28	24	17
Oral contraceptives	0	0	24	41
Suppositories, foam, jellies	8	3	6	7
Diaphragm	3	25	11	7
Rhythm Method	3	22	12	8
Other, or combination of methods	7	5	11	5
Intra-uterine contraceptive device	0	0	1	9

Sources:
Westoff, C. F. and Ruder, N. B. 'United States, Methods of Fertility Control 1955, 1960 and 1965'. *Studies in Family Planning*, **17,** 1, 1967.
Jaffe, F. S. *Science*, **174,** 119, 1971.
Westoff, C. F. *Family Planning Perspectives*, **4** (3), July 1972.

in their manufacture. The latex condom, in addition to being thinner and less liable to contain holes, was cheaper to manufacture, although standards of testing were introduced which were expensive and some manufacturers sold defective products. It was considered that by 1936, 105 million condoms per year, retailing at about 20 cents each, were sold in the U.S.A.; and proportional sales were made in other industrialized nations. These sales increased over the years and by 1965 had risen in the U.S.A. to about 700 million per year (Table **10/3**).

In 1955 a revolution occurred. In that year Pincus reported his experience with hormonal oral contraceptives at a meeting in Tokyo, and at the same meeting the Japanese reported their re-introduction of the intra-uterine contraceptive device. The latter had been used in the 1920s and 1930s, particularly by Grafenberg in Germany and Oppenheimer in Israel. However, as the device was difficult to introduce and was frequently followed by complications, such as pelvic infection, it had been condemned by gynaecologists and had fallen into disuse. From

Table 10/3

The sale of condoms (per year per adult male) in various nations 1955 and 1970

Country	*Condoms per year per adult male*	
	1955	1970
U.S.A.	12	7
Sweden	10	5
Japan	8	6
Britain	5	7
West Germany	5	4
Hungary	3	3
France	1	2
India	0·06	0·4

Sources:
Teitze, C. in *Advances in Sex Research*, Hoeber, New York, 1963.
Levin, H. in *Family Planning and Population Programs*, Chicago Univ. Press, Chicago, 1966.

1955 on these two methods, 'The Pill' and 'The Loop', became the predominant methods of contraception recommended. Estimates of the usage of oral contraceptives for the year 1971 showed that over 20 million women were using the Pill for contraception, and 10 million women have intra-uterine contraceptive devices in utero. The current methods of contraception, particularly the oral contraceptives and the intra-uterine contraceptive device (IUD) are considered in detail in the next section. Despite this stress on the Pill and the IUD, a careful randomized survey of sexual habits made in England and Wales in 1970 somewhat surprisingly revealed that over one-third of married couples used no contraceptive technique, whilst of those using some method, the condom was the most popular, particularly amongst couples of the lower socio-economic groups who lived in the north of England (Table **10/4**). Statistics of contraceptive usage in Melbourne, Australia, in 1970 are also given in Table **10/4** so that comparisons can be made.

It is interesting, and instructive, to compare these findings with a study made in Denmark, where sex education is stressed in schools, and where sex is not considered obscene. Amongst

Table 10/4

Contraceptive practice by married couples in England and Wales, 1969 and Australia, 1970

Contraceptive	*Per cent of all couples (England and Wales)*	*Per cent of those using contraceptives (England and Wales)*	*(Australia*)*
No contraceptives used	37		
Condom	29	46	9
Pill	19	31	38
Diaphragm }	6	9	5
Spermicide }			3
Coitus interruptus	5	7	19
IUD	3	5	8
Rhythm	1	2	14
Other	—	—	4

Sources: U.K. Gorer, G. *Sex and Marriage in England and Wales*, Nelson, 1971.
Sources: Australia. Caldwell, J. C. *et al. Studies in Family Planning*, **4**, 49, 1973.
* Based on interviews in Melbourne: 62 per cent Australian born, 17 per cent U.K. or Northern Europe, 2 per cent East Europe and 19 per cent South Europe.

Danes of all classes, there is far less prurience towards sexuality than there is in Britain. In a nation which has a rational attitude towards sex and contraception, preference for the newer, safer methods of birth control is marked. In 1970, 66 per cent of contraceptive users chose oral contraceptives, and the number choosing coitus interruptus or the condom had dropped to less than 10 per cent (Table **10/5**).

Since 1960, there has been an increasing awareness in Governments, International Agencies and individuals that control of population growth is essential, and that the most humane and desirable method is by the use of contraceptive techniques.

It is unfortunate that one powerful force, which could influence the attitude of millions of women, has failed to accept the need for the control of the growth rate of population, and has rejected modern, efficient, birth control measures. This is the Roman Catholic Church. It is not that the gravity of the

Table 10/5

The choice of contraceptives in Denmark between 1949 and 1970

(*Per cent of couples using each method*)				
	1949	1959	1966	1970
Coitus interruptus	29	10	3	—
Condom	11	34	28	10
Diaphragm	2	26	48	10
Oral contraceptives	—	—	12	66
IUCD	—	—	1	10
Others or none	58	30	8	4

Source: Oster, M. *Advances in Planned Parenthood,* **6,** 35, 1971; and personal.

situation had not been recognized. It is also accepted that many Roman Catholics use birth control measures, and, more seriously from a moral and a medical viewpoint, obtain illegal abortions. Opposition to human intervention in the reproductive processes initiated by coitus is found in many religions. It stems from the belief that procreation is sacred, and interference with it will bring down the wrath of God.

The concern of the great humanitarian pope, John XXIII, for the problems of exponential population growth, led to his appointment of an advisory commission. This commission was formalized, and enlarged by his successor, Paul VI. It reported in 1967 that in matters of birth control the final responsibility was the conscience of the individual. However, the advice of the commission, and a growing request for change by Roman Catholic laity was rejected by Paul VI. In his encyclical Humanae Vitae in July, 1968, he reaffirmed the traditional doctrine of Aquinas that all mechanical, or pharmacological methods of birth control were 'unnatural'.

Even amongst Roman Catholics changes are evident. At present these are voiced mostly by affluent women, but discussion is beginning at all levels, and in some instances is encouraged by Roman Catholic bishops and priests.

As a final note, it is perhaps ironic that the calumny and derision hurled at the pioneers who suggested that the knowledge of contraception, a desire to use contraceptive measures and the availability of contraceptive devices would improve the human condition has today been replaced by an awareness that their views were correct, their approach justified and their integrity unquestioned.

ELEVEN

The Technology of Contraception — I

There is no perfect contraceptive. That is, a contraceptive which will consistently prevent pregnancy, which is reversible, is easy to use and which is without side-effects. But modern technology has developed contraceptive methods which are highly effective, and which are available for use by men and women in a variety of cultural, intellectual and environmental circumstances. The concept of a choice of methods, one of which is most suited to a particular circumstance, is important. Doctrinaire belief in the superiority of one method, in all places and at all times, is self-defeating. In certain circumstances it may be preferable to recommend a less efficient method, which is more readily available and easier to use, than a more efficient method which is complicated to use, and likely to be discontinued by the user after a longer or a shorter interval. In this connection, the finding in several surveys in India that nearly half the women studied who chose the Pill had discontinued its use within twelve months of accepting the method is, to say the least, disconcerting.

In any examination of contraceptive technology it is useful to have some method of comparing the capacity of the chosen method to prevent unwanted pregnancies. In other words to be able to calculate its use-effectiveness. A method, which has been available for the past forty years, was devised by Raymond Pearl, and is usually referred to as the Pearl index. The index calculates the unintended pregnancy rate from the formula

$$\frac{\text{The number of unintended pregnancies}}{\text{Total months of exposure to pregnancy}} \times 1{,}200$$

The result is expressed as the *failure rate per 100 woman years*. The number of pregnancies in the numerator must include all known pregnancies, whatever the outcome. The factor 1,200 is the number of months in 100 years. The total months of exposure to pregnancy in the denominator is obtained by deducting all those months when coitus did not take place for reasons of separation, sickness or whatever. By convention, ten months is deducted for a pregnancy which reached 30 weeks, and four months for a pregnancy which ended before that time.

A valid criticism of the Pearl index has been made by Lasagna who had 'a harsh look at current practices', and concluded that the index has the disadvantage that it disregards motivation and the variability of couples in respect of their monthly risk of conception. It ignores the variables of the socio-economic group, and the ages of the subjects, on their coital frequency and conception risk. Finally, the index can be calculated in several ways. Lasagna claims that the index 'blithely assumes that the rates for groups of women under observation for different periods are comparable and can be lumped together'. He writes: 'One is reminded of the play which included a minister, a prostitute, and a man paralysed from the waist down so as to represent "a cross section of humanity".' Lasagna recommends a modified life table approach as proposed by Potter and termed the cumulative pregnancy rate. Unfortunately, the calculations are more complex, so that most investigators continue to use the Pearl index. For this reason it will be used in this book, but as well the range of estimates of use-effectiveness will be given, and the author supports Tietze's plea that cumulative rates should be utilized in future studies.

In any study it is important that the subjects investigated are representative of all the users, and that the trial is continued for a reasonable length of time. This is because higher failure rates are invariable in the early months since some subjects are careless, or poorly motivated. The minimum total number of subjects in a prospective trial is probably 100, who are exposed for at least 10 months. This gives a minimum of 1,000 months of exposure, but anyone initiating a trial should seek statistical advice.

In the following discussion, methods used by men will be discussed first, and those used by women will be considered second. In many cases, however, the decision about the method to be used will be a joint one, made by the couple after being given advice. An additional complication occurs in many developing nations. This is that in these male-dominated societies it is the husband who decides whether or not his wife will be permitted to use contraceptive measures, and which method she will use. In these societies, induced abortion, which appears to follow a decision made by the wife alone, is common. And it is dangerous.

Contraceptive Methods for Males

COITUS INTERRUPTUS

Apart from abortion and infanticide, coitus interruptus is probably the oldest method of birth control. It is used in all cultures and is known by a variety of names, 'withdrawal' and 'being careful' being the most usual ones. Coitus interruptus played an important part in the transition from a high to a low birth rate, which occurred in many European nations between 1820 and 1890, as was mentioned in Chapter 10. Its use has now diminished, even in Britain where it was previously popular, particularly amongst the lower socio-economic groups of the nation. A social survey into sex and marriage carried out in England and Wales in 1957 showed that coitus interruptus was the method of choice of birth control of 20 per cent of a random sample, but in 1969 the proportion using the method had fallen to 5 per cent.

The reliability of coitus interruptus, as a method of birth control, depends on the ability of the man to recognize the pre-ejaculatory phase of coitus, and his agility in removing his penis from the vagina before ejaculation occurs. It also demands that he directs the ejaculate away from the vulva, as pregnancy can follow sperm deposition in the vaginal introitus. Provided that the man can exercise this degree of control, coitus interruptus is relatively efficient. The method requires no prior preparation and is without cost, which is an advantage.

Claims that coitus interruptus is physically or psychologically injurious to either partner cannot be substantiated, although a woman with a high libido may fail to reach orgasm, and may become sexually frustrated, unless her partner brings her to orgasm by digital or oral stimulation of her clitoral area after he has ejaculated.

THE CONDOM

The history of the condom, its method of manufacture and the standards required, have been considered in Chapter 10. Modern condoms made of fine latex or plastic, prelubricated by adding silicone, and individually packed in hermetically sealed aluminium foil sachets, are efficient and hardly noticeable contraceptives. They have a store life of at least five years, and can consequently be made available through a variety of outlets. In Britain, for example, over 65 per cent of sales are made through pharmacies and men's hairdressers, a fact which has led Potts to state: 'This is a matter of considerable importance, and a possible reason for the continuing popularity of the condom, as it can be purchased without a prescription and from a variety of outlets, including the impersonal vending machine.'

The reliability of the condom is difficult to evaluate, for it depends on the technique used, although its simplicity should reduce this factor. In general, the condom is drawn on to the erect penis, which means that its use must be related to immediate coitus. The rolled condom is unrolled onto the penis, care being taken to remove air from the closed end, which may be teat- or plain-ended. There is no difference in effectiveness. If air is left in the closed end, its pressure, together with the ejaculated semen, may lead to the condom bursting. Although the risk is slight, couples using the method, for whom an inadvertent pregnancy would be disastrous, should also use a spermicidal cream, or pessary, introduced into the vagina prior to coitus.

As well as its ready availability, the condom has medico-social advantages. If the couple have only infrequent and unpredictable coitus, it is more logical for the man to use a condom than for the woman to use an oral contraceptive or the IUD. One such situation may be when the man is away from home for the greater part of the year, or if he returns unexpectedly. A condom should be used for preventive reasons if the man seeks coitus with a prostitute, although its protective value is by no means absolute. It should also be used if the woman has psychological or religious reasons against her using a contraceptive method. There are no clinical contra-indications to the use of the condom, and there is a complete absence of side-effects. Modern condoms are virtually undetectable by either partner during coitus.

Because of its ready availability, its cheapness, and its ease of use, the condom remains a very popular method of birth control, in the developed and in the developing nations. In the former, its use varies with the culture, the age and marital status of the user and his socio-economic group. More older men use condoms than younger men; and more men of the lower socio-economic groups than those of more affluent groups use the method. In the most recent survey in Britain, Gorer found 20 per cent of the married population habitually used the condom for birth control. In the U.S.A., the use of the condom has declined considerably since oral contraceptives became available, but sales continue to remain high. In Japan, nationwide surveys conducted in 1950 and 1959 showed that the use of the condom increased from 38 per cent to 58 per cent in the population studied. This increase coincided with a fall in the number of abortions performed.

The reliability of the condom, as an effective birth control method, is difficult to estimate because most surveys have been made on selected groups. Teitze has reviewed the available literature and has concluded that when used by parous couples, who were motivated to prevent a further pregnancy, the pregnancy rate calculated by Pearl's formula, was 3 per 100 women years. In most investigations, however, the pregnancy rate lies between 10 and 20 per 100 women years.

VASECTOMY

Vasectomy is now accepted as a highly effective, easily performed, permanent method of conception control. The operation is easier to perform than the standard tubal excision and ligation, and even easier than laparoscopic tubal cautery, and it requires no motivational follow up. It does require considerable motivation to induce men to accept it. This motivation must be linked with information, so that the many verbalized and non-verbalized questions asked by prospective clients are answered. Health workers must avoid the trap of assuming that the wealthy are necessarily more accurately informed about their reproductive system. Even amongst intelligent people, vasectomy is confused with castration, and a hidden fear is that a man's sexual powers will be reduced postoperatively. He needs reassurance that the operation will in no way affect his sexual desires or his sexual performance. Concern may also be expressed about the dangerous accumulation of spermatozoa distal to the cut vas deferens. The physician must explain that the accumulation of spermatozoa is minimal, and that most of the quantity of the ejaculate derives from secretions of the accessory glands. He may also explain that as spermatozoa accumulate in the testicles, spermatogenesis almost ceases, and macrophages eliminate sperm in the epididymis and tubules, but that the synthesis of androgens continues. The most successful method of convincing a prospective client is for him to meet a man who has had a vasectomy performed, and who is satisfied with the result.

The technique of the operation is shown in Figure **11/1**. In that figure it can be seen that local anaesthesia is used, 2 to 5 ml of 2 per cent lignocaine, with adrenaline (1:200,000), being injected after the scrotal skin has been cleansed with an aqueous antiseptic. Alternatively, the operation may be performed under general anaesthesia, but this limits its use to hospitals or clinics; whilst vasectomy under local anaesthesia can be performed in remote rural areas as an outpatient procedure, as has been demonstrated in India.

The vas deferens, which is about 2·5 mm in diameter, forms one component of each spermatic cord, together with the testicular artery, arteries to the vas and to the cremaster muscle, a pampiniform plexus of veins, the genital branch of the genito-femoral nerve and lymphatics. Rarely it is duplicated. It can be readily palpated as a cordlike structure, and isolated, by finger and thumb, at the junction of the scrotum and the body. The vas is lifted up in a fold of skin and held whilst the skin is infiltrated with local anaesthetic. A small incision is made, and a loop of spermatic cord is delivered through the wound. The sheath is incised and the vas is dissected from the other components. Two small artery forceps clamp a segment at least 1 cm long, which is excised. The cut ends are tied with 3/0 silk, and, in some techniques, are folded back on themselves. The remainder of the operation is shown in the Figure. It is most important to ensure haemostasis, or a small painful haematoma

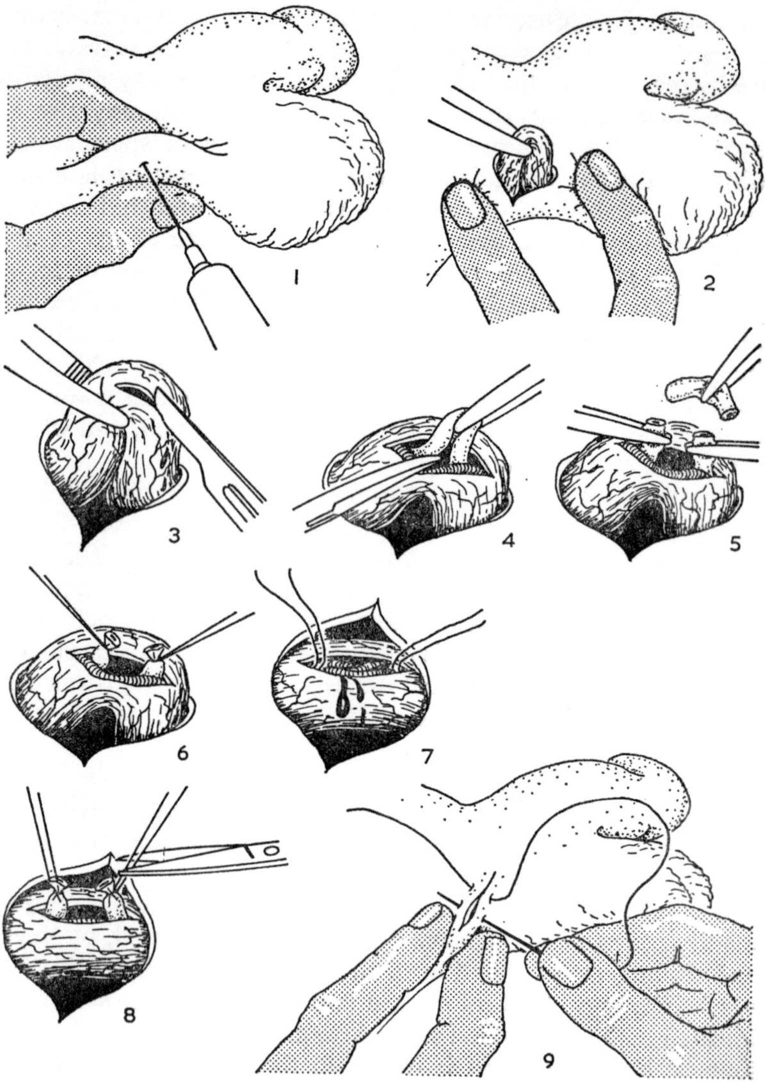

Figure **11/1** 1. Spermatic cord palpated and lifted in fold of skin.
2. Delivery of spermatic cord through scrotal incision.
3. Incision through sheath of cord (after infiltration with local anaesthetic).
4. Dissection of vas from other constituents of cord.

will result. The patient should wear a testicular support (a jock strap) to prevent discomfort. The sutures are removed on the fourth day.

Coitus may be resumed whenever the man wishes, but he, or his partner, must continue to use other contraceptive measures as he is not sterile until all the spermatozoa accumulated in the seminal vesicles have been ejaculated. This may require twelve ejaculations, and until a seminal appraisal has been made, the man is potentially fertile. Where it is not possible to do a semen analysis, the couple should continue to use other contraceptive measures until the man has had fifteen ejaculations.

The physical effects of vasectomy appear minimal. There is no evidence that vasectomy reduces the androgenic function of the testes after vasectomy. In fact in experiments in dogs, the total interstitial (Leydig) cell volume is increased (Kothari and Mishra), and in humans there is preliminary evidence of increased testosterone secretion.

The psychological effect of vasectomy has been studied in several nations. The consensus is that if the operation is socially and culturally acceptable in the society, and if the patient himself has been properly prepared for the operation, the effects are minimal. Those who are most disturbed are men who were psychologically unstable before the operation. Over 70 per cent of men interviewed claimed to have a more satisfactory sex life after vasectomy, and only 2 per cent were unhappy. There is no evidence to support the myth that vasectomized men become increasingly unfaithful to their wives.

In general, the operation should be considered irreversible, although it is possible to do a reconstructive operation, if too wide a wedge has not been excised. The technique is not difficult and the pregnancy rate is fair. In published series since 1960,

---

5. Crushing of vas in 2 places. Removal of intervening 1 cm (minimum) of vas.
6. Cut ends ligated with black silk.
7. Ligated ends of vas allowed to return to cord and cord to scrotum. Bleeding points checked.
8. Cut ends of vas delivered out and black silk ligatures shortened.
9. Closure of scrotal wound.

sperms are found in the ejaculate of 60 per cent of men (range 16 to 100 per cent) after reanastomosis, and pregnancy has followed in 30 per cent (range 10 to 66 per cent) of cases (Presser). A novel idea, as yet little developed, is for a man to deposit a quantity of his spermatozoa in a 'sperm bank' where it is stored under liquid nitrogen for use later should he wish for some reason to have a further child.

In Britain, vasectomy is now available at no cost under the National Health Service; in India, men who have had vasectomy performed are given a money grant so that they may take time off work; but in most nations the operation must be paid for.

Vasectomy is becoming increasingly acceptable in the developed nations of the world. The increase in the number of operations has coincided with concern about the effects of population growth, and over the side-effects of other contraceptive measures.

Contraceptive Methods for Females

In the following discussion the least effective methods will be considered first, and the most effective methods last. However, as in the discussion of contraceptive measures used by men, the method must be tailored, where possible, to the needs of the particular woman. In certain situations even relatively ineffective measures, which are easy to use, may be preferable to no contraception at all.

LOCALLY USED CHEMICAL CONTRACEPTIVES (SPERMICIDES)

In Chapter 10 it was pointed out that chemically impregnated intravaginal plugs have been used for contraceptive purposes by several primitive tribes. The plug delayed the spermatozoa's transit to the cervix, and the chemicals were spermicidal. The method had a period of popularity in Britain between 1885 and 1935 due to the persuasive (but discreet) advertising of Rendells cocoa-butter and quinine vaginal pessaries; and other chemicals have been suggested from time to time. Currently, there are over 50 suppositories, pessaries, gels, or foams available. The solid vagitories (to use the word recommended by the IPPF for pessaries and suppositories) use a spermicide in a base of soap, gelatin- or cocoa-butter, which is designed to melt at body temperature. The vagitory is inserted just prior to coitus. The gels are made up in a water soluble, gelatinous base so that they disperse easily in the vagina. They are usually used as an additional protection if the male uses a condom, or in conjunction with a vaginal diaphragm. The gel, or cream, is introduced high into the vagina via a plastic plunger applicator which is provided in the package. The foams are either in foaming tablet form or are made as 'Pressure-Pak aerosols' and are theoretically more efficient than other methods of application.

Used alone, locally applied chemical contraceptives are inefficient; but used in conjunction with condoms or occlusive diaphragms they add to the protection given by the occlusive measure. Their main advantage is that they are easy to buy, and easy to use, but against this must be set a failure rate of 40 per 100 woman years usage (range 18 to 48).

Even less effective is a post-coital vaginal douche, which usually contains vinegar, or some proprietary spermicide. Logic should confirm that to use a douche as a contraceptive measure in this way is unaesthetic, ineffective and stupid. Since the ejaculated spermatozoa begin their transit through the cervix within one minute of ejaculation, it is like washing the stable door with the sperm well inside.

THE 'SAFE PERIOD'

In a woman with a normal cycle, ovulation will occur approximately fourteen days before the anticipated menstrual period. The ovum can only survive for two days unless it is fertilized, and the ejaculated spermatozoa survive, and are able to fertilize the ovum, for four days at the most. It is obvious from these facts that if coitus is avoided for four days before ovulation, to six days after it has occurred, pregnancy should be prevented. The physiological concepts for this belief were independently observed in 1929 by Knaus in Austria, and Ogino in Japan, and the so-called Ogino–Knaus method was enthusiastically adopted by Roman Catholics who were not preventing conception, but were regulating births in a 'natural way'. The original observations have been developed in recent years but the principle is the same. That is for the couple to restrict coitus to times of physiological infertility. Unfortunately the method, despite improvements, requires considerable motivation, and is not particularly safe, as the average woman does not have an exactly regular cycle, and ovulation may occur at different times during the cycle, especially if the emotions are stirred.

Since the method is the only one permissible to Roman Catholics, it requires further consideration in its four modern forms—the 'calendar rhythm method', the 'temperature method', the 'mucus method', and the 'predictable ovulation method'.

The calendar rhythm method

If a woman is prepared to use a calendar, and over a period of six menstrual cycles to record the duration of each cycle, she can determine her own safe period by calculating the date of ovulation in each cycle, and then subtracting three days from that day in the shortest cycle and adding three days in the longest cycle (Figure **11/2**). Coitus should be avoided during the danger period, and if a woman has a cycle of less than twenty days, or if the duration of her cycle varies by more than ten days, coitus will be infrequent and sexual frustration likely. A careful study in Washington D.C. of 30,000 cycles in 2,316 women, showed that only 30 per cent of them would qualify for the calendar rhythm method on the basis of a cycle range of eight days or less. The cycle range varied with age, the smallest variation being in the age group 30 to 34, when 40 per cent had a cycle with a range of eight days or less. However, if the couple are prepared to accept that coitus takes place in accordance with the calendar, not with desire, then the method is reasonably successful.

The temperature method

This is a more accurate method of pinpointing ovulation. It is based on the physiological observation that when ovulation has occurred, progesterone synthesized by the corpus luteum causes a rise in body temperature (Figure **11/3**). A motivated woman has to be prepared to take her basal rectal, or vaginal, temperature each morning on waking and before she gets out of bed (which may be difficult for a woman with a young

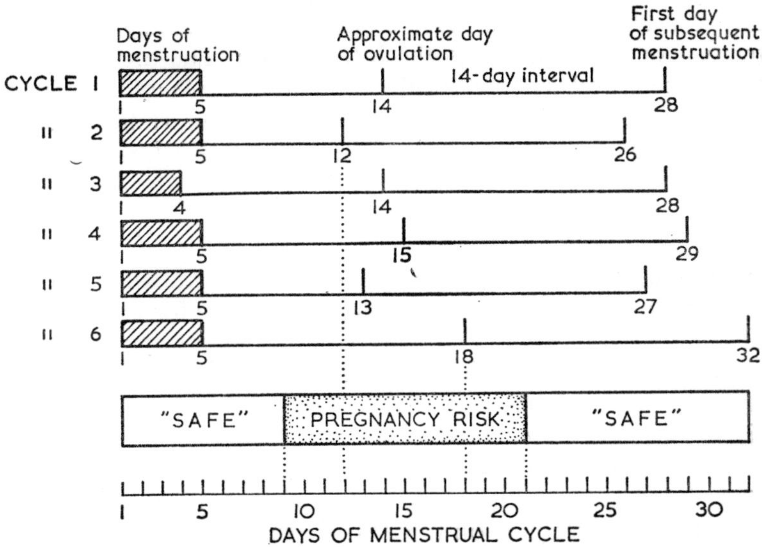

Figure **11/2** The Rhythm Method: calculation of the 'Safe Period'. In this example the shortest cycle was 26 days, the longest was 32 days. Ovulation in the shortest cycle was calculated to take place on day 12, in the longest on day 18. Three days each side of ovulation are potentially fertile (as the spermatozoa and ovum live for 3 days). For this particular woman, the days on which coitus should be avoided are from day 9 (i.e. the day of ovulation in the shortest cycle, less 3 days) to day 21 (i.e. the day of ovulation in the longest cycle, plus 3 days).

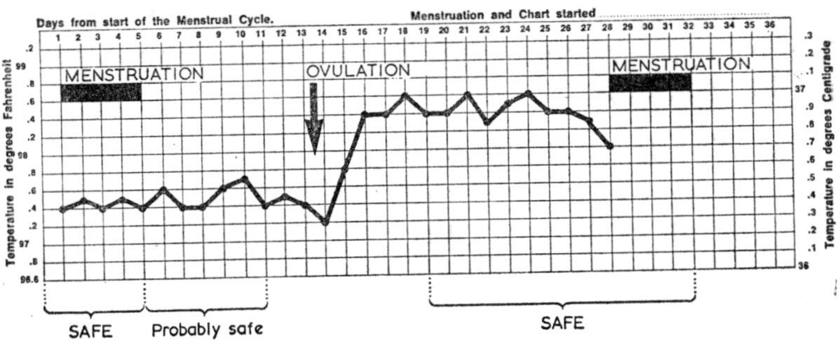

Figure **11/3** The temperature method of birth control.

family), or has any food or drink. From the daily readings she makes a chart, and can have coitus safely three days after the temperature rise indicates the luteal phase. The problems are that not all cycles show 'ideal' temperature rises and in 20 per cent of cases show a variant. In addition, intercurrent infection can invalidate the reading, and the method requires considerable motivation.

The mucus method

In this method, which was developed by an Australian physician, the patient learns to examine her vaginal orifice for the presence of mucus. Immediately postmenstrually the vaginal orifice feels dry. As ovulation time approaches, mucus can be detected. Initially this is cloudy and sticky, but as the level of oestrogen rises, the endocervical cells are stimulated to secrete more mucus and its character changes. It becomes clearer, strands stretch without breaking, and it 'feels slippery'. The peak of the clear mucus is reached on the day of ovulation, after which the mucus becomes cloudy again. The physiological concept of this sequence is correct, but the detection of mucus at the vulva requires considerable motivation, and perhaps the eye of faith. As well as this, vaginal secretions, either physiological or pathological, can confuse the issue. The motivated patient is given a chart and enters her findings each day using differently designed stickers for different types of mucus. Coitus is 'safe' when there is no mucus, and more than three days after the last day of the clear mucus. Between these times coitus should be avoided. Patients trained by Dr. Billings claim considerable success with his method, but the only reported study, which was made in Tonga by Weissmann, showed that the pregnancy rate was 25 per 100 woman years.

The predictable ovulation method

It will be appreciated that the safety of the 'safe period' depends on ovulation occurring on a predictable day during the menstrual cycle. Increased safety would be ensured if ovulation time could be regulated to within three days, and unexpected ovulation eliminated.

In this, there has recently been a break-through. If a woman takes conjugated equine oestrogen in a daily dose of 100 μg from day 9 to 15 of the cycle, ovulation will occur on day 13 to 17 in over 95 per cent of cycles (Boutselis). Coitus need only be avoided from day 10 to 20 of the cycle in these patients, and the woman does not need to take her temperature daily, or to inspect her vagina for mucus. Conjugated equine oestrogen (Premarin) is rapidly absorbed from the gut, and at this dosage rapidly stimulates pituitary gonadotrophin release. At the dose suggested, side-effects are minimal.

This method, if adopted, should improve the efficiency of the 'safe period' method of birth control for those women who are unable to use more efficient methods.

Conclusions

It will be appreciated that the 'safe period' method of birth control requires considerable motivation, whichever method is used to determine the 'safe' days. The method is now only used by those Roman Catholics who wish to avoid pregnancy and whose conscience does not permit them to use other contraceptive methods. Despite the fact that 'safe period' users are a select group, the pregnancy rate varies between 14 and 40 per 100 woman-years, depending on their motivation. In well-motivated patients, Marshall reports a rate of 5 to 19 per 100 woman-years.

In South America, where it was hoped the method would help limit the rate of population growth, it appears to have been a failure. Information from Bogota and Cali in Colombia, reported by Stycos, indicates that despite a large number of consultations, home visits, and short courses conducted by Roman Catholic Family Planning organizations, only 8 per cent and 3 per cent of the 1,800 and 2,400 women initially recruited in those two cities continued to use the method.

Diaphragms and Cervical Caps

The early birth control clinics, and the few physicians who offered birth control services, both in Europe and North America, adopted the vaginal diaphragm as the main method of contraception. The reasoning was good. If the spermatozoa could be prevented from being sprayed onto the cervix during ejaculation, and if they could be immobilized in the vagina, pregnancy would be prevented. The vaginal diaphragm or the cervical cap, combined with a spermicidal cream, did both things: insemination of the cervix was prevented by the diaphragm, and the sperms were eliminated by the spermicide, and by the hostile vaginal environment.

The enthusiasm of the workers in Family Planning clinics, who were mainly middle class, was matched by the enthusiasm of their mainly middle-class clients. For many years many middle-class women in the U.S.A., and in Britain, have used the diaphragm, although since the introduction of the Pill, its popularity has waned. Amongst the lower socio-economic groups it was never as popular, partly because of prudery, most women feeling it improper to introduce an object into the vagina, and partly because many of the women lacked a bathroom to enable them to insert the diaphragm with comfort and privacy.

In the developing nations, the lack of privacy was even more marked, and the diaphragm as a method of birth control was relatively unsuccessful.

Nevertheless, it is a good, and fairly efficient, method. Its advantage is that it is completely without side-effects (although some spermicidal creams cause vaginal irritation which disappears when the cream is changed). Its disadvantage is that for maximal efficiency it must be inserted each evening whether coitus is anticipated or not. The psychological problem to a sexually aroused couple of the female needing to go away to 'put in my diaphragm' is obvious. The instruction to the patient should be: 'Put in your diaphragm when you clean your teeth each evening.' In Australia and Britain, where dental health is deplorable, the slogan is even more brief: 'Put in your diaphragm when you take out your teeth.' Once inserted, the diaphragm must remain in for at least six hours after coitus.

There are basically three devices, although because of a falling demand, the last two are becoming increasingly difficult to obtain. They are the vaginal diaphragm (Dutch cap); the vault cap, and the cervical cap. The vaginal diaphragm is the easiest to fit, and to use, and is the most efficient as a protective against unwanted conceptions. It consists of a thin latex rubber dome attached to a circular flat, or coiled wire spring. Because of the varying capacity of different vaginae, the diaphragm is made in a series of sizes from 45 to 100 mm, usually in steps of 2·5 mm.

The technique of finding the appropriate size requires experience. The fitting is most usefully combined with a pelvic examination to exclude abnormalities and with taking a cervical smear for cancer detection. If the patient has a marked degree of uterovaginal prolapse, the diaphragm may not be readily kept in place and the vault cap may be more appropriate.

An estimate of the correct size is obtained from the vaginal examination. The distance between the posterior vaginal fornix and the symphysis pubis gives an indication of the appropriate size. This is then confirmed by introducing a range of diaphragms, from a fitting set, and finding the one which fits snugly behind the symphysis. The woman should not be aware that the diaphragm is there.

The patient is next shown how to introduce the diaphragm and how to remove it by hooking it out with her finger. Since it is mandatory that a spermicidal cream is used in conjunction with the diaphragm, she is taught to place a large blob in the centre of its upper surface and additional cream around the rim. This also makes its introduction easier. She is taught how to ensure that the diaphragm is in place, and to know she must feel her cervix through the rubber to be sure that it is (Figure **11/4**).

A woman generally needs to have some knowledge of her anatomy. Many women believe, quite incorrectly, that the vagina runs vertically upwards rather than upwards and backwards. The patient should practise introducing and removing the diaphragm at home. It is best she returns for a second consultation, when she can be reassured that her technique is good, and when her additional questions can be answered; but this is not always possible.

The International Planned Parenthood Federation's *Medical Handbook*, the textbook by Peel and Potts, and the pamphlets issued with each diaphragm by the manufacturers, give additional details, but the quickest way to learn how to instruct patients is to go to a session organized by a family planning association.

It will be realized that the complexity of fitting the diaphragm, the necessity for the patient to use intelligence in its insertion,

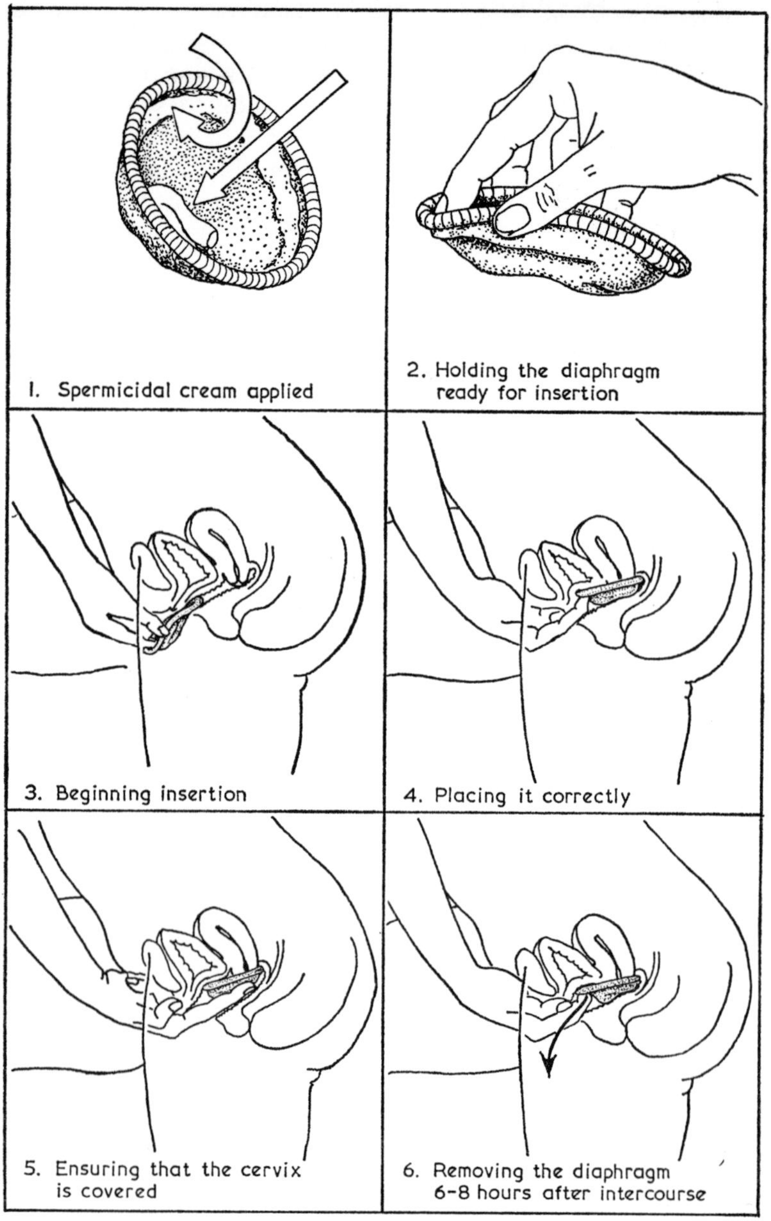

Figure **11/4** The technique of using the vaginal diaphragm.

and the need for her to be so motivated that she makes sure it is in place every time she expects coitus, has limited its popularity. Used properly, the pregnancy rate is 3 per 100 woman years, but the average pregnancy rate is 15 to 25 per 100 woman-years.

The place of the diaphragm in a birth control campaign should not be minimized, as it has no side-effects, is perhaps protective against cervical cancer (by barring mutagens from reaching the transitional cervical epithelium), and if maintained properly can be used for one to two years before being replaced.

TWELVE

The Technology of Contraception — II

Hormonal Contraceptive Steroids

The processes by which ovulation is initiated, controlled and regulated have been elucidated in the last fifty years. It is now known that the mechanisms are complex and that the various components are interconnected. The primacy of the hypothalamus has also been determined, as has its response to 'feedback' of ovarian sex steroids.

By the mid-1930s, the knowledge was sufficient to postulate an oestrogen feedback mechanism which would prevent the release of pituitary gonadotrophins, so that ovulation would be inhibited and conception controlled.

Synthetic oestrogens were developed in the mid-1930s which made conception control nearer, but its full realization had to await the discovery of a cheap source of synthetic progesterone-like steroids. This break-through came in the 1940s when Marker demonstrated that certain plants, particularly the Mexican yam, were rich sources of steroids from which orally effective gestagens could be synthesized cheaply. The combined oestrogen–gestagen product was tried out in Puerto Rico in 1954 by Pincus and his colleagues. It was found to be highly effective in suppressing ovulation in women. The era of the Pill had begun.

Since that day it has become apparent that lower doses of the synthetic oestrogens, ethinyl oestradiol and its methyl ether, mestranol, and of the synthetic gestagens, can be used without any loss of efficiency in suppressing ovulation, and since 1970 only low-dose oral contraceptives have been prescribed.

The Steroids in Oral Contraceptives

OESTROGENS

The oral contraceptives available today contain either ethinyl oestradiol or its 3-methyl ether, mestranol. Mestranol is pharmacologically, and biologically, a weaker oestrogen, at least so far as suppression of ovulation is concerned. In the body it is converted to ethinyl oestradiol before acting. The best estimate is that 80 μg of mestranol is equivalent to 50 μg of ethinyl oestradiol, and at these doses ovulation is suppressed.

GESTAGENS

The term gestagen is preferred to progestagen for the progesterone-like substances which are used in oral contraceptives. Two forms of gestagen are available, (1) those derived from testosterone by replacing the methyl group (CH_3) of the carbon 19 atom with a hydrogen atom (19-nortestosterone), and (2) those derived from 17-acetoxy progesterone.

1. *19-nortestosterone*

These compounds act mainly as gestagens, but have a weak 'androgenic' activity, thus stimulating weight gain and reducing menstrual flow. A minute amount ($<$0·02 per cent) of the compound metabolizes in the body to oestrogen. The 19-nortestosterones in use today are norethisterone, lynestrenol, ethynodiol diacetate and norgestrel.

The biological potency of the gestagens varies. Norgestrel appears to be the most potent gestagen, being about twice as active, weight for weight, as norethisterone, three times as potent as ethynodiol diacetate, and four times as potent as lynestrenol. Thus it is apparent that the milligram strength of the gestagen is no real guide to its biological potency. This must be remembered when assessing the value of new oral contraceptives.

2. *17-acetoxy progesterone*

These compounds are pure gestagens, which have no 'androgenic' activity and do not metabolize to oestrogen. Those in use today are megestrol acetate, chlormadinone and medroxyprogesterone acetate.

THE TECHNOLOGY OF CONTRACEPTION—II

Formulations

1. ORAL HORMONAL CONTRACEPTIVES

At present three formulations of oral contraceptive pills are available generally. These are (1) the combined pill, (2) the sequential pill, and (3) the gestagen pill.

(1) *Combined pill*

Both an oestrogen and a gestagen are taken from day 5 to day 25 of the menstrual cycle. The gestagen may be a 19-nor-testosterone derivative or a 17-acetoxy progesterone derivative.

(2) *Sequential pill*

The term is a misnomer. Originally, oestrogen alone, in a dose of 100 μg, was taken daily from day 3 or 5 for 16 days. From day 19 or 21 to day 25, a gestagen and oestrogen were given. This formulation was associated with an unacceptably high rate of unexpected pregnancies, and by marked mucorrhoea in some women. Recent formulations, which are retailed under the name of sequential pills, contain oestrogen in a dose of 100 μg, together with gestagen in a dose of 100 μg taken for 16 days from day 3 of the cycle. From day 19, oestrogen 100 μg and gestagen 1,000 μg are taken for 7 days.

(3) *The gestagen pill*

In this formulation a low dose of gestagen is taken daily without interruption. Studies have been conducted using daily doses of norethisterone acetate, 300 μg, chlormadinone, 500 μg, and norgestrel, 75 μg.

2. ONCE-A-MONTH PREPARATIONS

The need to take an oral contraceptive pill daily means that women have to make daily decisions to take the pill. In order to reduce the chance of omitting the pill, a study is being carried out using a single tablet of quinestrol 3 mg taken on day 1 of the cycle. Quinestrol is a long-acting oestrogen which is stored in body fat and slowly released. It is used in combination with a single tablet of a short-acting gestagen which is given on the 22nd day of the cycle. Little statistical information about the value of this preparation has been published, and only one reliable report is available (Claman).

3. LONG-ACTING INJECTABLE GESTAGENS

A further development is an injectable gestagen (in most studies medroxyprogesterone acetate) which is given at 3- or 6-month intervals.

A comparison of the various formulations is made later in this chapter.

Mode of Action

The mode of action of the oral contraceptive pill depends upon the actual component steroids and the ratio between them. In all formulations the oestrogen suppresses FSH secretion and reduces the release of LH, either directly in the pituitary or, more probably, by suppressing hypothalamic FSH and LH-releasing hormones. In this way, ovulation is usually prevented, and ovarian steroid synthesis is effected.

The gestagen (1) further suppresses LH release and prevents the 'peak' of LH which precedes, and appears essential to, ovulation, (2) alters the quality of the cervical mucus rendering it less penetrable to spermatozoa, (3) permits a gestagen 'withdrawal bleed' which is regular in onset, short in duration and light in quantity of blood lost, and (4) produces endometrial changes culminating in glandular exhaustion with pseudo-decidual stromal reaction. The degree with which these changes occur depends on the type of gestagen, the ratio of oestrogen to gestagen and on the duration of unopposed oestrogen action before the gestagen is given. For example, if oestrogen is given alone for more than ten days, and the gestagen then added, the endometrium will show a secretory pattern; but if a 19-nor-testosterone gestagen is added less than five days after oestrogen is started the 'glandular exhaustion' pattern occurs.

Biological and Physiological Alterations due to Hormonal Contraceptives

Both components of hormonal contraceptives affect the body's economy to some extent. Of the two hormones, oestrogen causes more alterations than does gestagen.

Hypothalamic–pituitary–genital tract axis

As mentioned, the mode of action of hormonal contraceptives is to suppress FSH and LH-releasing hormones, and thus the release from the pituitary of FSH and LH. In consequence, the ovaries are not stimulated, and appear quiescent with no follicle formation. However, ovarian response to gonadotrophin stimulation is unaltered, which indicates that the hormones act indirectly on the ovaries (Pujol-Amat). The uterine endometrium is affected by the levels of oestrogen and gestagen, and endometrial hypoplasia is usual. This is predominantly a gestagen effect. In formulations which are strongly oestrogenic (such as sequential regimens) cervical eversions may become more apparent and as the endocervical cells are exposed to the vaginal environment, mucorrhoea may occur.

Breasts

In some women the oestrogenic component of hormonal contraceptives causes premenstrual breast tenderness due to the stimulatory effect of the hormone on glandular development. At the same time the gestagen causes fluid retention in the tissues, and further glandular development. This manifests clinically as fullness of the breasts. These complaints are generally trivial. There is no evidence that hormonal contraceptives lead to the development of mammary malignancy.

Adrenal and thyroid

Although corticosteroid binding protein is raised, there is no evidence of disordered adrenal physiology; and the same applies to thyroid function. PBI, BEI and T_4 levels are raised; but thyroid function is not affected (Winikoff).

Liver

The effect of oestrogen on the liver is of particular importance, as the liver cells are stimulated to synthesize, and to release into the circulation a variety of serum binding carrier-proteins. This causes an elevation of circulating cortico-steroid binding protein, thyroxine binding protein, iron binding capacity, copper binding capacity, lipid binding capacity, plasminogen level, transferrin level and possibly others (Roman and Hecker). The raised carrier-protein levels in the blood alter tests of organ function which are based on measurement of the level of circulating hormones, and this must be taken into account when tests are carried out on women taking hormonal contraceptives. Oestrogen also induces the liver cells to secrete increased quantities of certain of the blood clotting factors, particularly Factors II, VII, IX and X (Poller). This would encourage blood hypercoagulability, were there not a corresponding increase in fibrinolytic potential, in the majority of women (Bick and Thompson). All changes revert to normal within 30 days of ceasing medication. Within the liver, oestrogen also alters the hepatic cell membrane permeability and inhibits the glucuronyl transferase system, leading to the retention in the cells of bilirubin, and of bromosulphthalein (BSP). The clinical effect is to decrease the rates of excretion of bilirubin and BSP so that raised blood levels are found. The raised levels do not indicate liver cell damage. They tend to return towards normal as the liver cells adjust to the new hormonal milieu, and become normal when the woman ceases to ingest oestrogen. A few women, with a genetic defect of liver cell function, develop cholestatic jaundice when using oestrogen-containing hormonal contraceptives.

Metabolic changes

Oestrogen appears to reduce glucose tolerance, although the degree of impairment depends to some extent on the age and weight of the patient, and on the dose of oestrogen. The younger the patient, the less she is overweight, and the lower the daily dose of oestrogen, the less is the glucose tolerance impairment. The oral glucose tolerance test shows that 30 to 60 per cent of women have a reduced ability to dispose of the glucose load. There is an impaired release of insulin from the pancreatic beta-cells initially, but this is followed by an excessive release (Spellacy). In addition, raised serum levels of lipids, triglycerides, cholesterol, non-esterified fatty acids, pyruvate and protein-bound cortisol have been found. The clinical implications of these findings are unclear, except in diabetic women who may require an upward adjustment of their insulin dose when taking oral contraceptives. There is no evidence that women on oral contraceptives have an increased risk of developing myocardial infarction.

Kidneys

Oestrogens tend to alter the renin-angiotensin system, but the details are not clear-cut, nor are the findings consistently present (Laragh et al.). It is believed that gestagen suppresses aldosterone release, and is naturietic, in contrast to oestrogen which is salt-retaining. In the few premenstrual days when no hormonal contraceptives are taken, a rebound release of aldosterone may occur, with salt and fluid retention.

Clinical Side-effects

The reason for using hormonal contraceptives is to prevent pregnancy. The use of a birth control measure occasions feelings of relief, or guilt, depending on the cultural background of the woman. If the latter, she believes she is doing 'wrong' in

Table 12/1

The 'side-effects' attributed to hormonal contraceptives

Oestrogen effects	*Gestagen effects*	*Combined effects*
Nausea and vomiting Fluid retention (i.e. transient weight gain) Pre-menstrual tension Headache Cervical 'eversion' Vaginal discharge Increase in menstrual flow ? Venous thrombosis	Premenstrual depression Appetite increase ? Weight gain ? Leg cramps Reduction in menstrual flow Disturbance in menstrual cycle (i.e. break-through bleeding, short or long cycles) Acne Greasy hair	Tiredness Irritability Breast fullness ? Decreased libido Vaginitis

hindering a 'natural' body function; if the former, she is delighted to be spared the risk of an unwanted pregnancy. These psychological alterations make the clinical side-effects due to hormonal contraceptives difficult to assess. As Goldzieher says, 'The burden of proof must now rest on those who claim that a given symptom is attributable to the contraceptive agent rather than to coincidence or psychic induction.'

The biochemical alterations previously described do have effects on the physiology of the woman, and side-effects additional to the main effect of birth control occur. Since oestrogen is implicated in more of the biochemical changes, it is also considered to be the cause of more of the side-effects (Table **12/1**). Most of them are maximal in the first few menstrual cycles, and cease as the body adjusts to the new hormonal milieu, but a few may persist. The side-effects may be beneficial or annoying. They are discussed in alphabetical order.

Acne

Acne is an inflammation of the sebaceous glands, associated with increased secretion of sebum. This secretion is controlled by androgens, and opposed by oestrogens. The oestrogen component of the oral contraceptive tends to improve acne; whilst 19-nortestosterone has the opposite effect because of its weak 'androgenic' component. The effect, however, depends on a variety of pre-existing factors. If a patient has acne, it is wise to use a sequential formulation, or a combined formulation in which the gestagen is a 17-acetoxy progesterone.

Cancer

The possibility that hormonal contraceptives might be carcinogenic has been raised because of observations on some experimental animals. However, in primate studies neither oestrogen nor gestagen has produced any malignancies. Indeed, in humans, gestagens in large doses are used to treat advanced, inoperable, endometrial carcinoma. It was noted earlier that hormonal contraceptives do not cause breast cancer (Fechner).

A report in 1969 from the Family Planning Clinics of New York suggested that an increased incidence of cellular change in the cervix uteri, resembling early malignancy, was found amongst women choosing oral contraceptives, when compared with women choosing the diaphragm (Melamed). Cervical malignancy occurs more frequently amongst women of the lower socio-economic groups, who begin coitus at an early age, and have several coital partners. Analysis of Melamed's population showed more such patients chose oral contraceptives, whilst more affluent women chose the diaphragm. The observation was confirmed in California where Stern showed that if cervical cytology was taken before issuing the Pill, more women with abnormal cytology chose the Pill as their preferred method of birth control.

Only 10 to 30 per cent of women with abnormal cytology will develop cancer of the cervix in 10 to 15 years after the initial observation. The epidemiological difficulties of establishing a cause and effect relationship with the ingestion of oral contraceptives are obviously great. The consensus is that the Pill does not lead to cancer of the cervix. This matter is considered in greater detail by Andrews, and in the IPPF Report.

Chloasma

Hyperpigmentation of the skin of the face may occur in susceptible women who have been taking a pill containing 17-acetoxy progesterone for more than two years, and is related to exposure to the sun. Treatment is to avoid direct sunlight, to change the oral contraceptive, and in certain cases to apply 2 per cent hydroquinone ointment. Despite these measures, the pigmentation often takes up to nine months to fade.

Depression, mood changes, reduced libido

It is almost impossible to make objective observations on the frequency with which depression and reduced libido are associated with the ingestion of hormonal contraceptives, as mood changes depend on a variety of external stimuli and internal changes, amongst which endocrine alterations may be of significance. In a study in Britain, Herzberg found that women who had premenstrual mood changes, and had a low sexual drive before starting oral contraceptives, were more likely to develop mood changes when using the drugs. In a large series reported from California by Kutner, no increase in depression or mood changes was found amongst nearly 2,000 pill users when compared with 1,700 controls. In a further study of 500 women, no evidence of impairment of sexuality was found. The overall findings are that it is unlikely that hormonal oral contraceptives increase depression, cause mood changes or decrease libido.

Dysmenorrhoea

Since dysmenorrhoea is unusual in anovulatory cycles, unless menstruation is heavy and clots are expelled from the uterus, hormonal contraceptives which suppress ovulation should relieve the condition. About 40 per cent of young women have dysmenorrhoea, and in 10 per cent it is severe. Combined oral contraceptives relieve dysmenorrhoea in over 90 per cent of cases, and although premenstrual irritability may occur, painful menstruation ceases.

Headaches and migraine

Headaches often occur amongst women who have mood changes, and tend to be worse premenstrually, perhaps because of aldosterone-induced fluid retention. Migraine may also be aggravated at this time. If a generalized migraine becomes focal, it is suggestive of vertebro-basilar occlusion and hormonal contraceptives should be abandoned (Salmon).

In a large-scale study of non-depressed women, Diddle found no increased incidence of headaches in treated women when compared with controls.

Hypertension

Hormonal contraceptives containing oestrogen may cause hypertension in a few women, particularly those who have a familial history. In addition, some hypertensive women taking oral contraceptives develop an increase in the level of the diastolic blood pressure. The aetiology is obscure, but may be due to an alteration in the renin-angiotensin system, as both plasma renin and angiotensin II levels rise. This may cause an increase in aldosterone secretion, and vasospasm (Lancet).

Amongst normotensive women, particularly those under the age of 35, the incidence is very low, and the diastolic blood pressure is not affected. The incidence in one large survey was 0·3 per cent amongst 9,000 women followed for one year (Chidell).

When facilities are available, the patient's blood pressure should be taken before starting oral contraceptives, and about six months later, but in many instances this will be impracticable. Women with known hypertension, or who were hypertensive in pregnancy, are more likely to be affected and require to have their blood pressures monitored more carefully, or to use other methods of birth control.

Menstruation

Most women are culturally conditioned to believe that in the absence of pregnancy or lactation, menstruation is essential to maintain normal genital tract well-being. Menstruation informs a woman that she is not pregnant, and reassures her that she can become pregnant. In fact, menstruation is unnecessary, and in areas where protein and iron intake is low it is a cause of anaemia. Given cyclically, oral contraceptives mimic a woman's normal menstrual cycle and permit menstruation whilst suppressing ovulation. Most women appear to prefer this.

Low dose combined oral contraceptives, using a 19-nortestosterone derivative as the gestagen, tend to produce a reduction in the quantity and duration of blood loss in over 50 per cent of women. In many the colour of the blood changes from bright red to dirty brown. Because of accumulated myths about the need for a good menstrual flow, women should be reassured that the colour of the blood loss is without danger. So-called sequential formulations are less likely to reduce blood loss, and preparations using a 17-acetoxy gestagen tend to increase menstrual loss.

For the majority of women, oral contraceptives ensure that menstruation occurs predictably on a known date. A few women, particularly in early cycles, or who are under emotional stress, develop blood spotting, or break-through bleeding, on an unpredictable day whilst still taking oral contraceptives. Spotting may be ignored unless it increases. Break-through bleeding may only occur in one cycle, but if it persists is due to insufficient gestagen. It can be controlled by increasing the quantity of gestagen in the oral contraceptive, by choosing a Pill which contains a higher potency gestagen, or by giving a larger dose (i.e. two pills daily). Break-through bleeding occurs in less than 1 per cent of cycles.

The patient who has menorrhagia before choosing oral contraceptives should not be given a sequential formulation, or a formulation containing a 17-acetoxy progesterone derivative, as the heavy periods may be aggravated.

About 1 per cent of women became amenorrhoeic when taking oral contraceptives. Since menstruation is of no importance, these women should be reassured that pregnancy will be prevented provided that they have not omitted to take the Pill each day (one missed day is probably safe, three missed days between days 5 and 12 is hazardous), and they should recommence the next course after an interval of 7 days, if the ordinary pack is used.

On ceasing to take oral contraceptives, two things occur. The majority of women experience a delay in ovulation of up to twenty days. If the woman is attempting to become pregnant, this must be taken into account, whilst if pregnancy occurs, the estimated date of delivery calculated from the last bleeding episode may be at least two weeks understated. Unless the patient is questioned about her use of oral contraceptives, fetal growth retardation may be erroneously diagnosed. A few women fail to menstruate on ceasing to take oral contraceptives, due to continued inhibition of the release of hypothalamic gonadotrophic releasing hormones. In the majority, menstruation restarts within three months; but in a few cases, amenorrhoea persists for twelve months. If this happens, investigations should be made to find the cause of the amenorrhoea, and if pregnancy is desired, ovulation should be stimulated using clomiphene citrate (Shearman).

Nausea and vomiting

Until the body adjusts to the ingestion of synthetic oestrogen, nausea, and occasionally vomiting, may occur. About 20 per cent of women experience nausea, and 2 per cent vomit, in the first cycle during which the Pill is taken. Tolerance develops rapidly and by the third cycle fewer than 2 per cent of women have any complaint.

Thrombo-embolic phenomena

As pointed out, most of the side-effects of hormonal contraceptives are either beneficial or only mildly annoying. One side-effect has been claimed to be lethal. The association between the use of hormonal contraceptives and thrombo-embolic phenomena is based on the known biochemical changes in blood coagulation factors, and on three retrospective studies. Two of these were made in Britain and one in the U.S.A. In these studies, patients with clinically diagnosed thrombo-embolic disease were questioned about their use of hormonal contraceptives; statistical calculations were made from these data, and from other data, of the estimated use of oral contraceptives in the community. In a 4-year period in Britain, Vessey and Doll collected 88 cases of idiopathic deep venous thrombosis, and concluded that the best estimate of risk of hospital admission for the disease was six to seven times higher in women taking oral contraceptives. In the U.S.A., Sartwell et alia collected 175 cases over a 3-year period, and concluded the risk of hospital admission for thrombo-embolism was 4·4 times as great for users of oral contraceptives as for non-users. The third study was made by the Royal College of General Practitioners in Britain. This study indicated that the risk was increased twofold.

The information led to investigations by the Safety of Drugs Committee in Britain and the Food and Drug Authority in the U.S.A. In the course of these investigations, evidence was given which purported to show that the risk was related to the dose of oestrogen and was lowest with preparations containing less than 75 μg of oestrogen. The British Committee on Safety of Drugs therefore recommended that, in general, formulations using no more than 50 μg of oestrogen should be used, and pharmaceutical manufacturers rapidly introduced new low-dose formulations. One point was neglected. Mestranol is converted in the body to ethinyl oestradiol so that its biological potency is slightly lower, approximately 80 μg of mestranol equating to 50 μg of ethinyl oestradiol. Yet the Committee advised no more than 50 μg of oestrogen be used. More recent evidence from Drill and Calhoun suggests that the Committee were incorrect, and that the incidence of thrombo-embolic disease is not increased at increasing dose levels of oestrogens.

The report of the Committee was released prematurely and received widespread press publicity. It occasioned very considerable concern to women using oral contraceptives. What was not made clear is that a retrospective study can only indicate that an hypothesis exists; it cannot establish a cause-and-effect relationship. For this a prospective study is required.

The supposed association between the use of hormonal contraceptives and the occurrence of thrombo-embolic disease has been put in doubt by an examination of reports of prospective studies of the incidence of thrombo-embolic disease amongst users of oral contraceptives by Drill. He concluded that there is no evidence from these studies that the incidence of thrombo-embolism is increased (Table **12/2**). Drill pointed out that if a cause-and-effect relationship existed (1) a higher proportion of cases would occur in the first months of use of the Pill, (2) larger doses should be more likely to cause the disease, (3) a higher incidence should be found in pregnancy when oestrogen levels are very high. The evidence is that none of the above occur.

Table 12/2

Venous thrombosis in women aged 15 to 44

	Women surveyed (1,000s)	*Rate per* 1,000 *women per year venous thrombosis*		
		Superficial	*Deep*	*Total*
Non-pregnant	?	0·99	0·31	1·3
Antepartum	350	0·31	0·36	0·67
Postpartum	288	5·3	4·5	9·8
Taking oral contraceptives	70	1·04	0·21	1·25

Source: Drill, V. A. *J. Amer. Med. Ass.*, **219**, 583, 1972.

Whether the Committee on Safety of Drugs or Drill is correct, it seems reasonable to state two things. Firstly, in general, oral contraceptives containing the lowest dose of oestrogen which suppresses ovulation should be used, as side-effects, possibly including thrombo-embolism, are less frequent. Secondly, if an association exists between thrombo-embolism and the use of oral hormonal contraceptives, the risk of death from the disease in women of reproductive age is low, and is much less than that due to pregnancy (Table **12/3**). In Britain, for example, pregnancy is seven times as likely to cause death as are oral contraceptives; whilst in the developing nations, where maternal mortality is considerably higher, the risk of death due to pregnancy is between 70 and 100 times more than that due to oral hormonal contraceptives.

Table 12/3

Mortality from venous thrombosis per 100,000 women in Britain

	Age of women	
	15–34	35–49
Oral contraceptives non-users	0·2	0·5
Oral contraceptives users	1·5	3·9
Pregnancy*	9·0	26·1

* Maternal deaths 1964–66 (Rep. *Public Health and Medical Subjects* 119, H.M.S.O., London, 1969.)
Source: Vessey, M. P. and Doll, R. *Brit. Med. J.*, **2**, 651, 1969.

Vaginal discharge and vaginitis

An increased vaginal discharge is usual, and is due to oestrogenic stimulation of the cervical mucus-secreting cells. The symptom is more marked in women taking sequential pills, as the anti-oestrogenic effect of the gestagen is less in the first 10 days. Leukorrhoea is of little clinical importance, provided that vaginitis has been excluded. Once this has been done, the patient can be told that the leukorrhoea is a normal event and signifies nothing sinister.

Monilial vaginitis appears to occur more frequently in women taking oral contraceptives, and smears should be taken to exclude the presence of this condition in all women who complain of an *irritant* vaginal discharge.

Weight gain

Transient weight gain is usual premenstrually and is due to fluid retention; it tends to revert when menstruation starts. The degree of transient weight gain tends to be increased amongst women taking oral contraceptives. In addition, gestagens have an anabolic effect, which only becomes apparent after a few months. Weight gain may be directly due to the hormone, or to increased appetite which occurs as a consequence of relief from the fear of pregnancy. Treatment is to explain the reason for the weight gain, and to prescribe a diet high in protein, and low in fats and calories.

Possible Harmful Long-term Side-effects

The situation at present can be summarized as follows:

1. There is no evidence that the long-term use of the oral contraceptives reduces fertility or causes chromosomal changes in the germ cells, and indeed fertility may be temporarily enhanced for a few months after ceasing to use the drugs, as coitus occurs more frequently in couples who have used oral contraceptives.
2. There is no evidence that the risk of endometrial carcinoma or breast carcinoma is increased.
3. There is no evidence that the incidence of diabetes or of liver damage is increased.

Prescribing Hormonal Oral Contraceptives

Oral contraceptives are the most effective and the most widely used method of family planning. Despite this, a large number of women abandon the method because of imagined fears, misunderstandings or sensational newspaper articles. The health worker should discuss possible side-effects with the prospective client, and must seek to reassure her. An educated woman may fear that the exogenous hormones will upset her natural hormonal balance. Less educated women, and particularly their husbands, have a variety of anxieties, based on misunderstood physiology, folklore and the fear that the drug will reduce sexual desire, activity or response. The particular fear varies from place to place and from time to time.

Hormonal contraceptives should not be prescribed until the client has been questioned about previous illnesses, particularly diabetes, hypertension, hepatitis, jaundice and deep venous thrombosis. She should be examined vaginally to exclude genital tract abnormalities, and pregnancy. When conditions are suitable, this examination may be utilized to take a cervical smear, so that the exfoliative cells may be examined cytologically to exclude malignancy. The patient's breasts may also be palpated, if cultural conditions permit, particularly in older women, to detect abnormal lumps. If possible, and particularly amongst older women, it is wise to take the client's blood pressure.

In the state of our present knowledge, certain women should be advised to use methods of contraception other than oral contraceptives. These include women who (1) have previously developed thrombo-embolism or cerebrovascular insufficiency, (2) have liver disease, (3) have blood dyscrasias, (4) have severe migraine, (5) have marked hypertension, or (6) during treatment develop transient cerebral retinal, or focal migraine attacks.

Present-day oral contraceptives are supplied in packs which make it easy for the patient to take the pills appropriately, and which hinder children inadvertently taking the drug. Directions for taking each formulation are given by the manufacturers, and should be explained to the client.

Although in the developed nations only qualified doctors usually prescribe oral contraceptives, there is no good reason why their distribution and prescription should not be in the hands of trained health workers.

Hormonal Contraceptives at the Extremes of the Reproductive Era

The age of puberty has declined from about 17 to about 12 in the past century. Girls are becoming physiologically, and sexually, mature earlier. Once a girl is at risk of becoming pregnant, it is likely that the effect of inhibiting hypothalamic-pituitary gonadotrophic function is without consequence. And, as is discussed in Chapter 14, unexpected, unwanted pregnancy in the young teenager is of considerable consequence. For this reason, a girl of 15 or 16 who is at risk of becoming pregnant should take contraceptive measures. The Pill is the only reliable method.

A question often asked is how long need a woman approaching the menopause take the Pill? The age of the menopause is about 50, and ovulation ceases a variable number of years before this age. The time of the menopause is individual for each woman and is unaffected by previous use of oral contraceptives. Oral contraceptives have two advantages in women approaching the menopause. Firstly, they protect her against a late, unwelcome pregnancy; and secondly, they assist in carrying her through the hormonal changes which precede the climacteric. A safe guide is that a woman should continue to take oral contraceptives until her fiftieth birthday.

Comparative Value of Different Formulations

The great majority of women will obtain a high degree of protection against unwanted pregnancies, with only minimal side-effects, using combined low-dose oral contraceptives. However, women with acne are best prescribed sequential preparations, or combined formulations in which the gestagen is a 17-acetoxy compound.

As has been mentioned earlier, certain groups of women should probably avoid using hormonal contraceptives containing oestrogen. If these women prefer to use hormonal contraceptives rather than one of the other effective measures, the use of low-dose continuous gestagen formulations, or of injectable formulations is indicated.

COMBINED ORAL CONTRACEPTIVES

Since over 20 million women are taking these formulations on any one day, they seem to be widely accepted, particularly amongst the more affluent sections of the community. There are at least twenty-five formulations currently available, each of which is claimed by its manufacturer to be the most effective, and to have the fewest side-effects. Unfortunately, few properly controlled studies comparing various formulations have been made. All combined pills, *if taken daily as prescribed*, are over 99·9 per cent effective in preventing unwanted pregnancy (Table

12/4). The variety of oral contraceptives available and the current concern about hazardous side-effects makes it difficult for the physician to choose the most appropriate pill. In general, it is best to become familiar with only a few formulations and to prescribe these. There appears little advantage in constantly switching the patient from one oral contraceptive to another in the hope of reducing the side-effects. But initially the patient should be prescribed the most appropriate formulation for her needs, and precautions must be instituted. For example, a few hypertensive patients develop a marked increase in the level of blood pressure when taking oral contraceptives. If they are prescribed, regular estimations of the blood pressure should be made and therapy suspended if hyperpiesis results.

Table 12/4
The effectiveness of oral hormonal contraceptives

	Cycles (in 1,000's)	*Pregnancies*	*Pearl Index (pregnancies per* 100 *woman-years)*
Combined orals			
a) 36 studies	325	17	0·07 (0·03–0·10)
b) Sweden, 1969	3,800	17	0·005
Sequential orals			
a) 17 studies	116	30	0·34 (0·20–0·56)
b) Sweden, 1969	187	73	0·47

Sources:
Teitze, C. *Advances in Planned Parenthood*, **6**, 117, 1971, Excerpta Medica.
Rutenskold, M. *Acta Ob. Gyn. Scand.*, **50**, 203, 1971.

SO-CALLED SEQUENTIAL FORMULATIONS

Except in women who have severe acne, or who have persistently scanty periods, and for cultural reasons wish to bleed each month, sequential formulations appear to have no advantages over combined formulations. The pregnancy rate is ten times higher than with combined pills, which is a disadvantage (Table **12/4**).

VALUE OF DIFFERENT FORMULATIONS

ONCE-A-MONTH PREPARATIONS

Little information has become available about the use of quinestrol since Claman's publication in 1970. Despite its ease of administration, it is necessary to take the gestagen on a precise day, and many women may forget to do this. In addition, it appears that heavy menstruation occurs in about 20 per cent of patients.

CONTINUOUS GESTAGENS

This method of contraception avoids the use of oestrogens, and consequently the patient has a low incidence of those side-effects commonly attributed to oestrogen. The biochemical alterations of blood-clotting factors, carbohydrate-lipid metabolism and liver function tests do not occur. Continuous low-dose gestagens cause a variable depression in the pre-ovulatory LH surge, with a variable suppression of ovulation (Orr and Elstein). Since ovulation occurs, the contraceptive effect of the gestagens is mainly due to an alteration of the cervical mucus, which renders it hostile to sperm migration, and to an alteration in endometrial receptivity to nidation.

In a double blind trial, over one year, norethisterone acetate 0·3 mg, chlormadinone acetate 0·5 mg, megestrol acetate 0·7 mg and norgestrel 0·075 mg were given to 378 women (between 70 and 80 in each group). Of the four gestagens, norethisterone acetate appeared the most effective. Its use was followed by the lowest accidental pregnancy rate, and the least disturbance to the menstrual cycle, although the gestagen side-effects of irritability, decreased libido and pruritus were noted (Vessey et al.). However, a study of the available literature suggests that in fact there is little difference in pregnancy rates, or side-effects, whichever continuous gestagen is chosen.

The main disadvantage of this type of oral contraceptive is the rather high incidence of break-through bleeding, which occurs in at least 11 per cent of women, and the frequency of short or long menstrual cycles. In 25 per cent of patients the bleeding pattern was quite unpredictable, which is a marked disadvantage of the method (Table **12/5**). Only 50 per cent of women using a continuous gestagen had a menstrual cycle of 25 to 31 days duration, compared with 71 per cent of women who used another, or no, method of birth control.

Table 12/5

Low dose gestagens taken daily as contraceptives

		Low dose continuous daily gestagens	
Drug		Chlormadinone*	Megestrol
Daily dose		500 μg	500 μg
Pregnancy rate		2·0–5·0	10–13
Break-through bleeding (cycle <18 days)	%	10–20	18
Short cycles (<24 days)	%	10–20	11
Long cycles (>35 days)	%	10–20	20

* Results for norethisterone acetate 300–350 μg; norgestrel 75 μg, and d-norgestrel 30 μg are substantially the same as those for chlormadinone.

Sources:

Martinez-Manautou, J. *Low level progestogens in Control of Human Fertility*. Ed. Diczfalusy E. and Borrell, J., Almqvist, Stockholm, 1971.

Vessey, M. P., et al. *Lancet*, **1**, 915, 1972.

The reported pregnancy rate is perhaps unacceptably high, but may well be lower in well-motivated women who remember to take the pill daily.

Perhaps the main advantage of the formulation is during lactation, as there is no reduction in the supply of milk in patients who use continuous gestagens, and indeed there may be an increase in milk flow (Hafnawi).

LONG-ACTING INJECTABLE GESTAGENS

The need for continuous decision-making by women would be reduced if a single injection of a slowly released gestagen or an oestrogen-gestagen combination could be given which would be effective for 3 to 6 months. Two depot-type formulations are currently under study. These are depot medroxyprogesterone acetate and norethisterone enanthate. In addition, research is taking place into the possibility of implanting four or five silastic capsules containing a gestagen (usually medroxyprogesterone acetate 20–30 mg) subcutaneously. The advantage of this technique is that there is a constant slow release of the hormone, whilst after the injected formulation high blood levels occur initially, which are well above those required for therapeutic purposes, and this is followed by a slow and unpredictable decline. The disadvantage of the capsule is that it must be removed after the contained drug has ceased to be effective. Current observations indicate that the patient is protected against pregnancy for 9 to 12 months if silastic implants are used.

The most experience of injectable gestagens relates to the use of depot medroxyprogesterone acetate. Although the method is effective in preventing pregnancy if the injection is given at the

Table 12/6

Long-acting injectable hormones used for contraception

Formulation	Medroxyprogesterone acetate[1]	Norethisterone enanthate[2]
Dose	150 mg every 3 months	200 mg every 3 months
Number of women	2,000	130
Pregnancy rate (per 100 women-years)	0·25	2·3
Discontinuation rate, end of year	37·0%	25·3%
Grossly irregular bleeding*	25–30%	35·0%
Shorter cycles (<24 days)*	25·0%	25·0%
Longer cycles (>35 days)*	No information available	12·0%
Amenorrhoea	28% (after 3 months) rising to 55% by 12 months	8·0%

* Estimated after 3 to 6 months (i.e. after one or two injections).

Sources:

1. *Upjohn Clinical Studies*, dated 3 March, 1972; Seymour, R. J., and Powell, L. C. *Obst. & Gynec.*, **36**, 589, 1970.
2. Zanartu, J., and Navarro, C., 'Fertility inhibition by an injectable progestagen'. *Obst. & Gynec.*, **31**, 627, 1968.

appropriate intervals (either 150 mg every 12 weeks or 300 mg every 24 weeks), menstruation is markedly disorganized (see Table **12/6**). In the first 6 months unpredictable uterine bleeding and spotting is common and affects more than 50 per cent of women. Thirty per cent of women develop amenorrhoea. As the months pass, the menstrual irregularity decreases, and an increasing number of women develop amenorrhoea so that by 12 months its incidence is over 55 per cent. On ceasing therapy normal menstruation resumes, usually after a 3 to 9 months' delay.

Long-acting injectable gestagens are suitable for those women who have tried, and abandoned for various reasons, other methods of birth control, and who are prepared to have injections at 3- or 6-month intervals. The pregnancy rate is about 0·24 per 100 woman-years.

THE 'MORNING AFTER' FORMULATION

As an emergency measure when unprotected coitus has occurred during the ovulation period, the administration of high doses of oestrogen, starting within 72 hours of the coital episode, is highly effective. In one study from the U.S.A., reported by Kuchera, 1,000 women were given stilboestrol 25 mg twice daily for 5 days, the first dose being taken within 3 days of coitus. No pregnancy occurred, although 40 might have been expected. Apart from nausea and vomiting, which can be very severe, side-effects were few.

The Intra-uterine Contraceptive Device

The idea that a foreign body, inserted into the cavity of the uterus, would prevent pregnancy, is not new. It is reported that the Arabs, at least five hundred years ago, introduced a small round stone, the size of a large pea, into the uterus of the camel, which then repulsed the advances of the male camel as if she were pregnant. This enabled saddle camels to be used for long journeys, without the possibility of them becoming pregnant, which made them difficult to manage.

The use of intra-uterine contraceptive devices (IUD) in the human female did not occur until the 1920s, when Grafenberg made devices of gold, silver and silkworm gut. He had a high success, with few adverse side-effects, but his imitators were not so lucky: both the pregnancy rate and complications (particularly pelvic infection) were unacceptably high and the method fell into disfavour.

Interest was revived in 1959, when Oppenheimer reported a series of 329 patients from Israel who had used Grafenberg's devices for up to 18 years with extraordinary success. In the same year Ishihama from Japan reported the successful use of metal (Ota) intra-uterine rings. These reports stimulated the Population Council to restudy the method as a means of offering contraception on a large scale. At about this time polyethylene devices, which provoke minimal tissue reaction, were made. The IUD had acquired a new respectability.

The Design of the IUD

A satisfactory IUD should remain in the uterus, thus preventing pregnancy; it should be easy to remove, and it should cause few side-effects. These conditions have led to the development of a variety of shapes and sizes of IUDs, but currently only five have proved superior. These are (1) Lippes Loop, (2) Margulies Spiral, (3) the M device, (4) the Dalkon Shield, and (5) the Copper-7 (or T) (Figure **12/1**). These devices are made of flexible plastic which regains its original shape once the stress is removed. This enables the IUD to be introduced by loading it into a narrow introducer. When it has been expelled into the uterine cavity it regains its normal shape. The devices are provided with nylon threads which project through the cervix, so that the patient can check that the device is still in the uterus. The addition of copper wire to a plastic shape is a recent advance. Early experience has shown that if the surface area of the copper wire which covers the stem of the device is between 120 and 200 mm^2, a lower pregnancy rate is obtained, and the side-effects appear to be reduced. The addition of a mixture of copper with a surface area of 30 mm^2 and zinc with a surface area of 47 mm^2 appear to give even greater protection against pregnancy, but this is still only experimental.

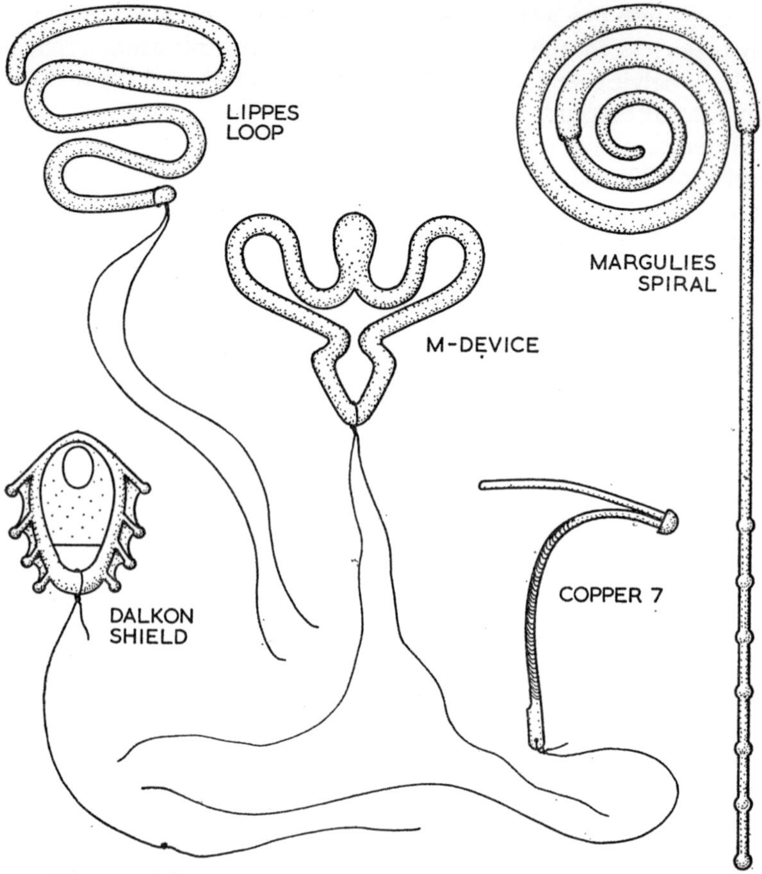

Figure **12/1** Commonly used types of IUD, actual size.

Mode of Action

Originally it was held that the IUD led to more active oviductal and uterine contractions so that the ovum reached the uterine cavity at a time when its zona pellucida was fully intact, which prevented nidation (Nakhlouf and Abdel Salam). This opinion has now largely been discarded, as oviductal activity has not been shown to increase consistently in patients with an IUD.

The current belief is that the IUD causes a marked allergic reaction in the endometrium, which results in a heavy infiltration by immunocytes and macrophages. The larger the surface area of the IUD, the greater is the reaction and the lower the pregnancy rate (Zipper). The immunocytes infiltrate possible nidation sites, the macrophages perhaps phagocytosing the implanting egg before it can establish a firm contact. They may also render the superficial endometrium 'hostile' to nidation (Sagiroglu et al.). However, in rats rendered leukopenic by giving chlorambucil, infiltration was minimized, but the IUD was still effective when introduced into one uterine horn, whilst 9 pregnancies occurred in the other horn of 15 rats (Marcus).

Neither of these hypotheses can be considered proven at present, and it is possible that both mechanisms, or other mechanisms, operate.

The devices with added copper have an additional mode of action. It is thought that the copper slowly ionizes in utero and that this further inhibits nidation. The use of a metal for this purpose has been criticized by Woolfers, and his comments echo the criticism made in the 1920s of Grafenberg's device. Woolfers claims that the lower pregnancy and smaller complication rates associated with the copper 'is too high a price for the small gains remaining to be made'. He notes that nothing is known of the effects of weak solutions of copper on the endometrium, the myometrium, the cervix or the penis, and that the 'introduction of pharmacologically active IUDs is gratuitous furor medicandi'. There are currently no objective data to support Woolfers, and his critics have pointed out that the other devices in fact all contain particles of barium—a heavy metal. It is true that as the copper ionizes, the device becomes less effective. Currently, it is given an effective life of 18 months after which it must be replaced. This would tend to limit its use in large-scale campaigns which have poor follow-up.

Technique of Storage

An IUD must be introduced into the uterine cavity under as sterile conditions as possible. The polyethylene devices cannot be sterilized by boiling as they lose their plasticity. However, they can be stored, almost indefinitely, in wide-mouthed, screw-topped jars containing benzalkonium chloride in a 1 : 750 to 1 : 1,000 solution. The sterilizing effect of benzalkonium is slow, so that devices must be stored for 24 hours before use.

In clinics where only few insertions are made, it may be more convenient to use iodine in a 1 : 1,000 solution. This will sterilize the IUD in 5 minutes. Increasingly manufacturers are providing an IUD with a disposable introducer in a sealed pack which has been sterilized by gamma radiation. This makes for considerable convenience.

Clinical Aspects

Interview

Before introducing the IUD, it is important that the patient is given information about her genital anatomy. The amount of ignorance and misinformation about this is considerable, and many women have a hidden fear that the IUD will 'get lost inside' or can 'move through the womb and affect the heart'. The health worker, or doctor, should demonstrate that such fears are groundless, using diagrams and models. The interview should also include an obstetric and gynaecological history, as recent pelvic infection, or recent menorrhagia, are possible contra-indications to the method, and certainly require further investigation. At the interview the patient should be told that she may have cramp-like pains after the insertion, which last for a few hours at the most, and that prolonged menstrual flow may occur in the first three to four cycles, but that this usually settles after this time. The possibility that the device may be expelled spontaneously should be mentioned, and the patient should be told that this occurs most often during menstruation. When custom permits, and no taboo prohibits it, the patient should examine the pads or vaginal tampons to make sure that the device has not been expelled, and she should be taught to feel for the threads which project through her cervix. She should make this examination after each period. It is also important to emphasize that the IUD has a 'failure rate', and that pregnancy occurs in 1 to 2 per cent of patients who use the IUD for 12 cycles.

Following the interview, the patient is examined pelvically, and when appropriate, or if desired, a cervical smear is taken for exfoliative cytology. The cost-benefit of this procedure is doubtful in many nations, and this is considered further on page 361. The use of the IUD is contra-indicated if the patient has myomata, which distort the uterine cavity, uterine carcinoma, an abnormal uterus (bicornute or septate), or if she is pregnant. If the pelvic examination reveals tubal masses, the method is contra-indicated, particularly if there is a history of gonorrhoea, as the infection has been reported to have been reactivated as long as six months after the symptoms have subsided (Morris and Edelstein). The pelvic examination also indicates the size and position of the uterus.

Insertion

The cervix is visualized with a bivalve speculum, and is cleansed with antiseptic. The health worker, who has scrubbed hands, and who is wearing sterile gloves, then decides whether it is necessary to introduce a uterine sound to determine the length of the uterus; or if it is necessary to hold the cervix with a tenaculum. The former may be required in insertions into nulliparous uteri, the latter if the uterus is retroverted or relatively inaccessible. If the cervical canal is narrow, it may be necessary to dilate it gently using a small Hegar dilator (number 2), but with the prepacked Copper-7 this is not generally needed. If the device is not prepacked, it is now removed from the antiseptic solution and loaded into the introducer. It is important to remember that the devices must be introduced so that they lie in the transverse plane of the uterus, and they should be loaded appropriately.

The introducer is inserted through the cervical canal so that its tip lies in the uterine cavity. The plunger is pushed forward slowly so that the device is expelled into the cavity. During this the patient is watched for signs of pain or shock. An error, which causes pain, is the failure to insert the introducer sufficiently, so that its tip lies in the cervical canal. Manufacturers mark the introducer so that this is unlikely to occur. The plunger is withdrawn and the introducer removed. The protruding threads are cut so that they project about 3 cm from the cervix.

The most appropriate time for insertion is at the post-natal visit, following abortion, or in the last days of a menstrual period, as at this time the cervical canal is more dilated and the patient is unlikely to be pregnant.

In the early studies it was considered that the IUD was

inappropriate in nulliparous women; the modern devices can be used with success in the well-motivated nulliparae.

Follow-up visits

Provided that the patient has been adequately informed, and instructed, at the initial interview, follow-up visits, either to the patient's home, or by the patient to the clinic or doctor's surgery, are not necessary. If side-effects occur, the patient will seek advice, and if she has none, the sole purpose of the visit is for statistical purposes and to ensure that the IUD is still in the uterus. Once the uterus has accepted the IUD, and provided that there are no side-effects, it may remain in utero until the climacteric without harm (WHO Report).

In programmes of family planning in developing nations, which rely mainly on the IUD, the importance of the pre-insertion interview and the availability of a friendly communicative health worker after insertion, has been noted. This person is available to explain the side-effects which may arise, and to reassure the patient when she hears of the imagined dangers of the IUD from misinformed neighbours. It appears that this approach has a higher cost-benefit than frequent home visiting of accepters by social workers. A study in Hong Kong by Chan showed that after 12 months no more women in the study group continued to use the IUD than those in a control group who were not visited but had access to health workers when they felt that they had problems.

Complications and Side-Effects

Mortality

The mortality from the use of the IUD is very low. The only valid statistical data is from the U.S. where 10 deaths from pelvic inflammatory disease were reported amongst over 2·5 million insertions (Teitze).

Bleeding and pain

In the first few months after insertion most patients report an increase in the amount and duration of menstruation. Whilst this is without clinical significance amongst affluent women, it can lead to increasing anaemia amongst undernourished women. No therapy reduces the blood loss, despite extravagant claims by various enthusiasts for Vitamin C, or other pharmaceuticals. Instead of attempting therapeutic prowess, all that is needed is to prescribe iron tablets, and to observe the patient carefully.

Menstruation tends to start one or two days earlier than usual. The blood loss is light initially, and then becomes heavy, when clots may be expelled. The heavy loss may continue for four or more days, after which the period ceases, or drags on with irregular bleeding and spotting for a few days. Usually menstruation becomes more normal in three or four months. Menorrhagia is significantly reduced if the Copper-7 device is used.

Apart from some cramp-like pains after the initial insertion, and some pain during menstruation when clots are expelled, pain is not common at other times. Its presence and severity depends to some extent on uterine sensitivity and on the patient's personality.

Bleeding and pain also appear to be related directly to the size of the device, and to the degree of endometrial compression and myometrial distension which it causes (Tatum). Pain and bleeding may lead to the patient's demand, during the first year of use, that the device be removed in about 10 per cent of insertions.

Expulsion

It has been mentioned that a defect of the device is that it may be expelled without the knowledge of the patient, who is, of course, no longer protected against pregnancy. The rate of expulsion is related to the size and type of the device, and to the parity of the patient. The currently used devices have a low rate of expulsion. At the end of one year about 7 per cent of Lippes loops (size D) have been expelled; and 10 per cent of Coils have been expelled; whilst the rate for Dalkon Shields is less than 3 per cent, and that for Copper-7 about 5 per cent. If the expelled IUD is replaced, its subsequent expulsion is much less likely to occur. Expulsion rates are also related to parity and there is some evidence that the higher the parity, the higher the expulsion rate (Bernard).

Infection

Pelvic infection following insertion of an IUD is not common, and is more likely to occur if the patient is promiscuous and consequently at a greater risk of contracting gonorrhoea. The diagnosis can be difficult, but uterine pain, tenderness and pyrexia are suggestive. If it is thought that pelvic infection is present, the device should be removed. The incidence of pelvic infection depends on the population studied, but at worst is less than 1·5 per cent per year.

Perforation

Perforation of the uterus may occur, either during the insertion of the device, or if it migrates through the uterine wall some time later. The modern devices have a low perforation rate, and this is usually silent. The patient or the medical attendant notices that the threads have disappeared, and pelvic radiography reveals that the IUD is extra-uterine. If this occurs it

Table 12/7

IUD—Results at end of 12 months' usage per 100 insertions

	The Loop (a)	*The Spiral* (b)	*The Shield* (c)	*The Copper-7* (d)
Women	2,500	2,500	2,000	4,743
Pregnancies	2·3	1·6	1·1	0·8
Expulsions:				
First	9·6	19·3	2·3	5·3
Later	3·9	5·9		
Removals:				
Bleeding &/or pain	8·9	14·3	11·0	7·6
Other medical	3·5	8·5		1·5
Planned pregnancy	0·8	1·1	0·4	2·0
Other personal	2·7	3·0	1·8	1·9
Continuation Rate	68·0	62·0	83·4	80·9

Sources:

(a) Teitze, C. *Brit. Med. J.*, **2,** 444, 1969; Rajab, M. I. and Sammour, M.B. *Amer. J. Obst. Gynec.*, **105**, 156, 1969.

(b) Teitze, C. *Amer. J. Obst. Gynec.*, **96,** 1043, 1966.

(c) Manufacturer's information.

(d) Stewart, W. C. *IPPF. S.E. Asia and Oceania Conf.* Sydney, August, 1972.

can be left in the peritoneal cavity. In most studies translocation of the IUD occurs in less than 0·1 per cent of insertions.

Pregnancy

Pregnancy can occur if the device has been expelled, if it has been translocated, or with the IUD correctly placed in the uterine cavity. The rate appears higher with small devices, but this is not statistically valid. In Table **12/7** the incidence of pregnancy and the various other complications are shown after 12 months' use of the IUD. In all reported cases in which pregnancy occurred with the device in situ, its presence did not interfere with fetal growth. This is because the device is extra-ovular, lying behind the placenta, or between the membranes and the decidua. It does not cause abortion, nor is it associated with any teratogenic event.

Postpartum IUD Programmes

Pregnant women form a 'captive' audience, who willingly receive information about family planning. This information is considerably reinforced if further information is given, and contraceptive appliances are offered, during their stay in maternity hospitals and clinics, or in their homes after delivery; at the postpartum visit; or at child health clinics. The postpartum IUD programme being tried in several nations is proving encouraging. It is important that information about contraceptive appliances should also be given to the husbands, for in studies in India and Hong Kong between 65 and 90 per cent of decisions for the women to use a contraceptive appliance are made jointly by husband and wife.

Since 1966, an evaluation of the postpartum approach has been in progress, and by mid-1971 information was available on 650,000 women in 30 nations. Analysis of the results by Sivin, in 1972, indicated a fair degree of success. Four years after the start of the programme a study showed that 46 per cent of women fitted with an IUD in the postpartum period continued to use the method, but only 13 per cent of women given oral contraceptives continued to use them. After careful statistical standardization, to eliminate the variables of age, and place of residence, it was confirmed that the IUD was more effective in mass programmes, in the developing nations, than were oral contraceptives. This may be a function of the need for women choosing oral contraceptives to make a decision daily, whilst the woman choosing the IUD has only one decision to make. The effectiveness of the postpartum programme in terms of reduced fertility, and natality, is shown by the reduction in pregnancy rates from 442 to 105 per 1,000 accepters and in the natality rate from 383 to 71 per 1,000 accepters. In other words the programme has led to a 30 to 40 per cent reduction in unwanted pregnancies. It is interesting to note that Sivin concluded that for the three-year observation period, ageing contributed 13 per cent of the observed decline in fertility, the initial cohort status to 21 per cent of the decline, increased abortion to 10 per cent and the use of the IUD to 56 per cent. However, 20 per cent of the accepters who had six or more children became pregnant within three years of joining the programme, although only 5 per cent expressed a desire for more children. The perfect contraceptive has not yet been found.

A technical point requires mention. In Thailand it was found that postpartum insertion of the IUD was followed in 30 per cent of cases by its expulsion within two or three weeks. It was argued that this was because the standard introducers placed the IUD in the dilated lower uterine segment, where it was more vulnerable to expulsion as the uterus involuted. A longer introducer was devised, and the IUD (usually Lippes Loop, size D) was provided with a longer tail. The expulsion rate was halved, and was only slightly higher than for insertions made six or more weeks postpartum (Rosenfeld and Varakamin).

Postabortion IUD Programmes

Immediate postabortal IUD insertions reach a female population which would otherwise be unlikely to use contraceptive services. In Chile, it has been found that only 20 per cent of women who were recommended to attend a contraceptive clinic after hospital admission for an incomplete (usually induced) abortion did so, but when immediate postabortal insertion was performed 80 per cent accepted the method.

Despite fears to the contrary, the method is safe and can be used even if the abortion was an infected incomplete one. Postabortal insertions have a lower expulsion rate than that of intermenstrual insertions. In a study in Santiago, Chile, the women had the IUD inserted whilst still in hospital and a follow-up assessment was made 30 days later. Experience from this study showed the lack of any serious complications in the first month, and the cumulative statistics were similar to those found in post-partum studies (Goldsmith).

The Place of the IUD in a Family Planning Programme

It must be realized that the modern methods of birth control are not in competition, but are complementary to each other. The decision to use a particular method will depend on the information which a client has obtained, either from health workers, or from satisfied neighbours; on prevalent custom; and on her particular needs. The IUD is particularly useful for women who dislike the idea of oral contraceptives, or are medically unsuited to use them, and who are not willing, or able, to use the diaphragm. It may be the method of choice for a woman who becomes muddled when taking oral contraceptives, since, once introduced, the IUD is no longer dependent on the client's daily decisions.

The IUD has the additional advantage that its cost of manufacture is low, it is readily transportable, and once inserted, and accepted by the uterus, it can remain in situ and prevent pregnancy for as long as the woman desires. Unfortunately, this idealistic sequence of events is marred by the disadvantages of the IUD. These are firstly, that insertion generally is required to be made by a doctor, although experience in Indonesia and Thailand has shown that nurses can be trained to insert the devices as efficiently and safely. Secondly, that certain events occur which induce the user to seek the removal of the IUD. These events must be examined before any conclusion about the place of the IUD in a Family Planning Programme can be assessed.

Experience from studies in many parts of the world since the introduction of the IUD have shown that of the earlier shapes, Lippes Loop D has the lowest incidence of pregnancies, and side-effects.

The results for a group of 10 investigators who had a 'good follow-up' of their patients were compared with 10 investigators with 'poor follow-up' and reported in 1969 by Teitze (Table **12/8**). The Table reflects the type of experience reported from many centres. It can be seen that at the end of one year about 2·5 per cent of the patients were pregnant, 14 per cent of the loops had been expelled, and 16 per cent had been removed for one reason or another. At the end of the first year about 67 per cent of patients were still using the device; 33 per cent had

Table 12/8

The Loop (size D): Follow-up to end of first year of use per 100 woman-years (cumulative rates)

Type of Event	*Good follow-up*	*Poor follow-up*
Pregnancies	2·3 (1·7–2·9)	2·6 (1·9–3·4)
Expulsions:		
First	9·6 (8·4–10·7)	9·0 (7·7–10·4)
Later	3·9 (3·1–4·6)	3·3 (2·4–4·1)
Removals		
Bleeding and/or pain	8·9 (7·7–10·0)	11·8 (10·3–13·4)
Other medical	3·5 (2·7–4·2)	3·9 (3·0–4·8)
Planned pregnancy	0·8 (0·6–1·3)	0·9 (0·5–1·3)
Other personal	2·7 (1·8–2·9)	2·3 (1·6–2·9)
Total closures at one year	31·7	33·8
Total number (woman-years)	27,412	18,978

Source: Teitze, C. *Brit. Med. J.*, **2,** 444, 1969 (letter).

ceased to use the IUD, and were termed 'closures'. By the end of the third year, the number of users had fallen to 45 per cent. This rather high rate of closures can be reduced by well co-ordinated follow-up activities. In Thailand, accepters are visited at home by trained nurses, about two weeks after the insertion and again at three months. At these visits problems are discussed and reassurance given (Rosenfeld and Varakamin). Continuation rates are higher too if the health staff are also motivated. This has been shown in the Pathfinder Fund's International IUD Programme which has involved centres in Europe,

West Asia, East and South East Asia (Bernard). The contributors were all physicians who were in fairly constant air-mail correspondence with the Fund's head office in New York. Unfortunately, Bernard uses a slightly different classification to Teitze, but it appears that amongst the study patients, only 13·6 per cent of women had ceased to use the method by the end of the first year and by the end of the third year, 60 per cent were still using the method. Expulsions were more likely to occur in older women of higher parity. The effect of previous abortions on the expulsion rate was not so clear, but it appeared that this was lowest if a higher parity patient had also had not less than two, but not more than four, abortions. It was observed that after expulsion of the device, the rate of re-insertion was higher, and that of closure lower in South and South East Asia than in West Asia and Europe. Analysis of this indicated that the re-insertion rate was influenced by the motivation of the physicians in charge of the clinic and their ability to induce the patients to accept insertion. This factor could well account for the difference in closure rates because of expulsions of the IUD.

As important medically, and more important socially, is the incidence of bleeding and pain. Unfortunately Bernard does not give statistics about this in his report, but in a personal letter he estimates the incidence to be 15 per cent. Bleeding and pain are of concern to the patient, to her husband and to her family, as in many cultures, particularly Hindu and Islamic, the woman who bleeds vaginally is restricted in what she may do. Cultural tolerance for the symptom varies between races and even within a race. In the Pathfinder study it was observed that the rate of removal of the IUD was five times higher amongst orthodox, than amongst other Jewish women attending the same clinic. Intermittent uterine bleeding is a particular constraint amongst Hindu women who can no longer cook or work in the field whilst they are bleeding. It is not surprising that bleeding and pain accounted for 10 per cent of closures in Teitze's series, and 5 per cent in Bernard's series. Apart from possible different cultural patterns amongst the patients, study of the documents suggests that if the motivation of the doctor to keep the programme going is strong, he or she will induce more patients to retain the device despite bleeding and pain, and the closure rate will fall. Of course, the doctor is influenced by the prevalent cultural pattern, and will be more ready to extract the IUD if he or she considers bleeding to be 'unclean' or against tradition.

It can be readily understood that this constitutes a major problem. No matter what shape, all devices so far made produce bleeding, or pain, in between 15 and 40 per cent of users. Although a motivated doctor can induce more women to continue to use the device despite the symptoms, the number of doctors available is limited, particularly in areas where family planning is most needed. Perhaps, paramedical personnel might replace doctors in campaigns for the use of the IUD, but this would require that medical organizations change their present attitudes and that the medical associates were very carefully selected and highly trained.

Tubal Ligation

When the couple decide that they wish to have no further children, or if a further pregnancy will endanger the life of the wife, permanent methods of birth control are preferable to temporary methods. Vasectomy was discussed in Chapter 11, and in this chapter tubal ligation will be considered.

The term tubal ligation is, in fact, a misnomer, as the recommended operations include the excision of a part of each oviduct, and the ligation of the cut ends. In India, the term bilateral partial tubectomy is favoured. Alternatively, the term sterilization is often used, although to non-medical people this word wrongly connotes castration.

In the past ten years, the number of tubal ligations performed annually has increased both in the developed, and in the developing nations, and an increasing number are being performed in the early puerperium.

Clinical Aspects

Tubal ligation should only be offered after the patient, and her husband, have had the opportunity to understand the nature and the consequences of the operation. As has been mentioned, many people, even those who are supposedly well-educated, are ignorant about their reproductive systems, and confuse tubal ligation with castration. The health worker, whether doctor or associate, must explain clearly that after tubectomy, the ovaries continue to function normally, and neither femininity nor sexuality is diminished. The fate of the ovum should also be explained as some women have a fear that the ova will accumulate in the peritoneal cavity like frog spawn.

It is also necessary to examine the patient vaginally in cases where tubectomy is performed outside the immediate puerperium. There are certain contra-indications to tubectomy. These are: (1) the presence of multiple myomata, (2) a history of menstrual irregularities which have not responded to hormonal therapy, (3) a marked uterovaginal prolapse, and other gross genital tract pathology. Patients with these conditions, who wish to have no further children, are best treated by total hysterectomy. However, hysterectomies are currently performed too often and often for too little reason. The operation is more painful, requires a longer convalescence, has a higher mortality than tubectomy, and has more sequelae. If the operation is performed after careful assessment, results are excellent; but this selection must be made. It is also advisable to establish that the patient is not pregnant, or the doctor may be accused of malpractice.

TECHNIQUE

Tubectomy may be performed after entering the abdominal cavity by laparotomy or by using a laparoscope.

Laparotomy

In the early puerperium the abdominal cavity is entered through a small subumbilical incision, and the uterus is manipulated to bring the oviducts into view. If the woman is not puerperal a small subumbilical midline incision, or a small transverse suprapubic incision, will give adequate access. This operation can be made easier by inserting a uterine cannula, so that the uterus can be manipulated and brought easily into the area beneath the laparotomy. Each oviduct is grasped by two light forceps, and a wedge of oviduct is excised (Figure **12/2**). The midportion of the tube is the most appropriate, and a non-vascular area of the mesosalpinx should be chosen. The cut oviduct, and its blood vessel on each side, are included in a transfixing suture, using a non-absorbable suture. The area is inspected for bleeding and the operation is repeated on the other oviduct. If the skin incision is sutured using a subcuticular absorbable suture, the patient need not stay in hospital for more than 36 hours. The operation is done under general anaesthesia. The total time for the procedure averages 20 minutes.

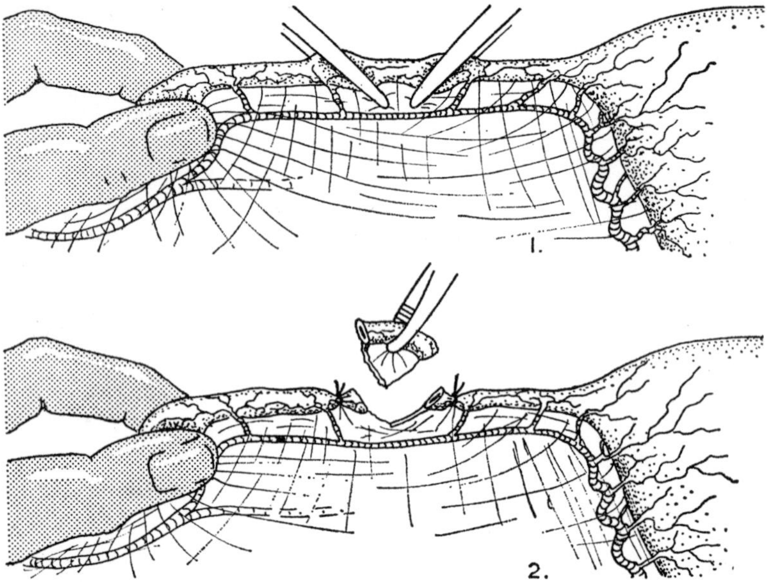

Figure **12/2** Method of tubal excision and ligation. 1. The oviduct is drawn taut and an area is isolated by two clamps. 2. A wedge has been removed from the tube. The uterine side of the tube has been clamped and tied using an unabsorbable suture. The lateral side has been clamped but not tied.

Tubectomy may also be performed at the time of a repeat Caesarean section, or following a therapeutic abortion. Evidence from Britain suggests that in the latter case the mortality is raised; but if the gestation period is less than 10 weeks, and the abortion is procured by using a suction curette, there is no increased mortality.

Unless the doctor is sure that he has excised the oviduct, he should send the specimen for a histopathological report. Some reported 'failures' of tubectomy are due to excision of a wedge of the round muscle (ligament) mistakenly thought to be the oviduct.

Laparoscopy

Tubectomy via the laparoscope is currently fashionable. The advantage is that the incisions are small, and after healing almost invisible, and that the patient can leave hospital after 36 hours, or sooner. Steptoe, who is a pioneer in the use of the laparoscope, describes his technique in his book *Laparoscopy in Gynaecology*. The procedure is performed under general anaesthesia. The cervix is inspected and a uterine cannula is introduced and fixed into position. A pneumoperitoneum is established using carbogen, about 3 litres being required. The patient is placed in a 40° head-down position and the laparoscope is introduced through a small transverse incision at the lower umbilical border. After inspecting the genital organs, a second incision is made in the skin about 5 cm from the mid-line, about half-way between the umbilicus and the symphysis pubis. By transillumination from the laparoscope, an avascular area is chosen. The trochar and cannula of the Palmer biopsy drill forceps is thrust through this lower incision, and the trochar is replaced by the forceps, which has first been tested to ensure that it will coagulate. The assistant manipulates the uterus to the left, and the inner portion of the right tube is grasped by the forceps about 1·5 cm from the cornu. The tube is lifted, and after making sure that nothing else is touching the forceps the coagulating current is passed for 2 to 5 seconds. The oviduct is then released and regrasped about 0·5 cm to 1 cm

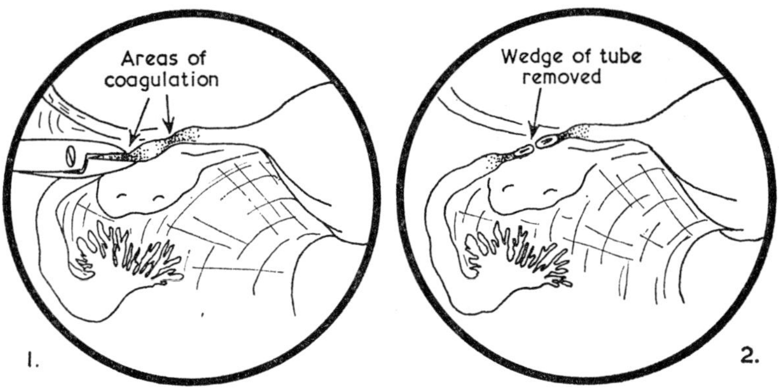

Figure **12/3** Laparoscopic 'sterilization.'
Source: Steptoe, P.

laterally and a further coagulation is performed (Figure **12/3**). Steptoe then severs the oviduct using the drill forceps at the centre of the coagulated area, but other gynaecologists feel that this is neither necessary nor desirable (Jordan). The procedure is repeated for the left oviduct by manipulating it to approach the drill forceps. Both oviducts are inspected to make sure there is no bleeding and the apparatus is withdrawn. The patient is returned to the horizontal and the gas evacuated. The incisions are closed with subcuticular absorbable sutures or a Michel clip. The average time for the procedure is 30 minutes. The patient lies flat for about 8 hours and may be discharged 24 to 36 hours after the operation, provided she has no pain or pyrexia. She can return to all her domestic duties within 5 days.

SIDE-EFFECTS

Mortality

If the operation is done by skilled surgeons, the mortality is very low. In most recent studies it is less than 25 per 100,000 cases (Presser).

Morbidity

The morbidity is difficult to compute, as different investigations use different criteria. It seems highest in the developing nations. Pyrexia complicates about 2 per cent of tubectomies, and superficial wound infection in about the same percentage.

Psychological

Investigations in the past 10 years show that over 99 per cent of women are satisfied by having had tubectomy performed. The degree of satisfaction is greater if the woman chose to have the operation than if it was suggested by her medical attendant, and is less amongst women who had psychosexual problems before the operation. Provided that the patient understands the nature of the operation, adverse responses postoperatively are few. The effect of tubectomy on libido has been investigated extensively. Despite the difficulty in interpreting some of the results, libido is unchanged in over 60 per cent of women, it is increased in 10 per cent and reduced in 20 per cent (Presser).

NON-SURGICAL TUBAL OCCLUDING PROCEDURES

Experiments are proceeding using quinacrine, with either metallic copper or zinc-chelating agents as a method of chemical 'sterilization'. Quinacrine introduced into the uterine cornua transcervically produces a granulomatous reaction which occludes the lumen of the oviduct. Early experience shows that the whole procedure is less traumatic and no more time-consuming than the introduction of an IUD. With the development of a hysteroscope the material would be more accurately placed. At present this technique must be considered purely experimental.

The Use-Effectiveness of Various Methods of Birth Control

It will be understood that the current trend is to offer a variety of birth control measures, depending on the socio-economic, cultural and environmental characteristics of the potential users. The use-effectiveness of the various methods in preventing pregnancy has been investigated, particularly by Teitze, and the salient facts are shown in Table **12/9**.

The Mortality of Pregnancy and of Methods of Birth Control

Every activity in life, even sitting in a chair, has some risk of death, although in most normal activities the risk is very low. A woman who has regular, fairly frequent, sexual intercourse is subject to additional risks, either as a result of pregnancy and childbirth, or else as a result of the measures she takes to avoid pregnancy. The risks of death due to pregnancy and childbirth are discussed in Chapter 19, and depend on the health of the woman, whether facilities for pre-natal care are available, whether she uses them, and on the standard of the obstetric services in the country where she lives.

In any assessment of the risks associated with contraceptive usage, the risks of pregnancy and childbirth must also be assessed, since contraceptives, used properly, reduce them to a significant degree. The more efficient the contraceptive technique in reducing fertility and natality, the less important in the

Table 12/9

Ranking of contraceptive methods by rate of effectiveness
(*as calculated from unexpected pregnancies per* 100 *woman years*)

		Rates
Group A	*Most effective*	
	Tubal ligation/vasectomy	0·005–0·04
	Combined orals	0·005–0·10
	Sequential orals	0·20–0·56
Group B	*Highly effective*	
	IUD	0·5–3·5
	Continuous gestagen	1·5–2·3
	Diaphragm or condom + cream	
	All users	2·0–18·0
	Highly motivated	2·5– 5·0
	Safe period	
	All users	10·0–30·0
	Highly motivated	2·5– 5·0
Group C	*Less effective*	
	Coitus interruptus	30·0–40·0
	Vaginal foam or cream	30·0–40·0
Group D	*Least effective*	
	Post-coital douche	45·0
	Prolonged breast feeding	45·0

Source: Tietze, C., in *Control of Human Fertility*, Almqvist, Stockholm, 1971; Tables in Chapters 10 and 11.

equation are the risks due to pregnancy. These matters require consideration, but only currently used methods of contraception will be discussed.

The method used will be to calculate the risk incurred by women at hazard from unprotected coitus, or from the use of contraceptive measures calculated on an annual basis. It is realized that this method of calculation fails to make allowance for the reduction of fertility as age advances, or for the fact that when a pregnancy is planned the patient ceases to use contraceptives, or for altering maternal mortality rates. Nevertheless it does give information about the effectiveness and risk of various contraceptive measures.

NO CONTRACEPTION

If a fertile woman uses no contraceptive measures, and has regular coitus, she has a 40 to 60 per cent annual chance of conceiving, depending on her age and whether she breast feeds or not. The two rates have been assumed, so that 40,000 to 60,000 of the cohort of 100,000 might be expected to conceive in any year.

COITUS INTERRUPTUS

Withdrawal before ejaculation is innocuous to the woman, and in all probability to the man. The method is without risk therefore, but since the method of conception control requires more precise timing to avoid ejaculation in the vagina, and to prevent spurts of spermatozoa spraying the vulva, the method is inefficient. About 35 pregnancies will occur per 100 women using the method each year. Since the mean maternal mortality (including abortion) in the developed nations is about 30 per 100,000 births, and in the developing nations about 300 per 100,000 births, the total risk of dying from an unwanted pregnancy is 10 per 100,000 users per annum in the developed nations, and 105 per 100,000 users per annum in the developing nations.

THE SAFE PERIOD METHOD

As with coitus interruptus, the rhythm method is without physical harm to either partner, although it may cause marital disharmony, as coitus is controlled by the calendar and not by desire. Unfortunately, ovulation may occur at times other than that calculated from the menstrual cycle. Collected evidence amongst users is that the safe period method has an average pregnancy rate of 20 per 100 women per year, although this is much reduced amongst highly motivated couples. If prevalent mortality rates are applied, the risk of death from an unplanned, and undesired pregnancy, is 6 per 100,000 women per year in developed nations, and 60 per 100,000 women per year in developing nations.

CONDOMS AND DIAPHRAGMS

The use of the condom or the vaginal diaphragm carries no risk to the user from hazards inherent in the method. The pregnancy rate following the use of the condom or diaphragm is difficult to calculate exactly, as it depends largely on the motivation of the couple to use the method properly. The modern condom is a highly efficient contraceptive, but may tear, releasing spermatozoa into the vaginal vault. The vaginal diaphragm is an effective contraceptive, but only if it has been placed properly in the vagina and covers the cervical os. Pregnancy rates are reported to range from 2 to 18 per 100 woman-years, the median being 10. If this rate is accepted, 10,000 pregnancies per 100,000 women will occur. The mortality rate per 100,000 users in developed nations is 3, and in developing nations 30.

LEGAL ABORTION

As will be discussed in Chapter 13, legally induced abortion is safe if it is performed prior to the 10th week of gestation and if a suction curette is used. Data from Eastern European nations indicate that the mortality from the method, if performed in this way, is 1·5 per 100,000 abortions. It is considered that in the developing nations a rate treble this would apply. However, a woman using this method is likely to require at least 2 abortions per year, so that the rate doubles. In the developing nations, the risk of legally induced abortion is three times that found in Eastern Europe, so that in these nations a rate of 9 per 100,000 applies.

INTRA-UTERINE CONTRACEPTIVE DEVICE

It is not known how the IUD works, but current suggestions are that it stimulates a marked foreign body reaction in the endometrium which hinders nidation. Hazards from the use of the IUD are that the device may penetrate and perforate the uterus, or that genital tract infection may occur. These hazards should not lead to death in more than 1 per 100,000 insertions in the developed nations, and double this in the developing nations. The pregnancy rate amongst IUD users appears to be about 1·5 per 100 women per year. If current maternal mortality rates in the developed and developing nations are applied to the 1,500 pregnancies per 100,000 IUD users, a total mortality of 1·4 and 6·5 per 100,000 users results.

TUBAL LIGATION

The failure rate of a properly performed tubal ligation is about 0·05 per cent, which gives an estimated pregnancy rate of 50 per 100,000 women per year. The mortality due to the operation is less than 25 per 100,000 operations. The average age of a patient deciding to have a tubal ligation is 30, and the operation will protect her against unwanted pregnancy over the remaining 15 years of her reproductive era. As the method is a guarantee of permanent conception control, the mortality rate should be calculated over an average of 15 years, so that it drops to 1·7 per 100,000.

ORAL CONTRACEPTIVES

The main hazard to life posed by the currently used oral contraceptives is the chance of the development of thrombo-embolic

Table 12/10

Annual pregnancy rates and mortality associated with various currently used methods of family planning in the developed nations

Method	*Pregnancies per* 100,000 *users*	*Deaths per* 100,000 *users*		
		Method	*Pregnancy (average mortality* 30 *per* 100,000 *births)*	*Total*
No contraception	60,000	0	18	18
Coitus interruptus usage failure = 35	35,000	0	10	10
'Safe period' method usage failure = 20	20,000	0	6	6
Condom & Diaphragm usage failure = 10	10,000	0	3	3
Legal abortion (up to 10 weeks gestation)	120,000	1·8	—	1·8
IUD usage failure = 1·5	1,500	1·0	0·45	1·4
Oral contraceptives usage failure = 0·07	70	1·5	0·021	1·5
Tubal ligation usage failure = 0·05	100	1·7	0·01	1·7

Usage failure = pregnancies per 100 women per year.

Table 12/11

Annual pregnancy rates and mortality associated with various currently used methods of family planning in the developing nations

Method	*Pregnancies per* 100,000 *users*	*Deaths per* 100,000 *users*		
		Method	*Pregnancy (average mortality* 300 *per* 100,000 *births*)	*Total*
No contraception	50,000	0	150	150
Coitus interruptus usage failure = 35	35,000	0	105	105
'Safe period' method usage failure = 20	20,000	0	60	60
Condom and Diaphragm usage failure = 10	10,000	0	30	30
Legal abortion (up to 10 weeks gestation)	100,000	5·4	–	5·4
IUD usage failure = 1·5	1,500	2	4·5	6·5
Oral contraceptives usage failure = 0·07	70	0·15	0·21	0·4
Tubal ligation usage failure = 0·05	100	1·7	0·01	1·7

disease amongst apparently healthy women. In affluent developed nations, thrombo-embolic disease is more common than in the developing nations, and in both the risk increases with increasing age. In the developed nations from which data are available (i.e. U.K. and U.S.A.), the chance of death occurring from oral contraceptive induced thrombo-embolism is about 1·5 per 100,000 users, if it occurs at all. Studies amongst obstetric patients in developing nations indicate that they have one-tenth the risk of developing venous thrombo-embolism as do obstetric patients in developing nations, and this rate can probably be applied to users of oral contraceptives. Amongst such women the death rate from thrombo-embolism would be about 0·15 per 100,000 users.

Oral contraceptives have a very low failure rate. It is less than 0·07 per 100 women per year, or 70 pregnancies per 100,000 users. Apply current maternal death rates in developed and developing nations to these pregnancies, and the chance of maternal death is 0·4 and 1·5 respectively.

THE HAZARDS OF CONTRACEPTIVES

The data just presented are summarized in Table **12/10**, which gives details for the developed nations, and in Table **12/11** which gives details for the developing nations. In both types of nation the superiority of oral contraception and the IUD, with legally induced abortion for contraceptive failures, and the increased adoption of permanent contraceptive measures when the desired family size has been achieved, is clearly shown.

THIRTEEN

Abortion

Abortion is usually defined by health workers as the termination of a pregnancy before the fetus has become capable of independent extra-uterine life, at which point it is said to be viable. In most nations, viability has been defined in terms of the period of gestation, or the weight of the fetus, and has been considered to occur at the end of the 27th completed week of gestation, which corresponds to a fetal weight of about 1,000 g. The reason for adopting this definition is based on the observation that few fetuses born earlier survive, and even in hospitals which have the facilities for intensive neonatal care, the number does not exceed 10 per cent of those born alive. However, because some do survive, many authorities have recommended a different set of criteria for viability. An additional reason for making this decision is because the clinical and aetiological factors associated with the deaths of infants weighing between 500 and 999 g (1 lb 2 oz and 2 lb 4 oz), relate more to those found later in pregnancy than those of the earlier weeks. The most comprehensive studies have been made by WHO expert committees who have recommended that the term abortion should be restricted to the process of expulsion of the fetus, and that the abortus should in future be termed an early fetal death. Most members of the scientific study groups have recommended that the upper limit for defining an abortion should be 20 completed gestational weeks, which corresponds to a fetal weight of 500 g (1 lb 2 oz).

It is appreciated that many nations will wish to retain the traditional upper limit of 27 completed gestational weeks and a fetal weight of 1,000 g (2 lb 4 oz) in their definition of abortion.

The choice of one or other of the definitions will influence perinatal mortality statistics. Although only 1 per cent of all pregnancies terminate between the 20th and 28th week, half of the infants are born dead, and may be termed intermediate fetal deaths, whilst of these babies born alive less than 10 per cent survive, so that if the 'extended' definition is chosen perinatal mortality rates will be higher. This is discussed in Chapter 18.

SPONTANEOUS AND INDUCED ABORTION

Quite obviously when abortion is under discussion, two entirely separate groups of events are being studied. The first is spontaneous abortion, which is the natural rejection of the conceptus, and the second is induced abortion, in which the conceptus is removed, or expelled, from the uterus by deliberate human intervention. Induced abortion, moreover, includes two populations—that in which the abortion is permitted by the laws of the country, and that in which the pregnancy is terminated illegally.

Spontaneous Abortion

The incidence of abortion remains a matter of considerable controversy. In the first place, embryological evidence from polytocous animals and some observations in the human suggest that by far the largest loss is of fertilized eggs prior to implantation or during the 10-day period after implantation. These losses will not be associated with any signs or symptoms and will consequently not appear in any statistics. The second reason for the controversy is that episodes of bleeding after a period of amenorrhoea may be considered due to abortion when in fact there is no evidence that the bleeding was more than a delayed menstrual period. Conversely for cultural, social or domestic reasons, spontaneous abortions may be understated, and illegally induced abortions may be reported as spontaneous.

The evidence, such as it is, suggests the estimate, made in 1954 by the Population Division of the United Nations that 10 per cent of pregnancies terminated by spontaneous abortion, was too low. The current estimate is that an overall ratio of 15 to 20 spontaneous abortions per 100 pregnancies is more accurate.

It is also known that in at least 65 per cent of early abortions, the pregnancy terminates because of genetic or developmental defects in the conceptus, and that abortion ratios, estimated at weekly intervals, fall from the first four-week period. In several studies of abortion, from different nations, the incidence of known spontaneous abortions per 1,000 pregnancies was highest during the 5th to 8th gestational weeks, and the frequency fell considerably after the end of the 10th week. In these studies over 75 per cent of the abortions had occurred before that time. (Figure **13/1**).

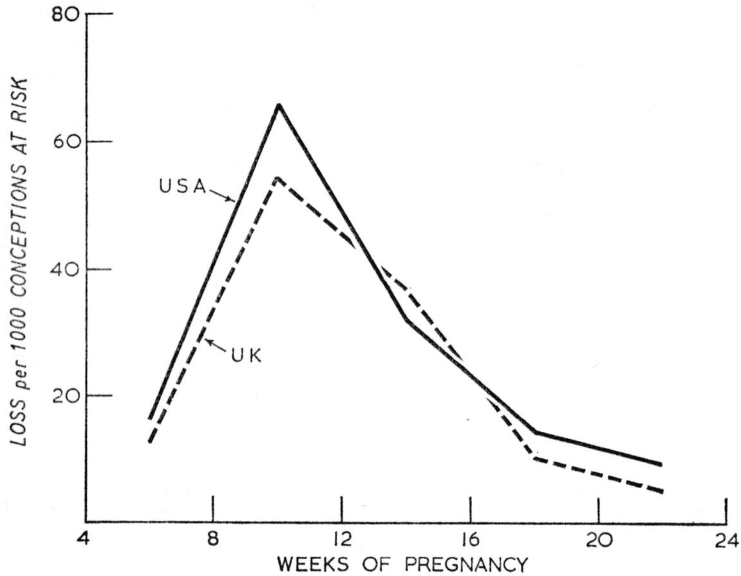

Figure **13/1** Fetal death rates by gestational week per 1,000 conceptions.

Sources: Stevenson, A., in *Trans. 5th World Congress Gynaecology and Obstetrics*, Butterworth, Sydney 1967; Shapiro, S. et al., in *Advances in Planned Parenthood*, Vol. 4.

SOCIAL FACTORS ASSOCIATED WITH SPONTANEOUS ABORTION

The medical aspects of spontaneous abortion are considered in some detail in *Fundamentals of Obstetrics and Gynaecology* and will not be written about here. But there are certain social factors which are associated with spontaneous abortion. Although the observations are limited, studies from Australia, Britain, Sweden and the U.S.A. indicate that the number of spontaneous abortions per 1,000 pregnancies increases with maternal age, with increasing parity and with the number of previous abortions. Evidence from Hungary suggests that the increase after previous abortions occurs whether they were spontaneous or induced. These associations, whilst independent of each other, reinforce each other.

Induced Abortion

Induced abortion is the oldest method of birth control and has been practised by women since people collected in groups for their mutual protection. When food was plentiful, pregnancy was welcomed; when food became short, either because of famine or population pressures, the unwanted pregnancy was a disaster. The world-wide distribution of induced abortion has been documented by Devereux, who found that amongst over 300 tribes or cultural groups studied, only one denied using induced abortion as a method of birth control. The exact frequency of induced abortion amongst women in primitive tribes is unknown, nor are the motives for using the method entirely clear. Anthropologists have identified two main patterns. In the first the abortion is induced for social reasons; for example, amongst Hottentot women, abortion is practised, as too frequent pregnancies would make their ability to work and to move from place to place difficult, and a new baby would displace an existing one at the woman's breast. In the second, the abortion is obtained for personal reasons. Shapiro quotes a report about Chagga women who seek abortion when they consider themselves 'too old to continue reproducing' and notes that amongst the Masai of Kenya impregnation by an old or unfit man is aborted, as the pregnancy 'may result in an enfeebled offspring'.

The ubiquity of induced abortion in all types of society, in all the continents of the world, and in all the nations, is well documented.

In recent years there has been a tendency for nations to permit legally induced abortion, and this has gathered momentum. One of the reasons for this is that studies from many nations show that the large majority of deaths attributed to abortion result from abortions induced by the woman herself, or by an unqualified person. In addition, in certain Latin American countries, where birth control information is restricted and appliances are difficult to obtain, statistics show that 25 to 50 per cent of all beds in maternity hospitals are occupied by women suffering from the effects of illegally induced abortion and from the after-effects of induced abortion. Illegally induced abortion is a leading cause of death of women of childbearing age in many nations.

Abortion has been legally permissible in Japan since 1949; in the U.S.S.R. and the countries of Eastern Europe since the 1950s; in China since 1954; in Scandinavia, on a restricted basis since 1939, and more widely since 1968; in Britain since 1968; in Singapore since 1969; in sixteen States of the U.S.A. and in South Australia since 1970; and in India since 1972. In 1973 the Supreme Court of the U.S.A. ruled that the States constitutionally were prevented from enacting laws which hindered a woman from obtaining an abortion. This, in fact, makes abortion legally permitted throughout the U.S.A. However, illegally induced abortion remains the most usual way of birth control.

THE ETHICAL AND RELIGIOUS ASPECTS OF INDUCED ABORTION

Since induced abortion involves ethical and religious questions, the currently accepted religious beliefs about its licitness must be stated briefly.

Communism

In most communist nations induced abortion is legal, subject to minor restrictions which vary from nation to nation. The principle is that abortion may be legally performed to further the emancipation of women, to enhance family welfare, and for humanitarian reasons to bring abortion under proper medical supervision, thus eliminating the hazards to the life and health of a woman from perilous illegal abortion performed by the woman herself or by unqualified abortionists. In pursuance of these aims, abortion is free, or almost free. It is rarely permitted after the 12th week of pregnancy and must be performed in a designated clinic or hospital by a qualified person. Following the abortion, instruction on contraceptive techniques is emphasized. In many nations, a second abortion is not permitted if a previous interruption has taken place in the previous 6 or 12 months.

Christianity

Roman Catholics accept the moral imperative that 'you shall not kill an innocent human being'. To be human implies the possession of a soul, and much discussion has centred round the moment of ensoulment of the fetus. Traditionally Roman Catholics hold that the soul enters the zygote at the moment of conception, although this has only been Roman Catholic dogma since 1869.

Until that time, and particularly after the Decretum of Gratian in 1140, the majority of Roman Catholic moral theologians held with Thomas Aquinas, that ensoulment did not occur until the conceptus had a human shape, and possessed basic human organs, for without human shape it could not be a human being. This view stemmed from the theory of hylomorphism, according to which the soul is the substance of man, whilst the human body is the result of the union of the soul with undetermined prime matter. This implies that an actual human soul can only exist in an actual, not a virtual, human body. The Council of Vienne, in AD 1312, further codified this view forbidding baptism of any birth which did not have a human shape, which in general was held to occur by the 12th gestational week.

In 1869 these views were finally reversed and ensoulment was held to take place at conception, or at the latest at nidation. By this time the basic facts of human embryogenesis had been observed, so that it was now realized that the fetus had no recognizable human shape until thirty days after conception, or the end of the 6th gestational week.

Liberal Roman Catholic moral theologians hold that a refined hylomorphic view is theologically correct; a spokesman, Father Donceel, S.J., stating that 'the embryo is certainly not a human person during the early stages of pregnancy, and that, consequently it is not immoral to terminate pregnancy during this time, provided there are serious reasons for such an intervention'.

In theory, therefore, induced abortion would have been licit in early pregnancy, although Roman Catholics also accepted the teaching of the early churchmen in the Didache, written about ninety years after the death of Jesus, that 'You shall not kill the child by abortion. You shall not kill what is conceived.' However, moral dilemmas did arise, and abortion or infanticide (since no theological distinction was made between the two) to save the life of the mother was considered to be lawful by most moral theologians. This view was based on a justification by Tertullian, in the third century AD, that 'sometimes by a cruel necessity, whilst yet in the womb, an infant is put to death, when lying awry in the orifice of the womb he hinders parturition; and kills his mother'. Cyril Means, discussing the Roman Catholic view, is also of the opinion that abortion for a social reason—in the instance quoted, rape—was licit up to the year 1890; and as can be seen the moral issue is still under dispute.

However, it must be recorded that the Papal Encyclical 'Humanae Vitae', issued in 1968, declared 'we must once again declare that the direct interruption of the generative process already begun, and above all directly willed and procured abortion, even for therapeutic reasons, are to be absolutely excluded as licit means of regulating birth'.

Protestant theologians differ considerably in their opinion as to the licitness of induced abortion, but most are more liberal than Roman Catholics. In 1962 the British Council of Churches decided that biological life became human life at the time of nidation, not of conception, and a year earlier the National Council of Churches (U.S.A.) approved induced abortion for the sake of the woman's health. This brought them into line with the Anglican conference, which, in 1958, had allowed abortion for 'medical necessity'. The position of the Anglican church is that it condemns abortion as murder since the fetus is a unique individual although utterly dependent on its mother for survival. But if the fetus threatens the life of the mother then abortion is licit, as the mother acts in 'self defence'. Parenthetically, the Anglican church encourages contraception as a way to prevent the birth of unwanted children. Anglican theologians point out that nowhere in the New Testament does Jesus state that procreation is the main purpose of marriage. The sexual relationship in marriage has a role to fill which is quite independent of the procreative need. Even Paul considered it important. In his first letter to the people of Corinth, when discussing sexuality in marriage, he wrote, 'Do not refuse one another, except perhaps by agreement for a limited time, to devote yourself to prayer; but then come together again.' The American Baptists in 1968 favoured abortion on request in the first 12 weeks of pregnancy, and upon medical indications after that time. However, despite these pronouncements, the Protestant churches in most instances have failed to take any stand, and the individual member of the church has had to form his own opinion, without real guidance. That the consensus of lay Protestant opinion favours a more liberal attitude to legally induced abortion for social as well as medical indications is demonstrated by the changes which have occurred in the predominantly Protestant nations of the North Atlantic seaboard since 1967.

Islam

Islam has consistently held that the fetus is unformed until 120 days has passed after conception, and that it 'is permissible to take medicine to procure abortion so long as the embryo is unformed'. However, Islamic attitudes differ from country to country, some taking the time when abortion is permissible to be before 40 days. This derived from the ancient Greek (Aristotelean) belief that life started at 40 days after conception, and this had been adopted by Islam in the old Turkish empire. Many Islamic jurists added that for abortion to be licit, a reason should exist. As an example of such a reason, the Grand Mufti of Jordan in 1964 quoted Ibn Abdin who had said 'like the mother who has a baby still unweaned and who becomes pregnant and thus her milk ceases and the father is unable to hire a wet nurse to save the life of the baby'.

Buddhism

In theory Buddhism holds all life, human or animal, to be sacred and consequently abortion is prohibited. But Buddhism recognizes that man is imperfect, and finds it hard to strive for the way, so that tacitly abortion is permitted, certainly when a medical indication exists.

Judaism

The Jewish belief is that the human soul is the one quality which distinguishes man from all other animals, and it is only discernible from the moment of birth to the moment of death. Most Jewish scholars from the time of the Talmud are of the opinion that prior to birth the fetus is simply a part of its mother and has neither individual life not personality of its own. The opinion of the nineteenth-century Rabbi Solomon of Skola summarizes the modern Jewish view. He indicates that there can be no objection of any sort to an abortion performed within the first 40 days after conception, and it may be done later if the fetus threatens the life or health of the mother.

Humanism

Since humanists reject the supernatural, they hold that all the positions taken about the time of ensoulment are matters of faith rather than of observation or empirical reasoning. To quote the distinguished embryologist, George Corner, writing in 1944: 'Looking through the microscope at the physical structure of embryonic man, I see no heaven-bound chariot of a soul, but only frail congeries of animal cells, fraught indeed with promise beyond all other embryonic creatures, but of necessity bound to grow and to organize itself as an animal if it is to be a man. Humbly employing such vision as may be granted to an embryologist, I declare my conviction that the spirit of man—all that makes him more than beast and carries him onward with hope and sacrifice—comes not as a highborn tenant from afar but as a latent potentiality of the body.' To a humanist, the decision for abortion must be to determine the potentiality of the fetus and the actual self of the mother. This must lead to the conclusion that birth control should be effected primarily by conventional methods, and abortion, in general, reserved for the failures; but once adopted it should be performed with efficiency, safety, and without affronting the dignity of a woman, by making her plead, or only after giving her moral strictures.

Illegally Induced Abortion

Accurate statistical data of the incidence of illegally induced abortion in a community and its annual incidence are almost impossible to obtain. The most acceptable data are extrapolated from sample surveys. The surveys are made of population samples, by analysis of the histories of obstetrical and gynaecological patients, by information obtained from family planning clinics, and the analysis of hospital statistics. Population surveys, made amongst randomly selected groups of women in different localities, give some information, but because of the belief by many women that abortion is a personal matter, and because of their fear of retribution, either by God or man, for having had an induced abortion, the numbers recorded tend to underestimate the true incidence by 10 to 40 per cent. Information from obstetrical and gynaecological patients gives a better estimate, because of the more intimate relationship between the health worker and the patient, but again estimates tend to be low. Many women claim an induced abortion was spontaneous, and, of course, only those women who are pregnant after a previous abortion, or who have a gynaecological complaint requiring attention will be questioned. It is believed that many women use induced abortion not to space children, but to determine the ultimate size of their family, so that either no further pregnancy occurs, or if it does, it is again terminated by an induced abortion. These women do not attend hospital or health clinics. What has been written applies equally to data obtained from family planning clinics, where a further bias is introduced as most women attending such clinics are more motivated to space their children by methods other than that of induced abortion. Hospital statistics represent only those women whose abortion requires admission to hospital, and miss the many women whose abortion does not. It would appear, then, that estimates of illegally induced abortion in various nations will never be accurately known, and such estimates as have been obtained, in general, understate the incidence.

The statistical analysis of the data poses a further problem. The abortion rate may be calculated as the number of abortions per year per 1,000 total population at mid-year. This crude abortion rate corresponds to other crude vital rates in vital statistics. A more refined measure is the general abortion rate, which is the number of abortions per 1,000 women aged 15 to 49. This is analogous to the general natality rate. Alternatively, abortion rates (or more properly, abortion ratios) may be

Table 13/1

Illegally induced abortion: estimated annual incidence and ratio per 100 live births in selected nations

Nation	*Year*	*Estimate* (*in* 1,000s)	*Abortion*/100 *live births*	*Source*
World	1964–66	20,000	30	a, b
Africa				
United Arab Republic	1969	180	21	a
America (North)				
Mexico	1966	—	20	b
U.S.A.	1968	1,000	30	b, f
America (South)				
Argentina	1964	500	100	g
Brazil	1964	1,500	25	b
Chile	1969	150	60	g
Colombia	1964–66	—	14	b
Peru	1965	—	15	d
Uruguay	1964	150	300	g
Asia				
India	1964–67	5,000	?20	b, d
Iran	1970	—	35	c
Israel	1959–60	—	8	a
Taiwan	1966	40	18	a
Turkey	1969–70	All 270	24	a
		Urban —	56	a
Europe				
Austria	1965–67	200	150	b, c
Belgium	1965–67	100	75	b, c
Britain	1965–67	100–200	15	e
Denmark	1940–55	20	30	d
France	1967	600	60	g
Germany	1967	1,500	150	g
Greece	1968	60	23	g
Ireland	1965–67	4		g
Italy	1965–67	600	75	g
Netherlands	1965–67	20		g
Switzerland	1965–67	25		g
Czechoslovakia	1965–67	3		d
Hungary	1965–67	5		d
Finland	1967	30	40	g

Sources:
(a) I.P.P.F. *Medical Newsletter.*
(b) Hall. *Abortion in a Changing World.*
(c) Mehlen, K. *Abortion on a Global Scale.*
(d) Geijerstam. *Annotated Bibliography of Induced Abortion*, Univ. Michigan, 1969.
(e) James, W. H. 'Incidence of Illegal Abortion', *Population Studies*, 327, 1971.
(f) Schwartz, R. A. *Comprehensive Psychiatry*, **9**, 99, 1968.
(g) Klinger, A. *Demografia*, **12**, 479, 1969.

computed per 100 live births or deliveries, and this ratio is most commonly used. Age-specific abortion rates may be computed, and are usually based on the age of the woman at the time of conception, or at the time of the termination. The method chosen can cause a substantial error, as has been pointed out by the WHO Scientific Group on Abortion. Their report should be consulted for further details.

Despite these problems, some indication of the widespread use of illegally induced abortion in various nations is given in Table **13/1**, which shows the estimated annual incidence of illegally induced abortion in the world is probably as high as 20–30 million. In Table **13/2** the percentage of women admitting to induced abortion as a means of avoiding unwanted birth is shown. This information has been obtained in a variety of ways and is probably a low estimate.

These two sets of data indicate the extent of the problem and underline the seriousness of illegally induced abortion as a

Table 13/2

The percentage of women in several nations admitting to illegally induced abortion

Place	*Reference*	*Facility*	*Total interviewed*	*Per cent admitting to induced abortion, (1 or more)*
Turkey (Ankara)	b	Hospital	6,325	40
Iran (Teheran)	b	F.P. Clinic	40,000	15–30
Chile (Santiago)	b	F.P. Clinic	15,467	43
Israel (Tel Aviv)	d	Hospital	N.S.	47
Greece Urban	c	Hospital	N.S.	40
Rural		Hospital	N.S.	31
All				35
Britain All	a	Random Survey	2,132	5
		F.P. Clinics		25
U.S.A. (New York)	c	Survey	N.S.	15–24
Korea All	d	Survey	N.S.	13
Urban				27
Rural				7

Sources: As in Table 13/1. N.S. = not stated.

public health hazard. The problem is not only one of potential, or actual danger to the mother, but one of economics. In addition to the cost to the mother herself, statistics show that the cost to the community is great. In a study in Egypt in 1970, it was calculated that the management of induced abortion consumed over 50 per cent of the maternity hospitals' budgets. In Chile in 1969, illegally induced abortion accounted for 35 per cent of all maternal deaths, 6·1 per cent of Chile's health budget and 17·8 per cent of its expenditure on maternal care.

Another approach to the problem of estimating the number of induced abortions has been made by Viel in Latin America. He points out that in the years before 1960 contraceptive measures were virtually unknown and induced abortion was illegal, as it still is. In communities characterized by a young population, a high percentage of whom marry under the age of 25 (which obtains in Latin America), the biologically determined birth rate would be about 50 per 1,000 population. If it is significantly lower, this must be due to abstinence of coitus in marriage, which is unlikely, to coitus interruptus, or to illegally induced abortions. Table **13/3** shows there is a marked deficit in the actual, as opposed to the theoretical, birth rate and that this is most marked in nations which are most highly urbanized. Other evidence indicates that induced abortion is relatively common in these situations. In the congested urban slum, the mother often needs to work outside the house, but knows that because of better paediatric facilities her existing children are more likely to survive to adulthood. And so when an unwanted pregnancy occurs she resorts to illegally induced abortion either by self-induction or by seeking an untrained amateur abortionist. Viel produces data which indicate that the fall in the infant mortality rate in Chile since 1935 has been paralleled by a rise in the illegally induced abortion rate.

THE SOCIOLOGY OF ILLEGALLY INDUCED ABORTION

In nations where induced abortion is illegal, abortion on medical or psychiatric grounds—the so-called 'therapeutic abortion'—can still be performed safely (both in respect of medicine and the law) by qualified physicians, provided that the patient is wealthy and has the appropriate contacts. It is true

Table 13/3

The actual birth rate related to the theoretical birth rate in Latin American nations

Country	*Birth rate per* 1,000 1965–70	*Difference from theoretical birth rate*	*Percentage urban population to total population*
Uruguay	22	−28	84
Chile	28	−22	74
Venezuela	46	− 4	76
Argentina	22	−28	71
Cuba	31	−19	58
Mexico	43	− 7	58
Colombia	43	− 7	55
Brazil	39	−11	54
Peru	43	− 7	46
Ecuador	46	− 4	38
Guatemala	45	− 5	37
Bolivia	44	− 6	25
Haiti	48	− 2	18

Source: Derived from Viel.

that many of the psychiatric grounds are spurious, and that in fact the abortion is performed for social reasons, but both patient and physician are protected against prosecution by this arrangement. In the period before legalized abortion was introduced in Britain, it was estimated that about five times as many therapeutic abortions were performed on the private service as on the public (National Health) service, although over 85 per cent of the population used the latter. Similar findings were obtained in a survey in the U.S.A. made in 1967 under the auspices of the American College of Obstetricians and Gynaecologists and the American Public Health Association. This showed the overall ratio of abortions to deliveries amongst private patients was 3·3 per 1,000, and amongst public patients it was only 1·1 per 1,000; but in areas such as New York the difference was tenfold to twentyfold. As will be shown later, the same pattern obtains in nations in East Asia and North Africa.

The real dangers of illegally induced abortions affect the poor, the under-educated, the under-privileged, and the fatalistic

Table 13/4

The constraints influencing acceptance of birth control, and the ease of obtaining an abortion in nations where it is illegal

Poor (Lower Socio-economic Groups)	*Affluent* (Upper Socio-economic Groups)
Limited sex education or knowledge of reproductive physiology	Some sex education or knowledge of reproductive physiology
Limited knowledge of contraception	Some knowledge of contraception
Limited access to contraceptives	Good access to contraceptives
Poor referral services for abortion	Good referral services for abortion
Complicated, time-consuming maze of medical system in public hospital	Early access to private gynaecologists
Hostile, punitive attitudes of staff, especially nurses	Absence of punitive attitudes
'Paramedical' or non-medical abortionists sought	Medical abortionists
Dangerous abortions; high incidence of sequelae	Safe abortions; low incidence of sequelae
Lack of money to obtain safe abortion	Sufficient money to obtain safe abortion
Absence of counselling after abortion	Availability of counselling after abortion

(Table **13/4**). From studies in the Americas, a stereotype can be made. In Latin America, the patient seeking an illegally induced abortion is aged 25 to 29, of the lower socio-economic groups, has three children already and has lived in an urban slum for about five years. She either tries to abort herself by introducing a caustic substance or a wooden (or metal) stick into her cervix, or she goes to an unqualified amateur who inserts some object into the uterine cavity. She has a considerable chance of developing infection, and in Brazil 20 per cent of maternity beds are occupied by aborting or aborted women; more seriously, she has a 1 in 100 to 1 in 200 chance of dying. This equals a mortality of 1,000 to 2,000 per 100,000 abortions.

In North America, particularly in States where induced abortion is still illegal, the stereotype is similar; but the death rate is much lower. Again reliable information is impossible to obtain, but a mortality of 50 to 100 per 100,000 abortions is likely, and induced abortion accounts for 20 to 30 per cent of all maternal deaths. In the U.S.A., in addition to married women, a considerable number of abortions are sought by single women, under the age of 25, who are prepared to go through marked indignities (including copulation by the abortionist) to prevent the unwanted birth.

In both areas, illegally induced abortions are common, but only the educated, the wealthy and the knowledgeable woman can obtain an abortion safely and with no loss of dignity. The poor woman is not only ill-informed about human reproductive physiology, but is also ignorant of contraceptive methods, and is discriminated against in her efforts to secure a safe abortion. As Beasley has written: 'Most of these women lack the sophistication to consider the possibility of a therapeutic abortion and the aggressiveness to pursue this through the institutions of medical care that are available to them.' The poor woman has only three choices: she may induce the abortion herself; she may submit to a cheap, crudely performed, dangerous, induced abortion; or she may continue the pregnancy and bear an unwanted child.

If she choses to procure an abortion she is particularly likely to develop the late sequelae of an unskilfully performed operation. The main problems result from infection, which may cause chronic pelvic pain, or chronic ill health and be followed by permanent sterility. In contrast, late sequelae following skilfully performed termination of pregnancy are uncommon, as will be shown later.

The effect of this economic discrimination is not only damaging to the woman, but if she fails to obtain an abortion and delivers an unwanted child may be damaging to it in that its health (in the WHO sense) is often impaired. A study in Sweden, which has excellent social services, by Forssman and Thuwe, of the children of 120 mothers who had been refused abortion in 1939–41, showed that the unwanted children were worse off than the controls in many respects. In this study the controls were the next, same-sexed children born in the same hospital. During the 21 years' observational period it became obvious that children who were born because their mothers were not allowed legal abortion had to face greater disadvantages and had an inferior station in life. They had more health problems, more psychiatric problems, were more likely to show anti-social and criminal tendencies and their educational attainments were poorer. All this 'indicated the handicapped position of the unwanted child'.

If this was the situation amongst affluent Swedes who have good educational and social services, the situation for unwanted children in less social-service-minded Western nations would be far worse. Of course, this would not apply in many nations in the developing world, for the child would be accepted from birth as part of the family group.

Legal Abortion

By 1970, about 30 per cent of the population of the world are living in nations, or in parts of nations, where humanitarian and social indications, as well as medical prophylactic reasons, exist for legally inducing an abortion (Table **13/5**). The exact conditions under which abortion may be obtained vary between the nations, but in the more advanced, abortion for social indications is restricted to termination before the 12th gestational week, by a qualified person, performed in a clinic

Table 13/5

Legal abortion

Nation	*Ratio per* 100 *live births*			
	1955	1960	1965	1972 *or latest*
Sweden	4	3	5	10
Denmark	7	5	6	12
Finland	4	7	6	12
Czechoslovakia	1	41	34	47
Yugoslavia	0	18	37	34
Hungary	17	111	136	127
Japan	21	68	47	36
Britain	—	—	1	16
U.S.A.	—	—	2	20

or hospital, and no further termination is permitted within 12 months. In addition, the women are given contraceptive advice. The reasons for these restrictions will become apparent later, but it must be recorded that in none of the nations mentioned has illegal induced abortion been eliminated. The numbers have dropped, but because of the restrictions, however minor they are to the educated, a number of the least educated, most harassed, poorest women still induce an abortion themselves or seek the services of an amateur abortionist. (It should also be noted that no nation has repealed all abortion laws, leaving the decision to the woman and her doctor.) The world-wide trend is to increasing liberalization of the abortion laws, usually in the interest of the health and dignity of the woman; and to emancipate her from perpetual childbearing. If this is indeed the aim, widespread contraceptive knowledge and facilities must also be made available to women. It is regrettable, medically and biologically, that in Britain, for example, over half the legal abortions performed in 1971 were on women who had not used any contraceptives. When questioned on this, the answer was almost invariably that the woman did not think that she would become pregnant. As Slome points out: 'What better indication is there that sex education is necessary, or that it is inadequate?'

MEDICAL INDICATIONS FOR ABORTION

In the years before permissive abortion laws were introduced, abortion was permitted in several nations if, in the opinion of the medical attendants, the continuation of the pregnancy would cause grave hazard to the life or health of the mother. In these cases, the medical reasons were clearly defined, and have been discussed in *Fundamentals of Obstetrics and Gynaecology*. The abortion to live birth ratio for abortions done for medical reasons was less than 1 per 1,000 live births. In addition, abortion was performed on psychiatric grounds more frequently, and this showed a positive correlation with the wealth and education of the patient. This finding, which has been documented in Australia, Britain, Canada and the U.S.A., led to the gibe that a wealthy woman who wished to terminate an unwanted pregnancy sought a psychiatrist and had a legal termination performed under safe conditions, but a poor, ill-educated woman sought an abortionist and had a dangerous, undignified abortion.

In nations with liberalized abortion laws, medical or psychiatric reasons which are genuine, account for a very small minority of all terminations of early pregnancy.

MORTALITY AND MORBIDITY OF LEGALLY INDUCED ABORTION

Experience in Eastern Europe has shown that the *mortality* from legally induced abortion should not exceed 1 per 100,000 reported cases if the operation is performed before the 12th, and preferably before the 10th gestational week, in a health institution, by a trained doctor. The mortality increases after the 12th gestational week particularly if the termination is combined with tubal ligation, or so reports from Britain would suggest. In the Registrar General's *1969 Supplement on Abortion*, the mortality rate attributed to abortion was eight times higher after, than it was before, the 12th gestational week, and fourteen times higher if tubal ligation was performed at the time of termination of the pregnancy.

The evidence that termination is much safer if performed before the 12th gestational week is shown in Table **13/6**. It should be noted that whereas 96 per cent of terminations were prior to the 12th gestational week in Hungary, the percentage was 74 in the U.S.A. and fell to just over 65 per cent in Britain. The reason for recommending termination only in health institutions is emphasized by experience in New York, where in 1970–71 the mortality rate for abortions 'in hospital circumstances' was 8 per 100,000, but in 'non-hospital circumstances' it rose to 38 per 100,000.

The conclusion drawn from these studies is that constraints on performing legally induced abortion (such as delays in referring patients, hospital abortion committees, review committees) must be eliminated, so that legal terminations may be made as early in pregnancy as possible, and usually before the end of the 10th gestational week.

The *morbidity* of legally induced abortion is less easy to determine and relates to the period of gestation, the method used, the place where the pregnancy is terminated, and the age of the mother. Once again the most accurate data come from

Table 13/6

The mortality of legally induced abortion

Nation	*Year*	*Number* (1,000's)	*Gestation period*	*Route of termination*	*Mortality per* 100,000 *reported abortions*
Hungary (a)	1968	201	0–12	Vaginal	1
Britain (b)	1969	31	0–12	Vaginal	6
		4		Abdominal	80
		10	13–28	Vaginal	38
		8		Abdominal	90
U.S.A. (c)	1970–71	73	0–12	Vaginal	1·8
			13–24	Vaginal + Abdominal	26·1

Sources:
(a) Klinger, A. 'Induced Abortion', *Int. J. Gynec. Obst.*, **8**, 680, 1970.
(b) *Registrar General Supplement on Abortion, 1969*. London 1971.
(c) Teitze, C., and Lewit, S. *Joint Program for the Study of Abortion.*

Eastern Europe, where almost all terminations are made prior to the 12th gestational week (Table **13/7**).

The morbidity rate rises with increasing duration of pregnancy. For example, in New York, 6·3 per 1,000 patients terminated before the 12th gestational week had immediate complications, and this rate rose to 30·5 per 1,000 when the operation was done after the 12th week.

Remote complications are even more difficult to assess, but there is undoubtedly a rising incidence of low birth weight babies in subsequent pregnancies, and the rate increases with increasing numbers of legal abortions. This finding has been reported from Japan, Hungary and Czechoslovakia. As well, an increase in the incidence of late abortion (15 to 20 weeks) in a pregnancy following a termination performed by the vaginal route after the 10th gestational week has been reported from England (Wright).

When abortion is performed competently, there is no evidence of any increased tendency to ectopic gestation or antepartum haemorrhage, although such sequelae have been mentioned in a few studies; nor is there any increased change in subsequent fertility compared with that following spontaneous abortion.

Table 13/7

Complications of legally induced abortions (*per* 1,000 *abortions*)

	Hungary 1968	*U.S.A.* 1970–71	*Britain (Oxford)* 1968–70	
Number	200,800	53,880	290	522
Gestation period (weeks)	<12	⩽12	⩽10	>10
Immediate complications				
Haemorrhage (>500 ml)	5·7	3·4	100	214
Perforation of uterus	1·1	3·4	3	24
Cervical lacerations	—	9·3	34	55
Infection, pelvic	3·8	2·9	26	40
Remission within 4 *weeks*				
Because of fever	4·5	1·3	} 13	} 44
Because of haemorrhage	8·3	4·7		

Sources:
Hungary: Klinger, A. (See Table 13/6.)
Britain: Stallworthy, J. A. et al. *Lancet*, **2**, 1245, 1971.
U.S.A.: Teitze, C., and Lewit, S. *Studies in Family Planning*, **3**, 97, 1972 (Table 25).

In nations which have a significant number of rhesus-negative women in their population, anti-D gammaglobulin 300 μg should be injected intramuscularly within 48 hours of the termination of the pregnancy, particularly when performed after the 10th gestational week, as a proportion of such women become sensitized and develop antibodies to Rh, which might affect a subsequent fetus.

Although legally induced abortions are not completely harmless, they are far less dangerous than illegally induced abortions, and in both Eastern Europe and the U.S.A., with increasing numbers of legal terminations, the numbers of cases of septic abortion and maternal deaths due to illegal abortion have fallen. In Britain, between 1961 and 1969, there were 3·0 deaths due to presumed illegally induced abortion per 100,000 total births; this had fallen to 1·5 deaths per 100,000 total births in the year 1970–71 when legal abortion was available.

In Yugoslavia, one gynaecologist has calculated that the mortality rate of illegally induced abortion in the period 1963–67 was about 118 per 100,000, whilst that of legally induced abortion was 0·4 per 100,000.

The introduction of legally induced abortion on social or socio-medical grounds has reduced the number of illegally induced abortions, but so far has not eliminated them.

In the initial period after the removal of the restrictive abortion laws, the total number of abortions—legal and illegal—increases, because some pregnancies which would previously be carried to term are terminated. Later the total number of abortions falls, illegal abortions falling more rapidly as increasing numbers of women—and men—use contraceptives.

PSYCHOLOGICAL SEQUELAE OF INDUCED ABORTION

In the period before legally induced abortion was permitted, only a few studies were made of the psychological effects on women recently aborted. Studies from the U.S.A. suggest that about one-fifth of women 'illegally' aborted have transient grief and one quarter have some degree of transient guilt, depending on the social and moral strictures about induced abortion in their cultural background; but the majority of women express great relief and have no regrets. Moreover, very few women develop postabortal psychiatric illness. Kummer, who has made one of the most thorough surveys, concluded that induced abortion 'far from being a precipitator of psychiatric illness, quite to the contrary is actually a defence against such an occurrence in women who are susceptible to mental illness'.

There is evidence from England that the degree of guilt and its duration can be influenced considerably by the attitude adopted by the medical attendants. If the patient is treated with odium and contempt by the nursing and medical staff; if she gets the impression that they consider her to be immoral and a nuisance, her guilt may be magnified—and the psychological sequelae increased. The medical attendants should treat the patients with sympathy and understanding and must avoid imposing their own moral standards on them.

In Sweden, information collated by Ottosson indicates that following legally induced abortion mental disorders (defined as impaired working capacity with sick leave or admission into hospital within a determined time period) were uncommon. In Sweden at the time of his study, abortion tended to be performed after the 12th gestational week. Because of this delay the mother was more likely to have a deeper image of her child and consequently to be more disturbed at its loss, and to have a greater guilt because of the complicated administrative procedures required. The relative paucity of mental upset in Sweden confirms that induced abortion has few psychological sequelae.

In South America where illegally induced abortion is common, Viel states that the less educated woman apparently does not associate abortion with the act of killing a human being and when she has an abortion she feels 'like a soldier killing an unknown enemy in an act of war'.

THE TECHNIQUE OF INDUCING ABORTION

The method used to terminate pregnancy depends on the gestation period, and it is usual to divide this into two segments: (1) termination before the 11th gestational week, (2) termination from the 11th week onwards.

WEEKS 0–10

Two methods are currently available. These are:
(1) evacuation of the uterus using a suction-curette, and
(2) the traditional method of dilatation and curettage.

The suction curette was originally used in 1958 in China, but was improved by work in the U.S.S.R., and a report was published in 1961. The principle is that a negative intra-uterine pressure is established which, by vacuum, strips the early conception from its attachment to the decidua, and by a system of tubes sucks it, and the superficial layer of the decidua, into a container. The patient is either anaesthetized, using thiopentone, or a paracervical nerve block is established. The cervix is dilated, with conventional rodlike dilators, until it is sufficiently wide to permit the introduction of the hollow metal, or glass, curette. For a gestation period of up to 9 weeks, a curette with a diameter of 10 mm is used, and for that of 10–11 weeks, a 12 mm curette is used. The curette is attached by transparent, strong tubing to the suction apparatus and a negative pressure of 0·5 to 0·7 atmosphere is established by an electric motor driving a rotary pump (Figure **13/2**). In China a much simpler apparatus has proved satisfactory, especially in remote rural areas. In this the vacuum is created by burning alcohol. Once the vacuum is established, the curette is gently moved within the cavity of the uterus, an injection of ergometrine 0·25 mg being given intravenously to enhance uterine contractility.

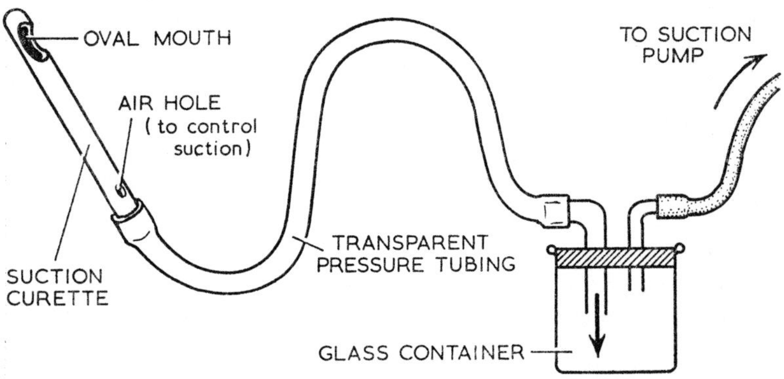

Figure **13/2** The suction-curette apparatus.
Source: Kerslake, D. and Casey, D. *Obstets & Gynec.*, **30**, 35, 1967.

There is no need for hospital admission if the gestation period is less than 8 completed weeks. In a series reported from London, the patient is seen by a doctor and a social worker. If accepted for abortion, she talks further with the social worker who is able to answer her questions, to talk about the value of contraception, and to discuss the explanatory pamphlet (Figure **13/3**). The abortion is scheduled to take place within a week of acceptance at the latest. On the date of operation the patient comes to the clinic and is shown by the social worker to the waiting room, and taken to the operating room by her.

In the operation room, the vagina and cervix are cleansed with povidone-iodine solution and a paracervical block is made using 1 per cent lignocaine which is injected in 4 ml amounts into the cervical tissues at the 12, 4 and 8 o'clock positions. The Karman suction catheter is used. This is a polyethylene tube with a rounded tip and two small eyes in series

Figure **13/3** Information for patients having 'ambulant' abortions. Source: Lewis, B. C. et al. *Brit. Med. J.*, **4**, 606, 1971.

IMPORTANT—PLEASE READ CAREFULLY

You have requested termination of your pregnancy at an early stage. Because of this it will be possible to perform the procedure on an outpatient basis. The method is simple but your co-operation and confidence in the doctor are important if it is to be successful.

When you come to the hospital you will be shown into a small sitting room. After a short discussion with a member of the staff, when you will be able to ask any questions, you will be taken to the examination room, and after getting onto a low bed you will be given a gentle internal examination by the doctor. In order to carry out the termination a plastic tube is passed through the neck of the womb, but it is unusual for you to feel this part of the procedure. You will then hear the sound of a suction machine which empties the womb. The suction may produce a cramp-like discomfort similar to having a normal period but many women have no discomfort at all. The whole procedure takes 5 to 10 minutes. Afterwards you will be able to lie down and you should be ready to go home within 2–3 hours. Coffee or a light lunch is provided.

If you have any anxieties before the termination please do not hesitate to discuss them with the doctor.

(Figure **13/4**). Because of its design a much higher negative pressure can be used safely compared with other suction curettes. The external diameter is 6 mm, so cervical dilatation is usually not required. If it is, the cervix is gently dilated to 7 mm. An intravenous injection of 0·25 mg ergometrine is given. The catheter is inserted and is connected by a transparent tube to an electric suction pump, and a negative pressure of 650 to 725 mm Hg is obtained. If the gestation period is less than 7 completed weeks, the abortion can be done using a Karman curette and a special 50 ml syringe. Karman and Potts claim that it is as efficient as when an electric suction pump is used. The catheter is rotated and moved up and down from the fundus to the cervical os until the cavity has been cleaned, the mean suction time being about three minutes. When the abortion is complete a 'rough' sensation is transmitted to the hands of the operator as the catheter is moved. If it is desired, a small curette can then be introduced.

The patient rests for two or three hours and then goes home, after being given a light meal. In a series reported from London,

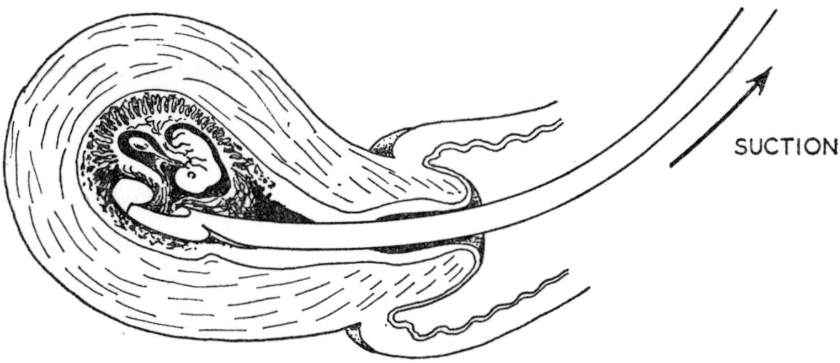

Figure **13/4** The Karman catheter used for terminating early pregnancy. The Karman catheter is a flexible length of polyethylene tubing closed at one end with a rounded tip immediately below which are two eyes placed in series. The eyes are so placed that if the catheter is pushed against the vault of the uterine cavity the tip will collapse rather than perforate the uterus. The catheter and its mode of action when suction is applied are shown in the Diagram. The products of conception are sucked in through the eyes; large portions of placenta or embryo are either compressed or broken up as they enter the catheter lumen. The upper edge of each catheter eye is convex and acts as a curette as the uterine wall is sucked against the catheter.

Lewis et al. (1971) found a mean blood loss of under 75 ml in 133 patients. No patient had excessive bleeding and only one required re-admission for infection. All the patients were interviewed 10 days after the operation and contraceptives supplied.

The advantages of the suction curette over conventional dilatation and curettage are: (1) the total blood loss is less, (2) the complications of uterine perforation and pelvic infection are reduced, (3) the trauma to the uterus is less (Table **13/8**). For example, a report from the U.S.S.R. shows that using the suction curette, fragments of uterine muscle were found in only 8–20 per cent of aspirated specimens, and only single fibres were detected. After conventional curettage, 40–60 per cent of the specimens showed uterine muscle fragments, usually in sheaves.

In 1972, a much larger study of ambulatory abortion was reported by Nathanson from the Center for Reproductive and Sexual Health in New York. This centre performs nearly 2,500 legal abortions each month. All the patients are referred by

Table 13/8

Complications of legally induced abortions using the suction curette and the conventional curette
(*per* 1,000 *abortions*)

Complications	*Suction curette*		*Conventional curette*	
	Yugoslavia	*U.S.A.*	*Yugoslavia*	*U.S.A.*
	10,500	47,618	7,800	3,077
Operative				
Uterine perforation	0·3	3·4	2·5	6·6
Haemorrhage (>300 ml)	1·1	3·4	2·4	5·2
Other injury, shock	0·8	9·4	2·1	9·2
Early postoperative				
Retained products	18·2	6·0	16·0	8·2
Pelvic infection	11·3	2·9	16·8	7·0
Bleeding	6·7	4·7	5·6	10·4
Total complications	38·4	29·8	45·4	46·6

Source:
Jurukovski, J., and Sukarov, L. *Int. J. Gynec. et Obst.*, **9**, 111, 1971.
Teitze, C., and Lewit, S. *Studies in Family Planning*, **3**, 97, 1972, Tables 13, 25.

Protestant clergymen or Jewish rabbis, and only women less than 12 weeks pregnant are accepted. On arrival at the centre the woman has a one-hour private talk with a trained female counsellor in which the reasons for the abortion, its psychological effect, and the technique used are discussed; and a review of birth control methods is made. The counsellor also accompanies the patient through the preliminary laboratory studies, and remains with her during the abortion and through the recovery period. After the initial discussion, if the patient wishes to have the abortion, she is seen by the physician who takes a medical history and performs a complete examination, including a pelvic assessment and a cervical exfoliative smear. If, in his opinion, the patient is fit for an ambulatory abortion, she is given premedication, and the pregnancy is terminated using a technique similar to that in London. After the abortion her vital signs and any vaginal bleeding are monitored for 2 hours by her counsellor, at intervals. After 2 hours she is again seen by the physician, and permitted to go home, having been given instructions to take her oral temperature twice daily for 5 days and to avoid baths and coitus for 14 days. She is told she may contact the centre at any time during this period, and a 24-hour service is provided.

Between July, 1970 and July, 1971, 26,000 abortions were performed with no mortality, and with a low incidence of side-effects (Table **13/9**).

Table 13/9

Ambulant induced abortions. Morbidity in 26,000 abortions performed in New York

Complications	*Rate per* 1,000 *abortions*
Operative	
Perforation or damage to uterus	1·4
Retained products (needing repeat curettage)	3·5
Early postoperative	
Infection (pyrexia 38°C) on two successive days	15·0
Haemorrhage	2·1
	22·0
Later	
Admitted to hospital within two weeks	7·0
TOTAL	29·0

Source: Nathanson, B. N. *New England Med. J.*, **286**, 403, 1972.

It is also significant that in the first year of the operation of the liberal abortion laws in New York, no death was reported from criminal abortion. In addition there was a remarkable decrease in hospital admissions for 'incomplete abortion'. In the first six months these dropped by 50 per cent, and were dropping at the rate of 15 per cent per month at the time of the report (Rovinsky). In Vancouver, Canada, a drop of 25 per cent in the number of 'incomplete abortions' was reported after the adoption of new abortion laws. Clearly the laws have dramatically reduced the number of dangerous, illegally induced abortions.

With increasing experience in many nations, it is becoming clear that terminations in the 11th gestational week and after, either using the suction curette or the conventional curette and ovum forceps, have a rapidly rising rate of complications, and the trend is to refuse to use this method after the end of the 10th gestational week.

WEEK 11 ONWARD

The consensus of opinion has established that two methods are safer and have fewer complications than the many others suggested. These are (1) the use of prostaglandins, and (2) the intra-uterine instillation of hypertonic saline. Both methods are more efficient if the pregnancy is permitted to continue to the 15th gestational week before the termination is performed. If termination is mandatory prior to this time, the methods may be tried, or hysterotomy performed, although this is much more time-consuming, costly and painful.

PROSTAGLANDINS

Prostaglandins were first identified as a physiological constituent of semen in 1935 by von Euler, but it is only since 1964 that their use in the induction of abortion has been studied. The substances are long-chain fatty acids and are found in a wide variety of mammalian tissues. One of their characteristics is to influence the contractile response of smooth muscle, particularly of the reproductive tract and of the gut. This effect is either a direct one, or caused by a prostaglandin-induced oxytocin release from the posterior pituitary gland. The fact that prostaglandins stimulate uterine contractions, at all stages of pregnancy, is the basis of their use in the termination of early pregnancy.

Variations in the configuration of the side-chains have led to the identification of at least 14 prostaglandins, and two of these, E_2 and $F_{2\alpha}$, have been used in gynaecology. PGE_2 is about ten times as potent as $PGF_{2\alpha}$ but is relatively unstable, so that most work has been done on $PGF_{2\alpha}$ or its 15-methyl derivative. 15-methyl $PGF_{2\alpha}$ is dose for dose about 10 times more potent than the parent compound, which makes it equivalent to PGE_2.

To induce an abortion, prostaglandins may be administered by the intravenous, the intra-amniotic or the extra-ovular route. The first is convenient, but is attended by severe nausea and vomiting in 40 per cent of patients, pain along the vein in 25 per cent and diarrhoea in 5 per cent of patients. It effectively induces abortion in the second quarter of pregnancy in about 80 per cent of cases, but in one-quarter of them the abortion is incomplete and the patient requires curettage to remove retained products of conception.

Both the intra-amniotic and the extra-ovular methods seem equally effective, particularly between the 15th and 19th week of pregnancy. The former is more painful and frightening to the patient, whilst the latter requires a more exact technique.

In the intra-amniotic method a fine needle is introduced into the amniotic sac through the abdominal wall, and the prostaglandin injected. We have found that the method is most efficient if the injection is made at 6 p.m., as prostaglandin appears to have a circadian rhythm of effectiveness, and is most active if the injection takes place at this time.

In a series of 111 patients who were all 15 to 19 weeks pregnant when terminated, 30 mg of $PGF_{2\alpha}$ was introduced into the amniotic cavity by thrusting a fine needle through the abdominal wall, after the superficial structures had been infiltrated with local anaesthesia. Care was taken to ensure that the tip of the needle was in the amniotic sac, and a fine polythene catheter was introduced through the needle, after which it was withdrawn. Prostaglandin was only injected if clear amniotic fluid was withdrawn through the catheter. The mean injection-abortion interval was 23·7 hours (range 5–61 hours). Gestational age made no significant difference, but the interval was longest in nulliparae. A repeat injection was required in 16 per cent of patients who failed to abort within 24 hours. Sixty per cent of patients vomited at least once, and 15 per cent had diarrhoea during the induction-abortion interval. Curettage for incomplete abortion was required in 40 per cent of patients (Shearman et al.).

Originally, the extra-ovular method required repeated

2-hourly injections of $PGF_{2\alpha}$ through a catheter introduced into the lower part of the uterine cavity via the cervical canal. This reduced the value of the method. The development of the 15-methyl analogue of $PGF_{2\alpha}$ has altered this. The 15-methyl $PGF_{2\alpha}$ appears to have increased potency and a more prolonged uterine stimulating action than the parent substance. This means that when given either intra-amniotically, or particularly by the extra-ovular route, it is more efficient and there is less need for the injection to be repeated.

If the extra-ovular route is chosen, the method is as follows. The patient is put in the lithotomy position and the vulva and vagina are cleansed. The cervix is exposed using a speculum and it is carefully cleansed. A Nelaton catheter (5F) or a Foley catheter, which is cut off just distal to the balloon, is introduced so that the tip of the former and the base of the balloon of the latter lies just above the internal cervical os. The balloon is then filled with about 10 ml fluid. The dose of prostaglandin (currently 800 μg 15-m-$PGF_{2\alpha}$) is mixed with 10 ml dextran and is injected slowly, any reflux being noted and estimated. Finally 2 ml of dextran is injected. The Nelaton catheter is removed, the Foley catheter left in situ under slight tension to prevent leakage. If contractions are not established in 12 hours, a further injection is given. The injection is quite painless. Between 75 and 85 per cent of the 41 patients, studied by Wiqvist, aborted within 24 hours, the mean injection-abortion interval being 15 hours. The mean number of episodes of vomiting or diarrhoea was 2, and 35 per cent of women required curettage for incomplete abortion (Wiqvist).

INTRA-UTERINE SALINE

The Swedish workers, particularly Bengtsson, have the greatest experience of this method. In general, it is advisable to wait until the period of gestation is at least 16 weeks when there is between 150 and 225 ml of amniotic fluid. The 20 per cent sterile saline is introduced into the amniotic sac after the equivalent amount of amniotic fluid has been removed. Under local anaesthesia a 14 gauge needle, 10 to 15 cm long, is introduced perpendicularly into the amniotic sac at a point midway between the uterine fundus and the symphysis pubis, and amniotic fluid, which may at first be blood-stained, is permitted to flow. When it is flowing freely, a 5F Teflon catheter is introduced through the needle and a further 15 to 33 cm into the amniotic cavity. The needle is then withdrawn over the catheter and as much amniotic fluid as possible is withdrawn. The hypertonic solution is then injected using a 50 ml syringe and a three-way stopcock. The amount injected should not exceed that withdrawn by more than 20 per cent, and no more than 200 ml should be injected. The injection should be made slowly, taking up to 30 minutes to complete. Since the injection leads to an increase in the maternal blood volume (up to 1,400 ml), to temporary hypernatraemia (up to 160 mEq per litre) and to increased osmolarity, the method should be avoided in patients with cardiac or renal disease, or with pre-eclampsia. The injection must be stopped at once if the patient complains of pain, headache, dizziness, tingling or numbness in the fingers or heat in the upper part of the body, as these signs indicate possible intravascular injection. During removal of the catheter it should be flushed with saline (or aqueous penicillin 1 million units) to avoid spill of the salt solution into the peritoneal cavity.

Blood clotting defects—consumption coagulopathy—may follow saline-induced abortion in a small, but unknown, number of cases. The condition appears to be due to damage to the placenta and the release of thromboplastins into the maternal circulation. Consumption coagulopathy is more likely to follow a short amniocentesis-labour interval, and is associated with haemorrhage. The defects remedy themselves spontaneously, without treatment, after the abortion is complete. Excess bleeding requires that the blood loss must be replaced rapidly, but the use of heparin, fibrinogen or EACA seems to be associated with serious complications.

The average time-lag between the injection and the onset of labour is 20 $\pm$ 10 hours and the injection-expulsion interval is 40 $\pm$ 15 hours. If labour has not started in 24 hours, a dilute oxytocin infusion may be set up. About 20 per cent of patients will require curettage to remove retained placental tissue if this has not been expelled spontaneously within 12 hours of the birth of the fetus.

Careful studies by Gustavii, working in Bengtsson's department, indicated that intravascular injection may be more common than usually stated. It has proved fatal in a small number of cases.

In order to reduce this hazard, Gustavii suggests giving the hypertonic saline by the extra-ovular route, and claims the method is successful from the 12th week of gestation. He uses a Foley catheter which has been shortened by cutting off the tip just distal to the balloon. The catheter is introduced so that the balloon lies just above the internal cervical os. The balloon is filled with 10 ml of fluid, and the catheter is pulled back so that the balloon acts as a 'plug' in the cervix. 7·5–10 ml of 20 per cent NaCl per week of pregnancy is injected slowly, taking 5 to 10 minutes. The patient is questioned about signs of intravascular injection. On completion of the injection the catheter is fixed by adhesive tape to the gluteal region, so that the 'plug' is leak-proof. It is removed after 2 hours.

The saline rapidly spreads between the decidua and the conceptus, and is apparently absorbed into the amniotic fluid and by the decidual cells within 4 hours. Gustavii believes that the damaged decidual cells and the placenta adjacent to the amnion release prostaglandins which in turn provoke uterine activity, and abortion.

ABORTION RECIDIVISM

Between 5 and 7 per cent of women whose pregnancy is terminated by induced abortion seek a further termination within 12 months. Many of these are unmarried, nulliparous women. These women are also more likely to fail to take prescribed oral contraceptives regularly. Experience has shown that IUD insertion may safely be performed at the time of pregnancy termination, and it is recommended that this method of contraception should be offered to women who are likely to be abortion recidivists.

The Effect of Legal Abortion on Health

The impact of systems of legal abortion on public health are difficult to gauge, and any results must be considered tentative. Experience from Eastern European nations indicates that after liberalization of abortion laws hospital admissions for other abortions declined.

The effect of legal abortion on neonatal and maternal mortality is even harder to determine. Neonatal mortality has been declining in most developing nations, and the introduction of legal abortion does not appear to have accelerated the trend. However, evidence from New York State shows that since 1971, when the new abortion laws were introduced, maternal mortality has dropped by 65 per cent to the lowest rate of maternal deaths ever recorded.

The Effect of Refusal to Grant an Abortion

Under the liberalized abortion laws adopted by many Western nations, between 10 and 20 per cent of women requesting, or being referred for termination of pregnancy, are refused. Since medical responsibility for the patient must not cease when the abortion is refused, it is important to know what counselling was given to these women and what was the outcome of the pregnancy. Two studies have been made in Britain to answer the question. The basis of refusal in most instances was that the only reason for the request was that the pregnancy was unwanted, and the physician could find no 'significant threat to the mental or physical health of the mother or her existing children', so that the request fell outside the provisions of the Abortion Act. In a study in London of 105 women who were refused termination, 10 per cent had a spontaneous abortion; 50 per cent accepted the decision and continued the pregnancy, and two of these women developed significant mental illness. The remaining 40 per cent obtained termination elsewhere, and 4 out of the 40 developed serious complications, one girl nearly dying from infection. In Sweden, between 1964 and 1966, when women seeking termination were required to be interviewed by a committee, and consequently termination tended to be after the 12th gestation week, 27 per cent of those seeking abortion were refused. Of them over 80 per cent continued with the pregnancy, but as had been noted, the child was at a handicap compared with his peers.

The Place of Legally Induced Abortion in a Family Planning Programme

In the past five years, significant changes have occurred in many nations in their attitude towards induced abortion. In nations such as Britain, and the States of the United States of America, where previously induced abortion was illegal (with a very few exceptions for 'medical grounds'), the change has been to a more liberal approach and to the virtual legalization of induced abortion on social grounds. This change has come about for several reasons. Firstly, it was realized that the law was being flouted, and despite the penalties a very considerable number of unwanted pregnancies were being terminated by the woman herself, or by resorting to unqualified abortionists. A law which proves to be consistently broken is a bad law. Secondly, statistical data increasingly showed that these illegal abortions were followed by a considerable morbidity due to infection and haemorrhage. Thirdly, safe induced abortion was available to the rich who, on considerable payment, were able to obtain the services of medically qualified abortionists; whilst the poor, whose need was greater, had neither the knowledge nor the financial resources to obtain safe abortion. This inequitable situation existed, and continues to exist, in many nations. For example, a report from Turkey in 1971, when induced abortion was illegal, indicated that 15 to 18 induced abortions were taking place for every 100 live births, but that the incidence was highest amongst the wives of professional and business men. This strong association between higher income and abortion was also reported from Iran, Iraq and the United Arab Republic where illegal abortions are ten times as frequently performed amongst women of the upper socio-economic groups than amongst needy and impoverished citizens.

Over the same period, several nations in Eastern Europe which previously virtually offered abortion on demand, have introduced restrictions in an effort to place abortion within the group of methods of birth control. Prior to the widespread use of the oral contraceptives and the introduction of the IUD, the available methods had militated against their use on a wide scale, and legally induced abortion had been introduced as a family welfare measure. However, now that modern effective contraceptive methods are available, restrictions are beginning to be placed on 'abortion on demand'.

There are several reasons for this. In the first place, statistics indicate that the morbidity following legally induced abortion increases with increasing frequency of termination in the same woman. Not only are immediate complications greater, but in subsequent pregnancies there appears to be a raised spontaneous abortion rate, possibly an increased chance of ectopic gestation, and a rising rate of premature births. Secondly, abortion on demand may lead to a neglect of contraception. Investigations in Canada (Claman) and New York (Rovinsky) showed that between 5 and 10 per cent of women who were aborted repeated the process within one year. Thirdly, induced abortion as the sole method to control the rate of population growth is inefficient. The interval between two consecutive pregnancies has three components: (1) the duration of the pregnancy itself, (2) the anovulatory phase after childbirth, which is increased by lactation, and (3) the re-established ovulatory phase, when the chance of pregnancy occurring in any one month varies between zero and 0·9, with a mean of about 0·8. Induced abortion, as a method of birth control, reduces component 1 from 40 weeks to 12 weeks and eliminates component 2, so that between 2 and 3 abortions are needed to avert one birth.

The WHO Technical Report on Spontaneous and Induced Abortion gives an illustration of this. In a population which has uncontrolled fertility, the annual pregnancy rate would be about the biological maximum which is 60 per 1,000 population. Since 10 to 15 per cent of pregnancies end as spontaneous abortion, the effective crude birth rate would be 50 per 1,000. To reduce the birth rate by half (to 25 per 1,000) by means of induced abortion alone, without contraception, would require between 50 and 75 induced abortions per 1,000 population, and because of the reduction in pregnancy intervals would increase the pregnancy rate to about 100 per 1,000 population (i.e. birth rate + spontaneous abortion rate + induced abortion rate). If, on the other hand, the population reduced its birth rate to 25 per 1,000 by the use of contraception, a further decrease to 20 would require only about 5 induced abortions per 1,000 population. This is clearly a much more satisfactory approach, but it requires an intensive and extensive campaign to disseminate the awareness of contraceptives, to make them freely available to men and women, and to motivate couples to use family planning methods.

Czechoslovakia has adopted this approach, and consideration is currently being given to: (1) increased sex education and 'education for planned and conscientious parenthood' (which will include knowledge of contraceptive techniques) in schools, (2) prohibiting induced abortion after the 10th gestational week, except for medical reasons, (3) extending the minimal interval between legal interruptions to at least 12 months (Kotasek, 1971). In Hungary where 95 per cent of legally induced abortions are on social grounds, and 92 per cent of them are performed before the 12th week, and in Yugoslavia, similar changes are under consideration.

In Britain, despite the Family Planning Act of 1968 which gave local authorities power to establish birth control clinics, by 1971 only a few had done so. Doctors, too, tended to offer moral advice when women, particularly young unmarried women, sought contraceptives. In 1968, the Abortion Act became operative and the numbers of induced abortions have risen from 58,000 in 1969, to 87,000 in 1970, and to 127,000 in 1971. The rise continues. Despite these measures, estimates by the Select Committee on Science and Technology in 1971 of unwanted pregnancies in Britain, show that they numbered between 200,000 and 300,000 each year. This is a disturbing figure for many will become unwanted children, at special risk of becoming antisocial adults. Furthermore, data concerning the legal terminations indicate more than 70 per cent might have been avoided by the use of contraception.

The answer does not lie in increasing abortions. The fault in Britain was that the liberalization of the abortion laws was not preceded by a campaign to encourage the attitude that unless a child is wanted, coitus without contraception is selfish and socially irresponsible, and by ensuring that contraceptives were freely and readily available.

Similar findings from countries with diverse political and philosophical attitudes place legally induced abortion in its proper perspective in relation to other birth control measures. The conclusions are: (1) Any nation introducing more liberal abortion laws or repealing all abortion laws to permit abortion on demand should concurrently introduce sex education, including education in sexual responsibility and contraceptive techniques, into schools so that children have knowledge and insight into human sexuality, sexual responsibility and contraceptive techniques within a year of puberty at the latest. (2) Facilities should be provided for *all* women to obtain contraceptive advice readily, without moral questions being asked, without financial hardship and preferably without payment. (3) A campaign of information should be mounted, in which the benefits of preventing conception and the irresponsibility of coitus without contraception, unless pregnancy is wanted, are detailed. (4) Legally induced abortion should be made readily and easily available for those women who become pregnant through ill-fortune, ignorance or ill-luck provided that, in general (the main exception being medical conditions), the termination is sought and performed prior to the 10th week of pregnancy. (5) Following the termination, the women should be expected to agree solemnly to use approved methods of birth control in the future, and to understand that the request for the termination of a subsequent pregnancy in the next 12 months is unlikely to be granted. As the Chairman of the British Abortion Law Reform Association, Madelaine Simms has pointed out: 'The law (in Britain) was reformed to assist those women who were the victims of great misfortune—the women whose mental or physical health would deteriorate if they had another baby, the women who were in danger of giving birth to a deformed child, the women living in dreadful housing conditions with sick or inadequate husbands and too many children already. The law was *not* reformed to enable foolish middle-class girls to dispense with birth control, or to replace rational behaviour with the most vacuous type of mindless femininity.'

Used responsibly, legally induced abortion has a defined place amongst the methods currently available for controlling population growth, for improving family welfare, and for preventing unwanted, unwelcomed births. It is clear, however, that the consensus is that it should generally be a 'back-stop' to deal with failure of contraceptive methods. A statistical model explaining this view is shown in Table **13/10**. Equally it is quite hypocritical to urge people to adopt family planning but to withhold help when such planning fails.

Table 13/10

Statistical model showing the annual pregnancy rates and death rates per 100,000 coitally active fertile women using various methods of birth control in the developed and developing nations

	Developing nations		*Developed nations*	
	Pregnancies	*Deaths*	*Pregnancies*	*Deaths*
1. No contraception, no abortion	40,000	120	60,000	12
2. No contraception, all pregnancies terminated by illegal abortion	80,000	320	120,000	60
3. No contraception, all pregnancies terminated by legal abortion	80,000	4·8	120,000	2·4
4. Highly effective contraception (orals)	(70)	0·3	(70)	3·0
5. Moderately effective contraception (12% failure), no abortion	4,800	14·4	7,200	1·4
6. Moderately effective contraception, all pregnancies illegally terminated	4,800	19·2	7,200	3·6
7. Moderately effective contraception, all unwanted pregnancies terminated by legal abortion	4,800	0·28	7,200	0·14

Notes:

The following assumptions were made:

1. In any given year, 60 per cent of sexually active, fertile women in the developed nations will become pregnant, but because of prolonged breast feeding only 40 per cent of women in the developing nations will become pregnant. In the absence of lactation pregnancy occurs between 4 and 8 months after the return of ovulation. (Line 1)
2. The maternal mortality (excluding that due to abortion) is estimated at 20 per 100,000 live births in the developed nations and 300 per 100,000 live births in the developing nations. (Lines 1–7)
3. The mortality associated with illegally induced abortion is 50 per 100,000 abortions in the developed nations and 400 per 100,000 abortions in the developing nations. (Lines 2, 6)
4. The mortality from legal abortion performed in hospital prior to the 12th gestational week is 2 per 100,000 abortions, and it is assumed that in the developing nations it will be three times as high, at least initially. (Lines 3, 7)
5. If a woman does not use contraception and seeks abortion within the first 10 weeks of pregnancy, the interval between pregnancies is assumed to be 10 + 4 weeks anovulation + 16 weeks ovulation before a new conception. She will therefore require to have, on average, 2 abortions per year. As

40,000 women in the developing nations become pregnant each year, 80,000 abortions will be needed; the number of abortions needed in the developed nations will be 120,000. (Line 2)

6. The number of pregnancies in Lines 5 and 6 is calculated by assuming that no women using the moderately effective contraceptives are lactating, and that 12 per cent of them will become pregnant (see Table **12/9**). But in Line 1, it was assumed that only 40,000 and 60,000 women respectively using no contraception would become pregnant. Therefore the number of pregnancies is 12 per cent of 40,000 and 60,000 (i.e. 4,800 and 7,200).
7. The mortality from thromboembolic disease associated with the use of oral contraceptives is 3 per 100,000 in the developed nations, and 0·3 per 100,000 in the developing nations. (Line 4)

Source: Derived from Tietze, C. 'Mortality with Contraception and Induced Abortion', *Studies in Family Planning*, **45**, 6 (Sept. 1969); and personal correspondence with Dr. Tietze.

FOURTEEN

The Campaign for Fertility Control and Family Welfare

The success or failure of a campaign to reduce the birth rate (and consequently the rate of population growth) will depend, ultimately, on the decisions made by many individuals within the constraints of their cultural and environmental background. Although, within limits, these decisions can be influenced by rewards and sanctions, the final choice is made by an individual woman and an individual man determining *not* to have further children. And since by far the highest proportion of the people who have to make the decision are poor, middle-class attitudes and values may be inappropriate. To a middle-class couple the reason for delaying conception, or deciding to have no additional children, is based on a reasonably informed opinion by people who consider planning a necessary factor in many aspects of life, and who have the capacity to wait for the gratification of a need. To many of the poor these attitudes are unaccustomed and luxurious. The women tend to be fatalistic, resigned and more concerned with the present than the future. They want immediate gratification as, all too frequently, calls for delay have meant that what they sought was never acquired.

In Western societies there is an additional factor. This is that an increasing number of pregnancies occur to single girls, and add a large fraction to the total of unwanted, unwelcome pregnancies which occur in the community.

In this discussion it is assumed that any limitation of natality will be voluntary, and that in present circumstances, no government, of whatever political philosophy, will introduce compulsory measures to reduce natality.

As I pointed out in Chapter 9, two concurrent approaches are required. The first is to induce new attitudes to the desirability of having many children, in other words to alter people's attitudes towards natality. The second is to make available birth control measures which, if used throughout the population, will ensure that every pregnancy is a wanted pregnancy, and every child is a wanted child. In this chapter those measures which seek to achieve the second aim will be considered, although I believe that the attitudinal changes engendered by the adoption of the norms of folk-heroes or trend-setters, and those induced by anti-natalist taxation, need to be more widespread if the goal of a zero population growth rate, or at least a markedly reduced growth rate, is to be reached. There is a difference between population control and birth control. Population control is the regulation of family size by a society; birth control only regulates the size of individual families. Until the attitude of society is changed so that women want fewer children (both in the affluent developed nations and in the hungry developing nations), progress to a markedly reduced rate of population growth will be slow; and those most likely to adopt the new attitudes are the more affluent women within a nation.

The Campaign for Population Control

Essentially there are three methods to achieve control of population growth: the first is nihilistic. It is to wait until social and economic change, by increasing the urban population and by more rapid industrialization, lead to a change in attitude to natality. This is what happened during the nineteenth century in the European nations. There is some doubt that there is time for this approach to be effective as the current rate of population growth is double that of a hundred years ago. In addition it increases the utilization of scarce mineral and water resources, and may produce increasing environmental pollution.

The second approach is to educate people so that their attitudes alter, and that an ideology glorifying small families is developed. This implies that the leaders of society take the lead in encouraging this attitude. Stycos has written about the problem in Latin America. He has pointed out that amongst the leaders of the 290 million people three main groups can be identified. The first are the conservatives, who are concerned with preserving existing society, and who hold that people make a nation strong. They reluctantly concede that social change must occur, but resist its onset, and are more concerned with suppressing any revolutionary tendencies. On rational grounds the conservatives might be expected to encourage family planning as this would reduce the social expenditure required for young dependants, without unduly diminishing the labour force of peasants and unskilled workers. The reality is different. The conservatives are split in their attitudes because of their identification with the hierarchy of the Roman Catholic Church. Although many of them use birth control measures themselves, they would oppose the dissemination of contraceptive knowledge, and appliances, to the mass of the people.

The second group are the revolutionaries who seek violent revolutionary change. If they fail to achieve this, they are anxious that the conservative status quo is maintained since it encourages revolution, as the expectations of the people are increasingly ignored. In their opinion social reform, by offering some amelioration of living for the mass of the people, will delay the ultimate revolution. In theory they should reject any population, or birth, control, but since most are marxist in philosophy, they support it to some extent, in so far as birth control leads to the emancipation of women.

The third group comprises the social reformers who wish to see social change brought about by peaceful means, but accept that if this is not possible, revolution is better than the status quo. This group is mainly middle class in attitude, and supports both population and birth control to a large extent, although their attitudes are influenced by the dicta of the Roman Catholic Church.

If the experience of Latin America can be extrapolated to other developing nations, considerable effort will be required to induce attitudinal changes amongst the leaders of many nations, although, as will be seen in the next section, attitudinal changes are occurring at an increasing rate amongst them and amongst women of all classes within the countries.

The third approach is not to seek to motivate leaders, or individual women and their husbands, but to make contraceptive technology so easy and the appliances so readily available that no motivation is required. Obviously increased research to produce the 'perfect contraceptive' is desirable even though the goal is unlikely to be achieved. But merely to rely on technology without inducing attitudinal changes is unlikely to be successful.

From this it would appear that the most successful approach is a multiple one. Efforts must be made to change the ideology of the nation's leaders, and of the people, to one of desiring small families. Concurrently, efforts must be made to enable women who have made the ideological change to achieve their new goals with the minimal inconvenience to their social and sexual lives.

Pro-Natal and Anti-Natal Attitudes

The psychological change to the desire to limit the number of children in the family is recent. Until about 1880 in the developed nations, and until 1930—50 years later—in the hungry developing nations, high natality was the desired norm. This was because high infant and childhood mortality reduced the number of children a woman would be able to rear to puberty. When, on average, one in every three children died in infancy and childhood, and when custom demanded two or more sons, a woman needed to have between six and eight children, which meant ten or more pregnancies. Today, when infant and childhood mortality has fallen to less than 100 per 1,000, a family can achieve its desires by having fewer children, confident that most will survive. Moreover, the introduction of compulsory education, at least to the age of 10, has reduced the economic value of numerous children. They are no longer potential producers, but are actual consumers.

That the attitudinal change to smaller families is slow, particularly in rural areas, is not unexpected as the requirement for large families is a product of 10,000 years of tradition.

There is fairly strong evidence that in the first 500,000 years of human differentiation man was a carnivorous hunter. Leakey's discoveries in Olorgesaillie in the Rift Valley in Kenya suggests that man's ancestor had developed weapons and lived by hunting. In discussing the implications of this, Ardrey in *The Social Contract* suggests that the short, light-weight, thin-skinned, small-toothed man could only survive if he formed co-operative hunting bands and carefully separated the duties of males and females. He believes that a hunting band consisted of 50 people at the most; and was made up of 9 to 11 male adults and sub-adults, the rest being women and children. The division was necessary, as of all the primates man is the only one which feeds its young after the time of weaning. The women looked after the boys too young to hunt, and the girls too young to reproduce. The men hunted. If the band became too large, one can speculate that infanticide was practised, or its survival would be in danger.

Then, some 10,000 years ago, man learned to cultivate grains and to domesticate animals. With settlement came territoriality; with territoriality came conflict with other tribes. Over the next 5,000 years, as more and better food was produced, more children survived (although the infant mortality must have been extremely high), and children became valued increasingly. The larger the tribe, the more hands there were to cultivate the soil and to herd the animals; the more males, the stronger the tribe was to resist attacks; the more females, the larger was the annual birth rate. A pro-natalist attitude had begun: children became valuable.

Today, as has been noted, conditions have changed dramatically. As a consequence of the impact of environmental sanitary engineering, the improvement of supplies of uninfected water, the better distribution of foodstuffs, the introduction of insecticides (which have reduced insect-borne diseases, such as malaria), and the effect of modern medical techniques, which include vaccines and antibiotics, few children die. Never before have so many children reached puberty and started to reproduce. This is unique in human history. It has led to the explosive rate of population growth, and to the acceptance by opinion leaders and key politicians that the pro-natalist policies of the past must be replaced by an anti-natalist, or at least a neutral policy in the future.

K.A.P. SURVEYS

This change in attitude has reached, and permeated, the more affluent sections of society, but has been slow to reach the underprivileged, the poor and the fatalistic. The I.P.P.F. and the Population Council have conducted surveys in many nations in which women are asked their ideal family size and their actual completed family size. As can be seen in Table **14/1,**

Table 14/1

The relationship between the actual family size and the 'ideal' family size, from K.A.P. surveys in several nations

Country	*Completed family size*	*'Ideal' family size*	*'Ideal' to completed (per cent)*
Ghana (urban)	7·0	5·3	76
Tunisia (national)	5·9	4·3	73
Korea (national)	5·4	4·2	78
Taiwan (urban)	5·5	3·9	71
Thailand (rural)	5·2	3·8	73
Turkey (national)	5·8	3·5	60
Colombia (urban)	4·8	3·6	75
Venezuela (urban)	4·3	3·5	81
Mexico (urban)	5·0	4·2	84
Panama (urban)	3·8	3·5	92
Brazil (urban)	3·3	2·7	82
Costa Rica (urban)	4·3	3·6	83
Japan (national)	2·0	2·8	—
Hungary (national)	2·5	2·4	96
France (national)	2·8	2·7	96
U.S.A.	2·9	2·4	83
Philippines	5·9	5·0	85

Source: Berelson, B. 'K.A.P. Studies on Fertility', in *Family Planning and Population Programs*, University of Chicago Press, 1966, p. 658.

most women want fewer children then they actually have, and in most of the surveys the actual number of children born exceed the desired, or ideal, number by more than 60 per cent. These figures have been obtained in K.A.P. studies in various nations. K.A.P. stands for knowledge, attitudes and practice in natality matters. K.A.P. surveys are based on questions asked of a sample of the population by trained interviewers, during interviews lasting between 40 and 80 minutes (Table **14/2**). One of the questions in K.A.P. surveys relates to attitude on family size. Berelson, who has pioneered such studies, admits that it is by no means easy to construct 'a valid instrument to measure' the items under investigation, and notes that the validity of the answers depends to a large extent on the ability

Table 14/2

Coverage of K.A.P. studies

Vital data: marriage age and duration, pregnancy history, live births, living children, fecundity.

Attitude on family size: desired family size, expected family size, ideal number of children, ideal pregnancy interval, desire for more children, discussion of family size with spouse and others, perception of others' attitudes on similar questions.

Attitude on family limitation: approval or disapproval of family limitation in general, of contraception, of sterilization, and of abortion; reasons for approval or disapproval, readiness to practise family planning, willingness to learn methods of family planning, approval or disapproval of government programme for family planning, attitude toward national population growth, source of influence on fertility attitudes, perception of others' attitudes on similar questions.

Knowledge: information about reproductive physiology, including time of conception; knowledge of contraceptive methods, general and specific; perception of recent trends in mortality, especially infant mortality.

Practice: ever, now, and expected practice of family planning by method, when started and sequence, sterilization of either spouse, experience of abortion.

Background characteristics: not only the usual demographic items such as age, education, literacy, religion, and occupation, but also rural-urban origin, household composition and facilities, family structure, interest in education, mobility, and other indices of modernized attitudes.

Source: Berelson, B, 'KAP Studies on Fertility', in *Family Planning and Population Programs*. (Ed. Berelson). Univ. Chicago Press, 1966.

of the questioners. He admits that in their answers they may be biased, but feels they give indications of broad tendencies, which is as much as can be hoped for. The question can also be posed in another way. This is to ascertain the percentage of women interviewed who want no children or no further children. The results, quoted by Berelson, are shown in Figure **14/1**, and indicate that there is a considerable desire to limit family size.

One of the most sophisticated studies is based on an analysis of the statistics of the United States National Fertility Survey (1965) by Bumpass and Westoff. The approach they used was rather different from that used in the K.A.P. studies. In the latter, a woman was asked how many children she would have liked to have, and how many she had had. From this her 'ideal' family size was computed. Her answer to the first question involved a value judgement and was influenced by her natality history, and on the adjustment she and her husband had made to it. Bumpass and Westoff point out that 'it is not at all inconsistent for a couple that has had a child that had been unwanted to state later, on the basis of a satisfactory (even beneficial) adjustment to the unwanted birth, that the size of their family is what they desire'. Because of this they asked a different set of questions, which sought to establish which of a

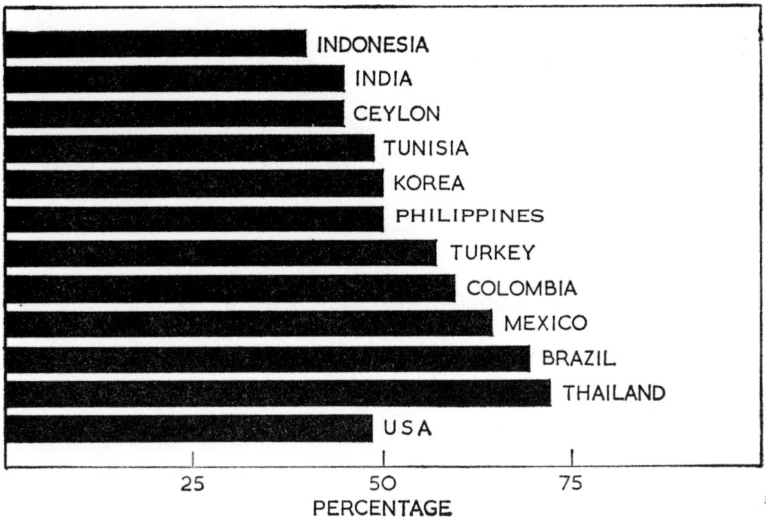

Figure **14/1** The percentage of women in several nations who were found to want no more children during K.A.P. surveys.
Source: Berelson, B., in *Family Planning and Population Programs*, Chicago University Press, 1966, p. 655.

woman's children had been unwanted at the time of conception. Using this method, they were able to infer the desired number of children by subtracting the number of unwanted births from the total number of births. This method indicated a considerably lower estimate of the 'ideal' family size. Whereas K.A.P. studies had shown the desired family size of American women to be 3·3, Bumpass and Westoff's estimate was 2·5. It was noticeable that the number of unwanted births was much higher amongst the poor than the non-poor, amongst the less educated than amongst the better educated, and amongst blacks than

Table 14/3

The percentage of children who were unwanted in the U.S.A. 1960 to 1965

	Percentage unwanted children (1960–65)
Socio-economic Status	
Poor	32
Non-poor	15
Educational Status	
Less than 12 years	26
College	13
Negro	36
White	17
All	19

Poor (and near poor) = non-farm families of 4 with net income less than $5,000 p.a. at 1965 prices.
Source: Bumpass, L., and Westoff, C. E., *Science*, **169,** 1177, 1970.

amongst whites (Table **14/3**). The number also increased amongst both groups, and in the two races, with increasing family size. K.A.P. studies in the countries shown in Table **14/1** indicate that this is a world-wide finding. The higher the income, the lower the desired completed family; the higher the educational level, the lower the desired completed family; and the higher the urbanization of a nation, the lower (on average) is the size of the completed family. Thirty per cent of fourth births, 44 per cent of fifth births and 50 per cent of sixth births or higher were unwanted in the U.S.A. between 1960 and 1965. Bumpass and Westoff calculate that if there was a perfect contraceptive, at least 4·7 million births would have been prevented, and 2 million of these would have been prevented in the 8 per cent of the population designated poor. This calculation is an underestimate, as the analysis was based on a sample of married women living with their husbands in 1965, and did not include births to unmarried women, those separated from their husbands, or those widowed.

A further study, made for the Commission in Population Growth and the American Future, and reported in 1972, showed the percentage of unwanted births increased from about 10 per cent to women with 'college education' to 31 per cent when education ceased before high school. Amongst the least educated women, 25 per cent of births to white women were unwanted, but this rose to 55 per cent amongst black women.

The importance of these analyses is that they indicate that in many nations there is a professed desire by women to reduce the number of children they give birth to, and if this desire can be stimulated and organized a considerable reduction in the birth rate should result. There is also evidence in the studies quoted, and in others made in India, Thailand and Indonesia, that the desire to limit natality is found as much amongst landless labourers as amongst the relatively affluent.

The studies indicate to national political leaders, to health and educational planners, to the media, to the health profession and to interested lay people (all of whose support is essential in any successful campaign for birth control), that the mass of women within a nation do wish to limit family size. The unresolved question is by how much.

FAMILY PLANNING AND FAMILY WELFARE

There is a tendency, currently, to emphasize the effect of the limitation of births on the welfare of the family. The main reason is that the concept of the need to limit population growth because of world, or national, problems it is causing is not readily understood by the great mass of the people. But the concept that high natality may adversely affect the welfare of an individual and his family is more easily accepted.

Family planning as a method of promoting family welfare should be concerned with several activities. In the first place family welfare is promoted by ensuring that all parents, and future parents, have some knowledge of the anatomical, physiological, psychological, social and ethical aspects of sexuality, and by educating them for parenthood. This education aims to show the connection between their reproductive behaviour and their own health and welfare, as well as the welfare and health of their existing children. In addition, family planning seeks to ensure that couples have the number of children they want. This applies as much to the couple who desire children, and have none, as to those who want to practise birth control measures because they have as many children as they desire. Family planning therefore includes the investigation of the infertile couple, and care of the wife throughout a pregnancy should this follow the investigations.

The main activity of family planning is in the area of birth control. As will be discussed, this involves workers in an educational campaign, to encourage individual men and women to start, and to continue, using contraceptive techniques. It involves workers in providing couples with advice about the health implications of childbearing, particularly if the interval between each conception is short, and the effect of this on family welfare. It also involves the worker in the provision of temporary or permanent methods of birth control, and in the continuing service to ensure that the method which the participant has adopted is effective, safe and convenient.

Finally, since family welfare is stressed, it involves the workers in the provision of maternity and child health care, which in the broadest sense includes education in nutrition, home economics and infant welfare.

Family Planning as a Part of Maternity and Child Health (MCH)

If the arguments just advanced are accepted, it follows that, logically, family planning should be integrated with maternal and child health services, although it should also be made available in other ways. This integration would ensure that all aspects of family welfare are emphasized. In the developing nations this means that MCH facilities should be available for family planning, and MCH personnel should be trained in family planning. In the developed nations it means that family doctors who care for mothers and babies should have received training in birth control techniques; and that family planning facilities should be part of the service offered by all maternity hospitals, and at all baby clinics. In both groups of nations the objective is to make family planning information easily available and contraceptive measures easily obtained.

Experience has shown, in several developing nations, that when family planning and MCH services are separate, both compete for scarce resources, particularly trained health workers and health educators, so that friction is likely. It is most important, too, that the health personnel, from doctors at the apex of the pyramid to the village midwives at the base, function as a health team if the greatest impact on family welfare is to be obtained. This arrangement produces a more complete service at a lower cost, by preventing duplication of facilities and employing scarce health personnel more fully.

The pre-natal period is one during which considerable information about the more reliable methods of birth control can be given to a 'captive audience'. In developing nations, and amongst the less affluent sections of the developed nations, such information needs to be supplemented with further information in the early puerperium and again some six to eight weeks later. This information is most usefully given in 'small group' or 'face to face' situations. The late puerperal visit is best made to the patient's home, when the husband is present, so that contraceptive measures for men can be discussed. Since this information is given by health educators or other health workers, their training programme requires careful organization as regards content and learned skills.

In addition to providing information, appliances—either condoms or vasectomy for husbands, and oral (or injectable) hormonal contraceptives or the IUD for women—need to be made available, and accepters need follow-up visits to reassure them, and to answer their questions. If the appropriate health worker is available the opportunity can also be taken to see the child and to give advice about its health care.

An additional facility which is offered by many private doctors, and some hospital clinics, in the developed nations is to take smears of exfoliating cervical cells from patients seeking family planning advice in order to detect abnormal cytology. Since the patients are usually young, the 'pick-up' rate is low, and it is questionable if the cost-benefit of the procedure justifies its establishment on a large scale, particularly in the developing nations. It would certainly be more rewarding in many nations to devote the time, and resources, set aside for such combined programmes to a campaign to eliminate anaemia amongst women of reproductive age, and to improve the nutrition of pregnant women and of children. Such a campaign would also further the aim of family planning, as the Director-General of the Food and Agricultural Organization stressed in an address to the First Asian Congress of Nutrition held in India in 1971. Mr. Boerma said '. . . if measures were taken to greatly increase the assurance of survival of, say, the first two children as a result of better nutrition, the parents would feel much less necessity to have further children, and would accordingly be far more psychologically receptive to the ideas and methods of family planning. . . . Malnutrition can wreak havoc with a country's growth potential. To look at it in the most cold-blooded way, the lives of children prematurely shortened by malnutrition—and malnutrition is a proven killer of young children on a horrendous scale—represent a severe economic loss to society. The resources that have gone into rearing them during their brief, pitiful passage through life have simply been wasted.'

Nutritional advice and child health instruction can be given in MCH programmes; if Mr. Boerma is correct, the integration of family planning in such programmes would lead to a greater acceptance of birth control, and would enhance family welfare significantly.

THE HEALTH TEAM

The many activities envisaged in a combined family planning and MCH programme, require that the services are offered by a team of health workers. Which person offers which service will vary, depending to some extent on the numbers of health personnel within the nation, on cultural attitudes, and on the funds available. Experience has shown that many skills currently reserved for qualified doctors can be learnt and applied by less well qualified health workers. For example, in Thailand, in Korea and in parts of the U.S.A., nurse-midwives are inserting IUDs with as much objective success as physicians. In many nations, women are not prepared to be examined vaginally by men. In these nations, nurses, or midwives, can be trained to perform a vaginal examination prior to the use of oral contraceptives, and can issue the contraceptive. Health educators and social workers have special skills to give to combined programmes, whether the patient is seen in the doctor's office, in a hospital clinic, a health centre or a rural clinic. Unfortunately, because of traditional opposition to change, many doctors, in the developed nations as much as in the developing nations, resent the use of 'paramedical' personnel to perform activities usually performed by qualified doctors, and resist change.

The Importance of Communication

The family planning organizer is analogous to the advertising agent. They are both trying to sell a product which they feel is needed. They both seek to inform people about a product and to induce them to try it. Unfortunately the selling of birth control involves sexuality and marriage. In many societies, divergence from accepted norms in such matters arouses ingrained prejudices, and makes the sale of family planning far more emotive, for example, than selling soap.

As well as this, there has been very little research into communication on sexual matters, particularly in the developing nations. Most communications research has taken place in the U.S.A., in universities on student groups, who were 'captive'—in that the exercise was part of a course in behavioural psychology—and concerned matters which were trivial and of low emotional content. These exercises have been supplemented by sociological interviews of selected groups of people, mainly for commercial reasons, with the objective of reinforcing, or activating, attitudes rather than changing them. An additional problem faces family planning campaigns. It is that family planning offers a variety of methods suited to a variety of circumstances. This involves the recipient with the need to make multiple decisions, and in the case of the condom, the diaphragm or the oral contraceptives with the need to make frequent decisions—to use or not to use, to take or not to take. Communications psychologists have pointed out that such multiple decisions are harder to make than a single decision.

Over the past few years, a certain amount of communication theory as applied to family planning has been accumulated. It has been shown that two types of information need to be utilized in any campaign. The first is information which aims to persuade people to abandon old, and adopt new, attitudes. The response to 'persuasive information' is to overestimate the power of the persuader, and to underestimate the audience's resistance to change.

The second kind of information is 'instructional information'. This type can only be used with an audience which is willing to be persuaded, or is captive in that it has been enticed to participate in an instructional session, and has a feeling of obligation to the communicator. The listeners to instructional information must anticipate that what the communicator tells them is incontrovertible and that it will help them reach a desired goal. As a final bait to their active participation in the instructional session, they must feel that they will be socially rewarded, rather than punished, if they adopt the advice suggested by the communicator.

The effect of these two kinds of information on the rate of adoption of, and continued use of, birth control methods will vary considerably with the nature of the society, with the nature of the approach, and with the type of family planning method proposed. If a society is modern and receptive to new ideas, the impact of a family welfare campaign will be greater than in a traditional type of society in which cultural norms are jealously guarded by people past their reproductive era. The nature of the approach will also affect the impact of the campaign. If national leaders are whole-heartedly behind a campaign, two target groups can receive instructional information. The first is the captive audience in schools, and the second is women during pregnancy. Thus it is of the utmost importance to persuade national and local leaders of the value of population control as an economic and social welfare measure. In most developing nations, and in some developed nations, the national leaders accept that family planning is vital to their countries, and this idea has been reinforced by the firm support of the United Nations and its agencies, particularly the WHO and the World Bank. The Declaration on Population Growth and Human Dignity and Welfare has been of considerable help in this respect. This Declaration was signed by the heads of State of 30 nations and issued on Human Rights Day, in 1967. Unequivocally and forcibly the Declaration states:

'The peace of the world is of paramount importance to the

community of nations, and our governments are devoting their best efforts to improving the prospects for peace in this and succeeding generations. But another great problem threatens the world—a problem less visible but no less immediate. That is the problem of unplanned population growth.

'It took mankind all of recorded time until the middle of the last century to achieve a population of one billion [*one thousand million*]. Yet it took less than a hundred years to add the second billion, and only thirty years to add the third. At today's rate of increase there will be four billion people by 1975 and nearly seven billion by the year 2000. This unprecedented increase presents us with a situation unique in human affairs and a problem that grows more urgent with each passing day.

'The numbers themselves are striking, but their implications are of far greater significance. Too rapid population growth seriously hampers efforts to raise living standards, to further education, to improve health and sanitation, to provide better housing and transportation, to forward cultural and recreational opportunities—and even in some countries to assure sufficient food. In short, the human aspiration, common to men everywhere, to live a better life is being frustrated and jeopardized.

'As heads of governments actively concerned with the population problem, we share these convictions:

> 'We believe that the population problem must be recognized as a principal element in long-range national planning if governments are to achieve their economic goals and fulfil the aspirations of their people.
>
> 'We believe that the great majority of parents desire to have the knowledge and the means to plan their families; that the opportunity to decide the number and spacing of children is a basic human right.
>
> 'We believe that lasting and meaningful peace will depend to a considerable measure upon how the challenge of population growth is met.
>
> 'We believe that the objective of family planning is the enrichment of human life, not its restriction; that family planning, by assuring greater opportunity to each person, frees man to attain his individual dignity and reach his full potential.

'Recognizing that family planning is in the vital interest of both the nation and the family, we, the undersigned, earnestly hope that leaders around the world will share our views and join with us in this great challenge for the well being and happiness of people everywhere.'

It is, of course, immediately apparent that such rhetoric is only likely to motivate leaders and intellectuals to adopt population control programmes. As has been pointed out earlier in this chapter, individual couples are not interested to any great extent in the population problems of society. They are very interested in the welfare of their own families. If they believe—as they do increasingly—that family planning will help them reach desired goals, all that they want is to know of the best methods, and to be able to obtain the appropriate appliance (whether condom, oral contraceptive, IUD or whatever) easily and cheaply.

Experience in the past decade has shown that the campaign for birth control must be tailored to appeal to the group approached, and to stimulate their interest to adopt the measures proposed. The variety of approaches needed, and its success cannot be accurately predicted from models; but with a knowledge of approaches already used, and a flexible, pragmatic attitude, a new campaign can succeed, and will avoid bogging down in academic sophistry.

Goals of a Birth Control Campaign

The goals of any campaign can be stated quite simply: they are to obtain maximum coverage at the minimum cost. In achieving this simple goal the campaign organizers aim to inform all, to motivate most, and to induce many to try and continue to use one of the methods which they have ensured are freely available. Several steps are needed to achieve this goal.

Acceptance by National Decision-Makers

The first essential is to obtain the support and encouragement of the Government and national leaders. In order to do this arguments to counter those supporting pro-natalist policies must be available, and different arguments are needed in different nations.

In some, birth control is offered as a means by which the true emancipation of women may occur. This approach is utilized in China, Eastern Europe and the U.S.S.R.

In other nations family planning as such is unacceptable, but is welcomed when it is offered in existing programmes of maternity and child health. The argument is that if births are spaced, both the health of the mother, and that of her last born child, are improved. This is particularly important in nations where the newborn child displaces the last born at the breast. If taboos exist about what foods may be eaten after weaning, the displaced child is at high risk of developing protein malnutrition, and kwashiorkor. Family planning, linked with maternity and child health care, implies family welfare in the broad sense. Family welfare is an acceptable goal of the leaders and people of several African nations, whilst birth control is not, and indeed is opposed on political grounds. This statement simplifies the African experience. In the Islamic nations north of the Sahara, family planning is accepted and acceptable, as it is in the independent nations which were previously under British colonial rule. In the former French and Spanish colonies, and in the existing Portuguese colonies, birth control is not permitted, but family welfare (including family spacing) is becoming an important concept. In the two nations of Africa which were never under colonial rule, Ethiopia and Liberia, family planning is accepted but not encouraged; whilst in the white minority dominated nations of Southern Africa, family planning is encouraged, but not fully accepted by the African majority.

In most Asian nations, family planning is encouraged as part of governmental policies to control the rate of population growth, and considerable efforts are being made to increase the number of accepters. In Singapore and Mauritius, for example, the free discussion of population dynamics and birth control is encouraged. In the majority of Asian nations a more direct approach to birth control may be made without shocking the cultural norms of the people.

In still other nations, the most suitable approach may be to seek to eliminate all unwanted births both outside and within marriage. Such an aim implies that widespread contraceptive knowledge and appliances are available for all women (and men) within the community, and that community standards of behaviour accept this concept. This is the currently favoured approach of those interested in population problems in Britain and in the U.S.A. In these two nations the reproductive growth rate is 0·5 and 0·9 per cent per annum respectively, implying a population doubling time of 145 and 85 years. And in both nations the reproductive growth rate is falling. Increasing numbers of women in the 15 to 24 age-group have determined to have no more than two children so that zero population growth has almost been achieved in this group. In 1972, the U.S. National Population Commission recommended that the Government should bring the growth of population to a gradual halt. The Commission found that a shift to zero population growth would not harm America's economic health and might improve it. They recommended that individuals should be able to avoid unwanted childbearing. It is evident that increasingly national leaders in both countries accept there is a need, and a desire, by the people to obtain a still lower reproductive growth rate. One way in which this might be achieved with little disturbance would be to eliminate unwanted pregnancies. In the U.S.A. it has been calculated that between 1960 and 1965 about 900,000 births each year were unwanted, and calculations in Britain showed that about 150,000 unwanted births occurred annually between 1965 and 1969. These figures may be underestimated. Jaffe, writing about the situation in the U.S.A., suggests that the majority of these births could have been prevented if several measures were intensified. These are: (1) to increase educational programmes on family planning, population dynamics, family life and sexuality in schools, (2) to remove the legal, administrative and cultural barriers which prevent birth control measures being provided to unmarried persons, (3) to ensure that such measures are readily and easily available through a network of family planning services to those married persons who desire them, and (4) to repeal anti-abortion laws so that abortion is available to those women who become pregnant by ill-luck or ill-management.

THE SPREAD OF INFORMATION

The second essential is to mount a programme of information in which the full use of radio and newspapers is made. In this campaign the advantages of family planning are stressed. This has the effect of making the whole programme legitimate and acceptable to traditionally conservative people. For greater impact, trained informed workers must start to talk to couples on an informal, person-to-person, basis. There is a distinct advantage in using existing communications networks. This means that, where possible, local people are involved, and local key people are activated to do the work. The information campaign requires to be repeated at intervals, but with variations, otherwise its impact is diminished.

In certain countries, a campaign to make talk of birth control acceptable needs to be mounted, as in many areas taboos surround talk on sexual matters. These taboos need to be broken so that education can also be given in schools, and community centres, about concepts of family welfare, and the relationship of population growth, human sexuality and family planning to it. The difficulties in the developed nations are considerable and in the developing nations immense. In the former the predominantly Judao-Christian ethic tends to regard sexuality as a forbidden topic for discussion in schools. The argument is advanced that sexuality, family life and family planning are matters for parents to tell their children, despite the obvious fact that the majority of parents are insufficiently informed themselves, or unwilling to communicate with their children. It is also held that teachers, in the last years of primary school and the first years of secondary school, are incapable of teaching such a 'delicate' matter, and this is the period when the information should be given to the children. This argument is, in part, true; but teachers' training programmes can be altered easily to include the subject, and 'in-service' courses can be arranged for graduate teachers without undue difficulty. Nor is the lack of appropriate teaching materials, particularly of textbooks, a bar. Such books can be developed.

A further argument is that the school is not an appropriate place for the transmission of such knowledge. Currently, the objectives of education appear to be to transmit a limited knowledge, and to enable the child to obtain some skills. Yet schools in many developing nations have additional objectives; one being to enhance the potential of the individual as well as helping society as a whole. Already in many nations, the elements of hygiene, nutrition and agricultural skills are taught.

Family welfare, including population dynamics and family planning, could be introduced with little difficulty, except that a curriculum already crowded would be filled still more unless some other subject was given less teaching time.

The argument that the curriculum is too crowded can also be answered, once the objectives of school education have been determined. If an objective is to promote a fuller, richer life for the individual, then family welfare should be included, and a more traditional subject given reduced time in the curriculum.

The final, persuasive, argument (to some) is that if children of 11 to 15 receive education in sexuality, and family planning, it will lead to promiscuity and vice. There is no evidence that this occurs. Children currently receive inaccurate information from their peers, outside the schoolroom. Promiscuity would certainly not be increased, and might be diminished, if accurate information on sexual responsibility were given in the schoolroom, if not by teachers, then by trained health workers. There is, in fact, support for the opinion that doctors and other health workers might supplement the information children receive from teachers, books, films and other materials.

In the developing nations the situation is more complicated. Not only is there a shortage of trained teachers, particularly teachers trained to conduct courses in family welfare, but not all children (and especially not all girls) obtain formal primary education, and only a few continue to secondary education. Since there is little pre-marital sexuality, it can be argued that the information would be forgotten by the time it was needed. Experience in the few nations which have introduced programmes suggests that this is not so.

Clearly, much thought must be given in each nation, by educational leaders and others, on the desirability of modifying existing curriculae to permit the introduction of courses of instruction in population dynamics, human sexuality and family planning in their relationship to family welfare. No outsider can help except in an advisory capacity, but indigenous doctors and other health workers in the field of family welfare can be of great assistance to educational planners. And it is likely that the effect of such programmes, in primary and secondary schools, will yield considerable benefits in making the concepts which lead to a reduced birth rate more readily acceptable.

GOALS OF A BIRTH CONTROL CAMPAIGN

The goals of such an educational programme do not necessarily include information about specific family planning methods, although they may. However, if the 35 to 45 per cent of the population under the age of 15 in the developing nations, and the 20 to 30 per cent in the developed nations, are made aware of concepts affecting family welfare, the technical information required later is more readily accepted, and the methods more readily adopted.

In the developing nations, particularly, the information obtained in schools needs to be supplemented by further information given in community centres to pregnant women during the pre-natal period and in child health care clinics. This is because so many girls fail to obtain schooling, or drop out before the information has been given.

During pregnancy the women are 'captive' and are more likely to accept instructional information because they are thinking about the care of their unborn child. In the developing nations, particularly in rural areas, the traditional midwife can play a valuable part in spreading family planning information, and in reinforcing information previously obtained. The importance of using child health clinics to inform mothers about family planning is emphasized by the finding that ten times as many mothers attend such clinics as go to post-natal clinics.

The purpose of all this educational and informational activity is to get the concept of birth control, whether for better family welfare or because of demographic problems, accepted and adopted by as many individuals as possible. Educational psychologists identify four stages in the process. Firstly, the aim is to arouse in the individual an awareness and interest in family planning, as something which would benefit the family as a whole. Secondly, if this aim is achieved, the individual will make the decision to seek further information. Thirdly, the additional information received will lead to a decision to try the method suggested. Fourthly, if the three preceding steps have been successful, a decision will be made to continue the use of the method. An excellent, and brief, source book in which the steps are discussed in great detail is *How to Improve Written Communication for Birth Control* by Donald Bogue and Veronica Herskanen.

The goals of the educational programmes outlined have been

stated with great clarity by Dr. Sloan Wayland in Berelson's *Family Planning and Population Programs*. I am indebted to Dr. Berelson and Dr. Wayland for their permission to reproduce this section, as I believe it important not only to teachers, but to doctors and other health workers, including health educators, in the field of family welfare.

'This list [of goals] is intended to be suggestive and not comprehensive. Furthermore, no effort has been made to differentiate between the goals for different levels of students or for different subgroups such as boys or girls.

1. For the individual's own personal behaviour patterns and attitudes
   a) Acceptance of the small family as a proper and desirable norm
   b) Understanding that uncontrolled reproduction is not necessary to ensure a desirable family size
   c) Understanding that the size of family can be controlled by deliberate planning
   d) Acceptance of marriage at a mature age as a desirable pattern
   e) Appreciation of the advantages of planning, including health and economic gains from spacing and limitation in total number of children, and of the health, education, and other opportunities for children that may be more adequately provided for in the small family
   f) Knowledge about the process by which human life begins
   g) Appreciation of an acceptance of community resources, such as family planning clinics, as legitimate agencies for use by married couples
2. For the individual's role as citizen and community member
   a) Understanding of the dynamics of population growth and of the current and projected characteristics of the population of his own country and of other regions
   b) Knowledge of the policy of his country and of others, and appreciation of the factors which have led to it
   c) Recognition that reduction in the rate of population growth is possible if the established agencies in the community are given support by community leaders and responsible citizens

d) Understanding of the ways in which uncontrolled growth makes difficult the achievement of the economic, education, and health aspirations of the nation
e) Understanding of the importance of accurate and complete vital statistics for planning in the nation
f) Appreciation of the possible courses of action open to an individual in the community who understands the social significance of family planning.

To this list may be added specific information about means of control where the cultural setting makes such an approach acceptable.'

THE IDENTIFICATION OF KEY PEOPLE

The third essential in any campaign to control fertility is to identify key people in an area who command the respect of the community, who are receptive to new ideas and who are prepared to spread the ideas to people around them and to encourage them to adopt them.

In traditionally conservative communities, the identification of key people is crucial if the campaign is to be successful. Local people respect their local leaders who can induce them to adopt measures which would be rejected if suggested by outsiders.

A particularly useful way of legitimizing and perpetuating a campaign is to reinforce the message spread by the mass media, and that of 'face to face' sessions, by public meetings at which films are shown and which are presided over by one of the local leaders.

PROMOTION BY 'SATISFIED CUSTOMERS'

The fourth essential of a successful campaign is to encourage the participants to promote the method they have adopted. This is most important. People are more likely to try a method if an acquaintance has already used it successfully. This method is encouraged if a well developed 'after sales service' is provided. Many women who have decided to use oral contraceptives or who have had an intra-uterine contraceptive device inserted experience side-effects and require reassurance that these will pass and that they are innocuous. Such women may become disappointed or dissatisfied participants unless they have the opportunity to discuss their problems with sympathetic, unhurried, uncondescending health workers. For a campaign to succeed it is essential that health workers involved in family planning programmes are trained in this area of communication. As the then Population Council Representative in Korea, Paul Hartman, wrote in 1965, 'In the most practical sense, service is our most important product.' It has been argued that this service should extend to problems of infertility and child health. There is considerable advantage, in many developing nations, to integrate family planning services in maternity and child health services so that a complete family welfare service is offered.

THE EVALUATION OF FAMILY PLANNING PROGRAMMES

Accurate evaluation of any activity demands knowledge of the objectives of the programme, accurate recording of data in a manner which permits it to be quantified, and facilities to check suspect data. The majority of programmes fail to meet all the criteria, so that evaluation is currently at best tentative. Lapham and Maudlin have listed criteria, both objective and subjective, and have analysed the progress of birth control programmes in 20 nations. The objective criteria are statistical measurements of accepters and users, and natality reduction measurement (Table **14/4**). The subjective criteria are certain procedural and supportive measures which may have some impact on increased acceptance. These are less readily quantifiable and include the following questions: (1) Does the Government have a population policy which includes a reduction in the birth rate? (2) Do national leaders speak favourably of, and obviously support, family planning? (3) Is the administrative structure adequate to provide birth control information and advice? (4) Does the Health Department carry out a vigorous effort to provide family planning services for all women of childbearing age, and for their partners, both in the post-partum period and apart from pregnancy? (5) Are contraceptives readily, easily and freely available throughout the country? (6) Are legally induced abortion services available? (7) Can every man and every woman desiring permanent contraception (tubal ligation or

Table 14/4 Evaluation of national birth control programmes

Criterion	*Comment*
1. Total number of first-time acceptors.	Although this gives an estimate of the number of couples using a birth control method for the first time, difficulties arise if the method is changed, as duplication may occur.
2. Acceptors as a percentage of permanently cohabiting (i.e. married, de jure, de facto or consensual) women of reproductive age (M.W.R.A.) usually 15 to 44 years or 15 to 49 years.	This is a better index. If more than 10 per cent of women are acceptors the programme is functioning efficiently.
3. Ratio of acceptors to net one year gain in number of 'married women' of reproductive age. The net gain is calculated by subtracting the numbers of women reaching 45 or 50, and adding the number of women aged 15 or more who have married in the year, to the total M.W.R.A.	The data is incomplete, or estimated in many nations. If the ratio is above that of previous year progress is being made; if below it may be because the level of acceptance is low and unchanging, or because it is low but is rising.
4. Percent of M.W.R.A. who are practising contraception.	This index is of value when compared with the data of earlier years.
5. Continuation rates *a*) 2-year continuation rate for each first method adopted *b*) average 2-year continuation rate, all acceptors, who may have continued with the same, or have changed methods *c*) percentage of acceptors who have not become pregnant in the three years following acceptance.	*a*) The information obtained from the data enables health planners to evaluate the success or otherwise of a particular method. *b*) This information indicates the overall success of the programme, but is not as useful as *c*) since avoidance of childbirth is the main objective of the programme.
6. Annual acceptor target and percent of annual target achieved.	It is usual to specify targets in the terms of number of acceptors per 1,000 M.W.R.A. However, it is a poor criterion as the target set may be low, when it will probably be achieved but will have little impact on the overall progress of the programme.
7. Cost per acceptor. This is calculated from the total expenditures on the programme divided by the number of first-time acceptors. This calculation is of more value than the cost of the birth control programme per head of population.	This information is difficult to obtain and to assess as so many variables are included. It is a crude measure for it omits costs' 'expended' in the continuing programme.
8. Evidence of declines in *a*) crude birth rate *b*) in age-specific birth rates, and evaluation of the amount of the decline attributable to the birth control programme.	The information, particularly of age-specific birth rates, is lacking in many nations, and the evaluation of the decline attributable to the programme is more subjective than objective in many instances as it has to be differentiated from changes due to changing age structures, and to changing age at marriage.

Source: Lapham, R. J., and Maudlin, W. P. *Studies in Family Planning*, **3**, 30, 1972 (This paper should be read for further details, and for a partial evaluation of socio-economic procedures and supportive measures. The authors note that these items are poorly quantifiable at present.)

vasectomy) obtain this legally, easily, openly and freely? (8) Does the mass media provide family planning information and motivation regularly, and is family planning literature readily available? (9) Do facilities exist for good record-keeping at clinic level, and for the provision of statistical summaries at regional or national levels of number of accepters, supplies distributed, effect on natality, etc? (10) Is the programme being constantly evaluated so that accomplishments can be rewarded, obstacles overcome, and changes to improve the effect made on factual information? These criteria and others are given in greater detail in Lapham and Maudlin's paper, but the examples quoted here indicate how difficult some are to quantitate, and how research is needed.

The indices mentioned by Lapham and Maudlin may be supplemented by the periodic use of K.A.P. studies, on the same population. The information may show, for example, that a significantly large number of women learned of a contraceptive method in the interval between two surveys; that a larger number were currently practising birth control; and it may give information about the type of method used (whether highly efficient or not, see Chapters 11 and 12).

The information can then be used to demonstrate to national decision makers the desire amongst the people for birth control, and can suggest more appropriate means of meeting that goal.

In addition to periodic reviews, the progress of a family welfare campaign needs continuing reviews to assess the progress made to goals which have been determined at the outset of the campaign. Such reviews may identify groups particularly vulnerable to conception, and their numbers, relative to the total population under examination.

Rosa has examined this by making certain assumptions. He has observed that in most nations pregnancy is relatively uncommon before the age of 17 and after the age of 40, although the fertile age range is usually stated to be 15 to 49 years. It is also known that between 10 and 15 per cent of the couples are involuntarily infertile. Rosa further observes that in nations in the stage of early demographic transition, the number of potentially fertile married couples accounts for 15 per cent of the population; and of those about half will have had three or more pregnancies. Since the ideal family size is 3 children in many nations, about 8 per cent of the population are likely to be interested in family planning. In addition, each year about 2 per cent of the population reaches the age of 17, and half of these are women. From these data it is possible to construct a population model (Table **14/5**).

Table 14/5

Population model showing potential family planning needs

	Total population	1,000,000
	Women	500,000
	Women aged 15–49	200,000
	Women potentially fertile and exposed	150,000
less	Women currently pregnant	40,000
less	Those with fewer than 3 children	30,000
	Women with 3 or more children	80,000
plus	Women annually completing desired family size	10,000
	Couples currently in need	90,000

Source: Rosa, F. W. *Organization of Family Planning*, Informal Document, WHO 1971.

In this model it can be seen that about 10 per cent of the population are likely to seek family planning advice if sufficiently motivated to do so.

The whole matter of the evaluation of family planning programmes is discussed at greater length in the World Health Organization's *Technical Report on Health Aspects of Family Planning* to which the reader is referred.

The Model of China

The degree to which nations have effectively met the criteria mentioned varies considerably. One nation has succeeded in making use of all methods available. That nation is China. Because of its relative isolation from other nations until recently, the Chinese experience in family planning has not been widely reported. Yet, as China is the world's most populous nation, her experience is of exceptional importance.

The objective of China's national family planning programme is to secure healthy mothers and healthy children, to create time during which women can work and study, to provide facilities for the education of all children, and to regulate family size because of its impact on the economy.

Because it was realized that the earlier the age of marriage, the higher the natality, efforts have been made to raise the age at marriage. In China, as a whole, the mean age of women for marriage is now 25 in the urban areas, and 23 in the rural areas. Before marriage, there is considerable mingling of the sexes, but without any obvious sexuality. Companionship appears to be possible without copulation and conception.

To delay, or to prevent pregnancy, China has made available a whole range of birth control devices, and has widely publicized their use. The people have the knowledge that their leaders, from Chairman Mao Tse-Tung down, approve of family spacing. The Chinese have also ensured that the contraceptives are readily, and easily, available to all who want them. These services are provided free.

Condoms are available at no cost from family planning workers, or can be purchased. Oral hormonal contraceptives and IUDs are widely available at no cost, and widely used. Injectable hormonal contraceptives are being offered increasingly. Abortion is available with certain restrictions, in the urban hospitals and in each of the 70,000 commune hospitals. Most are performed using the suction curette which, as was mentioned in Chapter 13, was developed in China. For couples who wish for permanent methods of fertility control, vasectomy and tubal ligation are available, often under acupuncture analgesia.

What marks the outstanding nature of China's family planning programme is the strong emphasis given to the initiative and self-reliance of the people themselves. The programme relies on an infrastructure of education, considered rational discussion and the free availability of all the methods. There is no element of compulsion in the programme, nor have the sanctions mentioned in Chapter 9 been required.

The self-reliance of the programme has been emphasized by the I.P.P.F. Western Pacific Regional Secretary who visited China in April, 1972. Mr. Katagiri points out that the clinical investigations, and adoption of new techniques are based on studies made in the major hospitals. In many cases the doctors, nurses and social workers (over 90 per cent of whom are women) have been the first to try the new methods. 'This method of testing new techniques is both a socially responsible one, because this group of people will be best trained to observe adverse side-effects early, and is also of great motivational significance because it means that the methods which are passed on to the community have been tried by the workers, and they themselves have confidence in them.'

Perhaps even more significant, in a predominantly rural nation, is the unique corps of health workers, 'the bare-foot doctors', who are recruited from the community in which they will work. They are given training in health techniques, including birth control. As they belong to the community they are readily able to communicate with their neighbours. They initiate educational sessions, and do 'face to face' motivation. They have contraceptives available for immediate distribution, and have been trained to introduce IUDs to those women who choose the method. In addition, they counsel the patients, and assist the qualified doctors in induced abortions, in sterilizations and in introducing IUDs. They are always available to answer questions and to reduce doubts about family planning.

The success of China's campaign cannot yet be fully assessed, because of lack of data, but it seems that considerable progress has been made to reach the target of a less than 1 per cent per annum population growth rate by the year 2000.

Mr. Katagiri said on leaving China, 'Under the guidance of Chairman Mao, more than 700 million people in China are doing an experiment never before attempted in human history, an experiment not only in family planning, but also in every aspect of human existence. Mankind awaits the results.'

There can be a no more appropriate way in which to end a chapter on the campaign for fertility control and family welfare.

PART III

Social Obstetrics

This is not a case. This is a patient, who is thirty-four years old, who is pregnant for the first time, whose husband has deserted her and who has toxaemia of pregnancy. She is a person who has had much misfortune and it is your duty as a doctor to treat the patient not only the disease.

Professor LEYLAND ROBINSON,
Professor of Obstetrics and Gynaecology,
University of Liverpool,
to the author, when he was an obstetric
resident in 1946.

FIFTEEN

Social Factors in Reproductive Efficiency—I

Better nutrition in childhood appears to be the main factor in the earlier age of menarche (see Figure **15/1**). In all European countries for which there are records, the age of menarche has fallen from between 16 and 17 years in 1840, to between 15 and 16 years in 1880, to between 14 and 15 years in 1920, and between 12 and 13 years in 1970. This earlier sexual maturity has coincided in the past 10 years with what is believed to be a greater sexual permissiveness in the U.S.A. and Canada, in Western European countries and in Australia and New Zealand. The greater sexual permissiveness has not been preceded by better sex education (including education in sexual and family responsibility), or by better and more accurate knowledge of contraceptive practice. The result has been an increase in teenage pregnancy.

In this connection 'teen-age' is taken to cover the period of years between menarche and the eighteenth birthday, as by the latter date physical maturity is largely complete, and intellectual maturity well advanced, although emotional maturity may not be reached for some years. Moreover, in the countries under consideration, 18 is now legally the age when adult responsibilities are accepted.

Statistics from the U.S.A. and European nations show that increasing numbers of teenagers are becoming pregnant. For example, in 1960, 189,000 U.S. girls aged 13 to 17 gave birth; by 1965 the number had risen to 196,000; and by 1970 to over 200,000. In the same year, nearly 10 per cent of all births were to girls under the age of 17 and a significant proportion of these births were to unmarried girls. Statistics from the United Kingdom and Australia show a similar pattern (Table **15/1**).

However, before these data are interpreted as indicating a

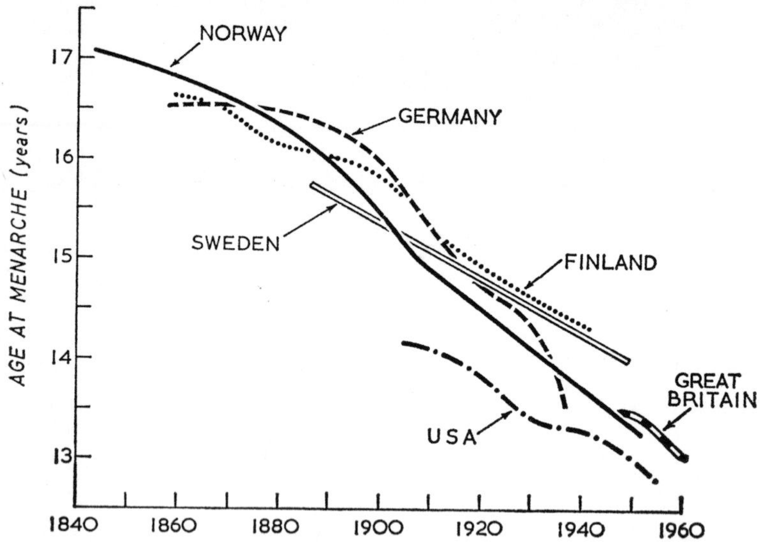

Figure **15/1** The secular trend in the mean age of the menarche in several nations.
Source: Tanner, J.

gross decay in traditional Judao-Christian moral standards in Western affluent nations, greater scrutiny is required. The crude data make no allowance for the increasing number of teenagers. For example, in the U.S.A., the number of young people, aged

Table 15/1

Extramarital pregnancies. The percentage in women aged 19 or less and 20 or more at the time of the birth in four nations

Nation	*Age of woman*			
	Less than 20 *years old*		20 *years or more*	
	1950–55	1960–65	1950–55	1960–65
Canada	38·7	46·5	61·3	53·5
England and Wales	36·0	48·0	64·0	52·0
Finland	12·0	26·6	88·0	73·4
U.S.A.	41·0	41·8	59·0	58·2

15 to 19, increased from 13·2 million in 1960 to 19·0 million in 1970. A better index of teenage pregnancy is to calculate age-specific natality rates (Figure **15/2**). These, it will be recalled, are the ratio of pregnancies per 1,000 females in the age-group. This shows that there has been a slight decline in the rate for American girls under 18 years of age in the decade 1960–70.

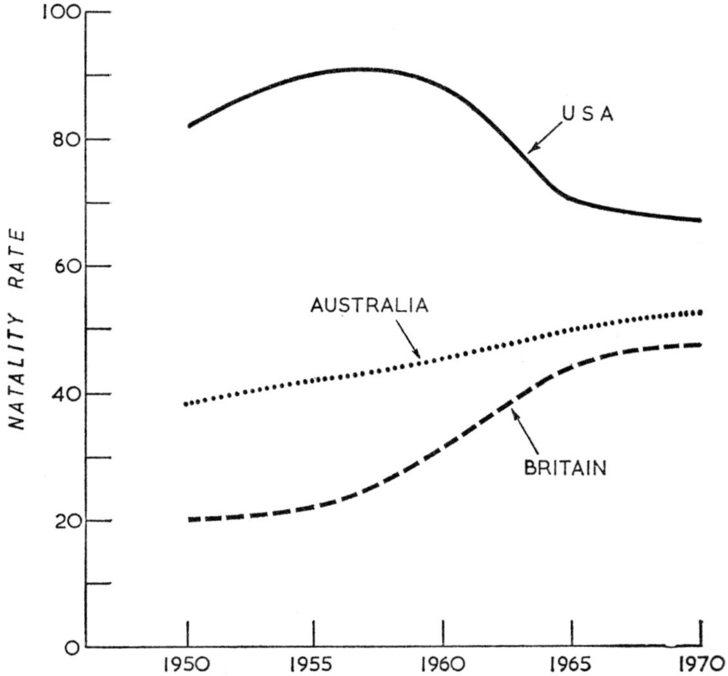

Figure **15/2** The age-specific natality rates of women aged 15 to 18 at the time of the birth.

This finding is the opposite of that in Britain and Australia, where age-specific natality rates show an increase in natality of girls under the age of 18. However, in all three nations the number of births to teenagers has risen proportionately in relation to the total national birth rate, because of the rather rapidly declining age-specific natality rates for older women, due to the greater use of contraceptive measures in these age-groups.

Professor Helen Wallace has summarized some of the social

problems of teenage pregnancy and marriage in the U.S.A., and there is no reason to suspect that her findings are much different from those in Europe or Oceania. Basing her findings on the 1960 census, Wallace found that about 25 per cent of the teenage mothers were unmarried and that between 40 and 60 per cent of marriages of teenagers were because of premarital conception, which had to be followed by a hasty marriage. Many of the marriages were 'forced' by parents to avoid the scandal of illegitimacy and without the adolescents having established any real relationship with each other. The effect of this is shown by the U.S. divorce rates in the age-group 15 to 19. In the United States about 25 divorces or annulments occur for every 100 marriages each year. The divorce rate in the 15 to 19 age-group is three or four times higher than that of older age-groups. In Australia in 1971, 38 per cent of marriages in which the girl was less than 20 years when she married ended in divorce. These harsh statistics emphasize the instability of teenage marriage and stress the necessity for sex education (in the broad sense of instilling sexual responsibility), and for information about contraceptives to be given preferably just before, or just after puberty. They also stress the need for marriage counselling services to be made easily available to the particularly vulnerable group.

The Obstetric Aspects of Teenage Pregnancy

In the past 20 years, some 30 papers have been published about teenage pregnancy in Western nations. The majority of these have come from the U.S.A. which has the additional problem that most of the pregnancies occur to black Americans, who tend to eat a worse diet and to obtain less obstetric care during pregnancy. Many writers have commented on this and have identified three main problems in teenage pregnancy. The first is that the pregnancy is likely to be concealed for as long as possible, so that antenatal care is not sought until the second half of pregnancy, if at all. The second problem is that teenage diets tend to lack adequate quantities of protein. An investigation in Chicago of the diets of 1,000 girls who had conceived at the age of 16 or less showed that nearly 45 per cent were classified as having 'poor' diets, and only 30 per cent ate 'good' diets, in which the protein, carbohydrate and mineral content was balanced and adequate. One American gynaecologist has complained that too many teenaged Americans eat diets which consist of potato chips, hamburger buns, Coca-Cola, hot dogs and pizza! Such diets are not particularly beneficial to proper fetal growth in utero. The third problem is that complications of pregnancy and labour are found disproportionately amongst unmarried teenagers (when compared to all pregnant teenagers), particularly if the girl is in a lower socio-economic group, has a low intelligence, has left school at the earliest permissible age and is occupied in unskilled work.

Since the incidence of pregnancy complications is directly related to the quality of pre-natal care received, it is obvious that the social agencies must expand to meet this problem and try to change opinion, so that people regard concealment of pregnancy a greater social stigma than the occurrence of conception.

PROBLEMS IN THE ANTE-NATAL PERIOD

The main problem is that the incidence of *pre-eclampsia* is increased.* In primigravidae aged 20 to 30, the incidence of pre-eclampsia ranges from 5 to 12 per cent; amongst teenaged primigravidae it ranges from 9 to 21 per cent. In a study amongst patients in Sydney, the incidence of pre-eclampsia was related to ante-natal care. Amongst those girls who sought ante-natal care before the 20th week of pregnancy the incidence of pre-eclampsia was 5 per cent; whilst amongst those who only sought ante-natal care in the last weeks of pregnancy, or were admitted to hospital in labour, it was 12 per cent and the pre-eclampsia tended to be more severe and fulminating in nature. In studies from the United States in the 1950s, *anaemia* was identified as a problem, particularly amongst black American teenagers. Amongst the 3,995 patients aged 14 to 19 investigated by Israel and Wontersz in 1963, 17·2 per cent had a haemoglobin level of less than 10 g per 100 ml compared with 10·9 per cent of controls. However, it was noticeable in this series that white American teenagers had a higher incidence of anaemia than black American teenagers, suggesting that the anaemia was due

*In the studies pre-eclampsia is defined as a blood pressure greater than 140/90, with or without proteinuria, after the 20th week of pregnancy.

to inappropriate diet rather than pre-existing blood loss at menstruation. In studies from Australia, Britain and South Africa, the incidence of anaemia was no higher amongst teen-aged primigravid patients than amongst those of older age-groups.

PROBLEMS OF LABOUR

The adult shape of the female pelvis and its stability is established within one year of the menarche, so that the pelvis is structurally and functionally adult by the age of 14. In none of the investigations reviewed was contracted pelvis a problem, nor was the incidence of cephalopelvic disproportion or mal-presentation of the fetus higher in the teenage parturient when compared with her older sister. *Premature labour*, or at least the *birth of a low birth weight baby* was more common in teen-aged patients. Amongst the controls in several studies (usually primigravidae aged 20 to 30) the 'prematurity' rate was 8 to 12 per cent; amongst teenagers it ranged from 8 to 19 per cent. Once again the influence of ante-natal care was apparent. If the teenager sought pre-natal care early, she had a reduced likelihood of delivering a low birth weight baby. Several studies suggest that labour tends to be prolonged in teenaged patients. Investigations of this point indicate that the increased duration is more likely to be due to a reluctance of the obstetrician to intervene, and so to spare the young girl, particularly the un-married teenager, an operative delivery. In fact, in all the studies the Caesarean section rates amongst primigravid teenagers was about half that amongst primigravidae aged 20 to 29.

The teenager is not more likely to develop post-partum haemorrhage, nor is there a higher perinatal mortality amongst infants born to teenaged mothers.

THE REPRODUCTIVE EFFICIENCY OF THE TEENAGE PATIENT

The preceding paragraphs and Table **15/2**, indicate that provided pregnancy is not concealed and that pre-natal care is sought as early as possible, pregnancy and labour in the teen-age patient is likely to be uncomplicated. Adolescence is, in fact, a safe time for pregnancy, and the teenage patient is obstetrically efficient—in many respects even more efficient than the slightly older patient. As long ago as 1922, Harris observed this when he stated that the ideal age, obstetrically, for a woman to have her first baby was 16. This opinion is perhaps too dogmatic; but all reliable evidence indicates that the optimal age period for pregnancy is 18 to 25 years, or from 16 to 29 to take the extremes.

Table 15/2

Young teenaged primigravidae, aged 17 or less. Complications in pregnancy and labour (per cent)

Complications	*Age of patients*	
	12–17	20–29
Pre-eclampsia	10–16%	4–8%
Prolonged labour (more than 24 hrs)	4–7%	2–5%
Low birth weight babies	6–9%	2–5%
Perinatal loss	4%	2%
Caesarean section	0·05–1·5%	1·5–2·5%

Source: Completed from studies reported by Utian, with additional information from Sydney, Australia.

Psychological Problems

The psychological problems of the teenage pregnancy are closely related to the patient's knowledge of pregnancy and the birth process, to the support she obtains from her family, and to whether or not she is married. The less knowledge she has, the less support she has, the less well is she able to adjust to the changed hormonal and physical climate of pregnancy, and the more are psychological problems likely to occur. These factors are compounded if the girl is unmarried, as now she may fear that she is guilty of breaking a moral code, and is often treated with hostility by her parents, who are more afraid of neighbours' comments and criticism than with the need to give the child the required love and comfort. Questions, of course, do arise. If the girl is at school, technical college or university, should she continue or should she leave? Should she seek to obtain a legal abortion if the pregnancy is extra-marital? Should she be sent from home to a neutral atmosphere where her 'shame' can be hidden? The discussion of these questions in the heightened emotional atmosphere of the home may seriously disturb the girl, and counsel from social workers is often welcomed, and is indeed necessary.

The main fears of the adolescent parturient seem to be, firstly that as she is young, her pelvis is not mature, so that labour will be painful and difficult, and possibly she will be damaged or die. Secondly, she fears the isolation of pregnancy, because during it she is cut off from her friends and their activities. The degree of the threat of this isolation is related to the support she receives from her family and to her emotional maturity. There is some suggestion that the emotionally immature fail to make the needed adjustment to pregnancy. This is a move from self-interest (which is manifest in the first half of pregnancy) to interest in the baby and its welfare which becomes important as the end of pregnancy approaches. The emotionally immature, who are often, but need not be, adolescents, fail to make the transition, and tend to treat the baby as a living doll rather than a child.

There seems to be an increased risk of suicide amongst such girls, according to Gabrielson, particularly if they are unmarried, are Roman Catholic and have poor support from their families. In his study the last factor was most often found if the girl came from a well-off suburban area.

It is clear that teenaged parturients, and especially unmarried teenagers, require considerable psycho-social and obstetric support from as early in pregnancy as possible. This remedial therapy should be given by obstetricians, nurses and social workers—all of them must avoid explicit or implicit moral strictures when dealing with the girl.

Extramarital Pregnancy and the Unmarried Mother

The social problem of the unmarried pregnant woman is largely confined to nations which are predominantly Christian in religion and Judao-Christian in ethos. Even this generalization requires modification, for consensual unions are not uncommon in Central and South America (Table **15/3**). This was investigated by Mortara, who found that in the decade 1940–50 only one nation in Middle and Tropical South America had less than 20 per cent consensual unions per 100 marriages. It is probable that the percentage is declining, but consensual unions still formed a significant proportion of marriages in those nations in 1970. Legally the children of such unions are illegitimate, but because the culture includes any such children

Table 15/3

Ratio of consensual unions to marriages in Latin American nations with populations exceeding 4 million in 1950

Nation	*Population* (1970) *in millions*	*Consensual unions in* 1950 *per* 1,000 *persons married*	
		Men	*Women*
Middle America			
Mexico	50·1	24·1	25·8
Guatemala	5·2	213·2	213·1
Caribbean			
Cuba	8·3	50·5	54·7
Haiti	5·2	276·6	314·7
Tropical S. America			
Colombia	20·8	22·4	24·4
Peru	13·2	46·4	56·3
Venezuela	10·4	62·4	71·9
Equador	6·0	28·1	30·9
Bolivia	4·5	19·1	22·4

Source: Mortara, G. 'Les Uniones Consensuelles dans l'Amerique Latine', *Proc. Int. Pop. Conf.*, New York, 1961.

in the family group, problems are minimal and neither mother nor child suffers social ostracism.

In the non-Christian nations of Africa and Asia, unmarried mothers form only a minute proportion of all pregnant women, because the cultural traditions of Hinduism and Islam have strict laws against extramarital loss of virginity and most, if not all, girls are married within two years of puberty. Only those families who have received a predominantly Western orientated, Christian education, or who are Christian, do not follow this procedure. Moreover, amongst Hindu and Islamic nations, the culture insists on chastity in girls, and sexual permissiveness amongst females is uncommon, although males may and do have recourse to prostitutes. Similar attitudes relate to the Buddhist nations of South-East Asia. In China it appears that a relationship between young people is possible without emphasis on sexuality. The Chinese recommend late marriage (26 years for men, 23 for women), make contraceptives available to delay the birth of the first child, induce couples to have no more than three children, and have made abortion available on demand. With the social attitudes and public health measures available, extramarital births in China are unusual.

Such evidence as there is indicates that in all these so-called 'developing' nations, the problem of the unmarried pregnant woman is minimal, and such women as do become pregnant are absorbed into a family group, the pregnant woman being treated as would any other in the group.

The influence of the teachings of Aquinas on orthodox sexual attitudes in Roman Catholic countries, and that of Calvinistic puritan ethics in Protestant countries, places the unmarried mother at a considerable disadvantage in many developed nations, whilst the putative father suffers far less condemnation. It is true that a high proportion of conceptions are followed by a hasty, forced marriage, which has been shown to have a high chance of being succeeded by marital disharmony, or at least indifference; or in countries where divorce is permitted, by a high divorce rate.

In the U.S.A., Canada, Australia and Western Europe, between 4 and 10 per cent of all births are to unmarried mothers, and in the past decade the proportion has been increasing (Table **15/4**). When the age of the mother is taken into account the increase has been more marked amongst teenagers. This trend has been observed, for example, in England and Wales, between 1950 and 1965, the proportion of extramarital pregnancies rose from 5·1 to 7·5 per cent of all births (Russell). When the extramarital pregnancies were computed by age of the mother, a startling rise amongst teenagers and especially young teenagers was noted (Figure **15/3**).

It is clear that the statistics must be interpreted with caution.

An increasing number of young people are reaching the reproductive era and are consequently at risk of becoming pregnant. As well as this, increasing use of contraception by married couples, together with a marked motivation towards smaller

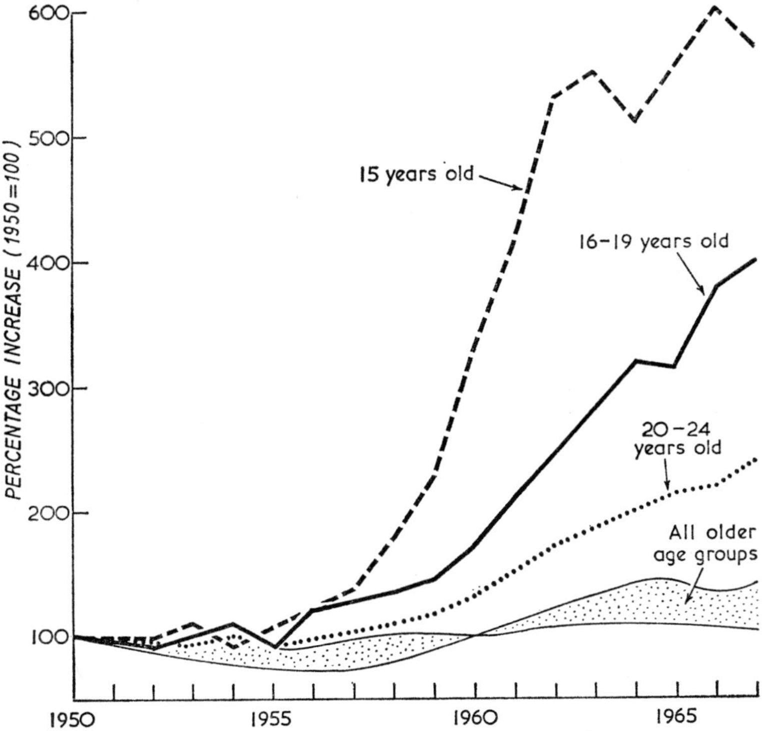

Figure **15/3** Extramarital births related to the age of the mother 1950–67 England and Wales, plotted as the percentage increase over 1950.

Source: Russell, J. K., *Practitioner*, **204,** 401, 1970.

families, has reduced the total number of births, with the result that extramarital births have increased disproportionately.

In Scandinavia and in Eastern Europe, the trend to an increasing proportion of extramarital births is not apparent. For example, in the Scandinavian nations the rate ranged between 8 and 11 per cent between 1930 and 1950, but since that time has declined. In Finland, the extramarital pregnancy rate (the 'illegitimacy rate') was 9·3 per cent of births in 1940, but had

Table 15/4

Live births to unmarried mothers as a percentage of all live births in selected nations

Country	1945	1950	1955	1960	1965
Austria	25·5	18·3	14·4	13·0	11·0
Belgium	4·2	2·6	2·1	2·1	—
Canada	4·5	3·9	3·8	4·3	6·0
Denmark	9·9	7·4	6·6	7·8	—
England and Wales	9·3	5·1	4·1	5·4	7·5
Finland	7·0	5·2	4·2	4·0	4·5
France	10·5	7·0	6·4	6·1	5·9
Netherlands	3·5	1·5	1·2	1·3	1·7
Norway	7·4	4·1	3·4	3·7	—
Sweden	9·6	9·8	9·9	11·3	13·1
Switzerland	3·5	3·8	3·6	3·8	—
U.S.A.	4·3	4·0	4·5	5·3	7·7
West Germany	—	9·5	7·7	6·1	4·8

Source: *Demographic Yearbooks*, U.N., New York.

fallen to 4·5 per cent in 1965. Sweden, which has a much more rational attitude towards pregnancy outside marriage, alone has moved against the trend.

The reason for the decline in Scandinavian nations and the increase in other 'Western' nations has been investigated by several authors, notably Wimperis and Paavola. Paavola comments that 'increasing enlightenment, especially sex education, and the ensuing increasingly common use of contraceptives have generally contributed to the decrease in the number of illegitimate births'. It is also clear that legally induced abortion in Scandinavia and particularly in Eastern Europe, has played a part in the decline. In Finland, for example, the proportion of legal abortions in unmarried women rose from 10 per cent in 1951 to 30 per cent of all abortions in 1965. In Britain since the introduction of the Abortion Act in 1968, about 48 per cent of the terminations have been in unmarried women. But despite a more liberal attitude to abortion, over 70,000 births occurred to unmarried mothers in 1969, and a further 70,000 pregnancies are known to have been conceived before marriage. This is probably a low estimate.

PREGNANCY AND THE UNMARRIED MOTHER

One of the disconcerting aspects of the study of pregnancy in the unmarried is that in all countries the proportion of unmarried girls under the age of 20 who are pregnant is increasing, and adolescents form a considerable proportion of the unmarried mothers. This applies to Scandinavian nations, to Western Europe and even more to Canada and the U.S.A.

For example, in the U.S.A. in 1960, 42 per cent of all births which occurred amongst women under the age of 20 were extramarital, by 1965 the proportion had risen to 44 per cent, and by 1970 to over 50 per cent. This rise is mainly because fewer adolescents are married than women in the older age-groups. In fact the unmarried adolescent girl is less likely to give birth extramaritally than the woman aged 20 to 24. Both in Britain and in the U.S.A., extramarital pregnancy rates were highest in women aged 25 to 29, when they were four times as high in Britain, and twice as high in the U.S.A. as those of women aged 15 to 19.

One reason for this finding may be that if the adolescent does become pregnant, she tends to get married before the child is born. In a study of births occurring between 1964 and 1966, Kovar found that one-third were conceived premaritally. However, 54 per cent of these girls married before the birth, and only 46 per cent were unmarried at delivery. When the ages of the mothers conceiving extramaritally, but marrying prior to delivery, were analysed, it was found that 42 per cent of infants born to mothers aged 15 to 19 were conceived extramaritally. In the age group 20 to 24, the figure was 14·5 per cent; 25 to 29, 3·7 per cent and after the age of 30 it had fallen to 1·8 per cent.

There is little information about the sociology of extramarital conceptions, but such as there is suggests they are related more to sexual ignorance than to sexual permissiveness. In one study in Finland, quoted by Paavola, no sex education had been received by 58 per cent of 100 pregnant girls aged 16 or under; and in Canada 44 per cent of 150 unmarried parturients had received no sex education.

The lesson is clear. Factual education in sexual matters, including sexual responsibility, and information about contraception should be given in all schools. The subject of human reproduction should be part of a course of human biology, which should largely replace currently taught biology. Concepts of sexual differences and descriptions of human reproduction should be taught to children aged 8 and over, and information about human sexuality, sexual responsibility and contraception should have been discussed within one year of puberty at the latest.

Obstetrical Aspects of Pregnancy in the Unmarried

Since so many of the patients are under the age of 20, the main obstetrical problems are those of teenage pregnancy. This is confirmed by Paavola's investigation. Of the 1,064 patients investigated, 87 per cent had never married, 10 per cent were divorced and 3 per cent widowed. Although the divorced and widowed women required social support, most of the medico-social problems arose amongst the unmarried. The incidence of obstetrical and social complications is directly related to the concealment of the pregnancy for as long as possible, to the lack of adequate pre-natal care, and to some extent to the necessity for the unmarried mother to continue working for as long as possible. In Paavola's study, for example, whilst over 90 per cent of married parturients had attended for pre-natal care before the 20th week of gestation, only 43 per cent of the unmarried parturients had sought pre-natal care by this time. Similarly, by the 36th week of gestation, whilst 67 per cent of married expectant mothers no longer worked, only 52 per cent of the unmarried expectant mothers were not working. A survey in Britain by Cholmondeley confirmed that the unmarried mother tends to avoid seeking ante-natal care in the first half of pregnancy.

In all studies, obstetric complications amongst the unmarried pregnant women are similar in incidence to those found in married controls with two exceptions. These are an increased incidence in severe pre-eclampsia and in anaemia. This increase is directly related to inadequate pre-natal care, and to the fact that a high proportion of the patients are teenaged primigravidae.

Labour is no more likely to be prolonged, nor to require operative delivery, than amongst married women of the same age and parity, but it may cause a considerable emotional upset. The degree of this is related to the support the girl has received in pregnancy from her family, or from the social worker assigned to look after her, and to the kindliness given by the attending obstetric staff in the hospital.

The one main obstetric complication is that unmarried parturients tend to give birth to low birth weight babies more frequently than married controls. The rate is increased between 1·5 and 2·5 times that of the married parturients (Table **15/5**),

Table 15/5

The percentage of low birth weight babies (2,500 g or less) in married and unmarried women

Year	*Country*	*Per cent of births which were low birth weight*	
		Married	*Unmarried*
1947	Finland	5·1	15·7
1948	U.K.	4·3	9·7
1961	Germany	6·9	15·0
1961	U.S.A.	7·2	11·6
1961	U.S.A.	7·2	7·4*

* Most received good pre-natal care.
Source: Paavola, A.

and because of this the perinatal mortality tends to be higher. The reason for this increase is not the unmarried state, but the lack of adequate pre-natal care, ignorance or neglect of dietary measures, perhaps smoking and the need to continue work after the 30th week of pregnancy.

Psychological Aspects of the Unmarried Parturient

Between 1930 and 1955, most writers about 'illegitimate' pregnancy tended to take the view that the parturients were emotionally immature, were 'oversexed', had suffered a lack of maternal love and had been brought up in a deprived environment. Even as late as 1952, Bowlby could write 'In a Western Community it is emotionally disturbed men and women who produce illegitimate children of a socially unacceptable kind. The girl who has a socially unacceptable illegitimate baby often comes from an unsatisfactory home background and has developed a neurotic character, the illegitimate baby being in the nature of a symptom of her neurosis.' Young, working in the U.S.A., concluded that although unmarried mothers came from all socio-economic groups and had a wide range of intelligence, they had similar mental problems. The main problem was that in most cases the girl had had a highly unsuccessful relationship with her mother, a poor relationship with her father, and there was frequently domestic disharmony. However, Young gave no information about the background of a group of controls, so that her conclusions cannot be validated. All these opinions must be criticized today, when sexual permissiveness is more common and extramarital pregnancy increasing. Should all those who have extramarital sexual relations be considered neurotic or 'oversexed', for if so this will include over 50 per cent of all males and 40 per cent of all females aged 19 or more in Britain and the U.S.A.? Or should only those who fail to marry after extramarital conception be considered neurotic? Or perhaps only those who fail to prevent pregnancy, by using contraceptives or obtaining an abortion, should be considered neurotic? And if the background of the unmarried parturient is so unsatisfactory, is this due to environment or to a poor genetic inheritance? If it is the latter, great concern should be felt as between 30 and 50 per cent of all babies born to unmarried parturients are adopted.

In a study in Sydney, Australia, no evidence could be adduced that unmarried parturients were more neurotic, were 'oversexed', had a greater degree of childhood instability, or had a higher degree of sexuality than married parturients. The only factors which seemed of importance were that the unmarried parturients seemed to have had less sex education from their parents or at school, and the parents' attitudes to sex seemed to have been more rigid and strict. It was also apparent that although the girls had heard of contraception, the information was frequently erroneous, and most had not used reliable contraceptive measures, or had left 'protection' to the male partner.

Similar findings were reported by Weir in Scotland, where of 228 unmarried mothers investigated there was no preponderance in any particular social class, promiscuity was unusual and venereal disease rare. That the mental stability of the mothers was not disturbed can be deduced from the fact that 65 per cent of the mothers kept their babies, and on follow-up have proved to make good parents.

The problem which faces the unmarried expectant mother is the scorn which conventional society places on her, her fear of reproach, her fear of shame, and the anxiety that pregnancy may hold dangers because she has contravened convention. In 1950, Marchetti and Manaker wrote 'we are convinced from our observations that the most important consideration needed to be given to the young pregnant girl lies in the management of her antepartum course. There are psychic as well as physical changes that must be borne in mind.' If the girls are unmarried as well as young, the need for counselling and support is even greater. Although this should be given by the medical attendants, by the example of their general attitude, additional support from trained social workers is of crucial importance.

Indeed informed opinion concludes that today's society is failing to meet the fundamental needs of adolescents, and as was stated at a conference on *Mental Health of Adolescents and Young People* held in Stockholm in 1969, it was not they who were maladjusted, but rather it was society that had not adapted. It is difficult to ask teenagers to develop responsibility when society seems to be fragmenting, traditional values are being discarded and when national leaders are seen to be intellectually dishonest. It is particularly difficult for young people to maintain sexual responsibility when the mass media constantly emphasize that the relatively affluent adolescent should instantly gratify his or her desires, and much of the advertising uses pseudo-sexual motivations to encourage sales. Cobliner has observed that current social and cultural changes have had a marked impact on the number of teenage pregnancies. He notes that family and school have relaxed their control over the activities of adolescents and that now they have much more leisure time, but no knowledge of how to fill it. Since sexual permissiveness is a cultural trend, many experiment in sex, and seek to emulate group heroes who boast of their sexual exploits.

The group of sexually active school children studied by Cobliner were of normal intelligence and had good scholastic performances, but lacked 'accurate information on sexual matters', a finding he considered conducive to extramarital pregnancy.

THE ROLE OF THE SOCIAL WORKER

The place of the social worker in counselling the unmarried mother-to-be, particularly if she is a teenager, is crucial. In writing this section I am most grateful to the social workers of the Women's Hospital, Sydney. Their experience is considerable, as over 1,200 pregnant unmarried girls are cared for each year; and their comments are cogent.

Firstly, the social worker is able to reduce the impact of the stigma of 'illegitimacy' placed on the adolescent by family and neighbours, or if the girl leaves home for the anonymity of the city, from her landlady. The social worker is a link with normality and friendliness, and can do much to reduce the 'shame' of being pregnant. She can help make the girl feel a worthwhile person. Since between 40 and 50 per cent of unmarried mothers-to-be keep their baby, much counselling is required so that the girl can take a relatively 'dispassionate view of what is likely to be the best course in the child's longterm interest' (Crellin). But, as a social worker in Sydney points out, the girl must make the decision herself. It must not be made by the girl's parents. Many parents feel that extramarital pregnancy indicates that the girl is immature and incapable of making any decision. This must not be permitted, or a long-lasting period of instability may result.

Secondly, the social worker can ensure that the unmarried mother obtains financial support and, if living away from home, suitable accommodation. In this aspect her counselling can be invaluable.

Thirdly, she can help educate the girl in human sexual relationships and in contraceptive technology. One social worker reported 'There is an alarming degree of confusion, superstition and ignorance regarding the nature, function and availability of contraceptives. This is reinforced by newspaper and magazine articles. This educative function is of great importance in preventing a recurrence of extramarital pregnancy. The social worker can also help to resolve the confusion the girl feels by the conflicting values of her peer group, who may, and I think often do, condone premarital sex and the values of her parents, who usually take a moralistic view of it.'

The Prevention of Unwanted Pregnancy

Social workers in Sydney, Australia, and the British authors of *Born Illegitimate* comment that educative measures need to be aimed at adolescents. This means that school curricula should include a course in human relationships, including sexuality and child development. This is especially important as many of the girls come from families which lack love, are broken, or where the parents are in conflict. To quote one social worker 'Better sex education, I believe, means not only giving information about physical bodily functions and contraceptives, but also discussing the responsibilities one has in a relationship with someone else.'

The second measure is to make sure that contraceptive advice and facilities are readily available for young people. There is no evidence that this leads to promiscuity. And if the measure is not taken it means that unwanted children will continue to be the real victims of extramarital pregnancies. Some will grow up unloved entirely; the majority will 'be reared in adverse environmental conditions which may then have longterm detrimental consequences in later life. As a result an (at present unknown) number will grow into alienated adults or inadequate parents of tomorrow' (Crellin).

The Child of the Unmarried Mother

The majority of children born out-of-wedlock are first children born to young mothers, and most are the result of unwanted pregnancies. The effect of being unwanted on the child has been considered (p. 325) where the results of a Swedish study were reported.

In recent years increasing numbers of unmarried mothers keep the child and attempt to rear it in a censorious cultural environment. In Australia, for example, about 45 per cent of unmarried mothers keep the child.

The effect of being 'illegitimate' on the child has been

examined in Britain by Crellin and her colleagues. These investigators have followed the progress of children, born extramaritally, over the first seven years of life. Comparisons were made between children retained by their single mother, those adopted and a 'control' group of children of two-parent families. The results are disturbing. To support themselves, most of the single mothers were forced to go out to work, and the quality of the foster day care varied considerably. As well as this, the mothers tended to have a high mobility, changing jobs and housing frequently. Housing conditions were usually inadequate. Over-crowding was common, and decent domestic facilities lacking. The children had a higher mortality rate than the adopted or control children. Although there was no difference in physical growth, they were less advanced at the age of seven in all aspects of ability and attainment. Speech patterns were less advanced, the children were more clumsy and had a poorer reading ability. In these early school years the children were backward in ability compared with the average, and were more often rated as unsettled or maladjusted by their teachers. Their mothers showed little or no interest in their educational progress. The authors of the study state that although contraception is now more generally available in Britain, single girls will continue to become pregnant, and this fact may only be an early sign of persistent social failure. Adoption of the child may be in its best interests, but there was no evidence in their study to show that the unmarried mother was incapable of successful child-rearing if she was given adequate social and financial support, rather than being treated as a 'fallen woman' deserving to be punished. Enlightened changes in the law regarding 'illegitimacy', and an improved social policy to help the unmarried mother who decides to keep her child, are needed.

The Older Primigravida

Earlier in this chapter it was stated that the ideal age obstetrically to become pregnant, for the first time, was from about 17 to 29. After this time complications of pregnancy and labour increase progressively as the primigravid patient approaches the end of the reproductive era. Because this increasing hazard is known, obstetricians have tended to designate a particular age above which the patient should be considered at greater risk and should receive more intensive care. Most writers have taken the age of 35 as the 'cut off' point and have considered a woman above this age to be elderly obstetrically. For this reason she has been called 'the elderly primigravida'. Not only is the term somewhat insulting to the woman, but because of earlier marriage 'elderly primigravidae' are becoming less frequent. In a study in Malaysia, Llewellyn-Jones analysed a series of primigravid pregnancies and found that a more appropriate age, after which increasing obstetric care was needed, was 30. He concluded that a primigravid patient aged 30 or more should be termed an older primigravida, although he conceded that the age was arbitrary, and that increasing problems occurred with increasing age. In most studies, fewer than 10 per cent of primigravid patients are aged 30 or more, and fewer than 2 per cent of all births fall into this category.

Obstetric Problems

COMPLICATIONS IN PREGNANCY

The incidence of pre-eclampsia and of hypertension complicating pregnancy increases amongst older primigravidae to between two and three times that found amongst primigravidae aged 17 to 29. Ante-partum haemorrhage appears slightly more common amongst older primigravidae than those under the age of 30, although this association is not found in all studies. No other complication of pregnancy, apart from a higher incidence of myomata, shows a significant difference in the older age group.

COMPLICATIONS OF LABOUR

Investigations in Aberdeen, Scotland; London, England and Kuala Lumpur, Malaysia, show that prolonged labour is more common amongst older primigravidae, and the incidence of forceps delivery and Caesarean section rises considerably with increasing age. These events are not due to increasing infant birth weights with increasing maternal age as was once thought. Kane, in a very large series, has shown that the mean birth weight does not change as the primigravida becomes older, and although older primigravidae do have a greater chance of delivering a low birth-weight baby than their younger sisters, the difference is not sufficient to materially alter the mean infant birth weight.

Table 15/6

The comparative obstetric efficiency of the younger and the older primigravida
(*per cent incidence of complications*)

	Malaysia		*Scotland*	
	Under 30	30 *and over*	*Under* 30	30 *and over*
Pre-eclampsia	6·1	13·8	10·0(4·6)*	30·0(5·0)*
Prolonged labour	3·7	11·9	35·0	60·0
Forceps	8·2	19·5	11·0	35·0
Caesarean section	2·5	11·2	2·0	4·3
Perinatal mortality (per 1,000)	20·1	47·9	37·0	70·0

* Figures in parentheses are those who had severe pre-eclampsia; pre-eclampsia probably also includes some cases of latent hypertension.
Source: Baird (1958), Nelson (1955), Llewellyn-Jones (1965) and unpublished.

The details of complications of labour from three studies are shown in Table **15/6**. The Malaysian patients were all from the lower socio-economic groups and those in Aberdeen from all socio-economic groups. The studies show that labour has three times the chance of lasting more than 24 hours in older primigravidae. Since this is not due to cephalopelvic disproportion, it must be considered due to a greater chance of inefficient or abnormal uterine activity. This was investigated by Stewart and Bernard in Scotland who found that uterine dysfunction as a cause of prolonged labour rose from 13·9 per cent in primigravidae aged 20–29, to 37·1 per cent in primigravidae over the age of 30. The older primigravida has three times the chance of being delivered by forceps and four times the chance of being delivered by Caesarean section. She also has twice the chance of having a postpartum haemorrhage in excess of 500 ml, unless the third stage of labour is actively managed. Even more significant is the fact that the perinatal mortality rate is raised.

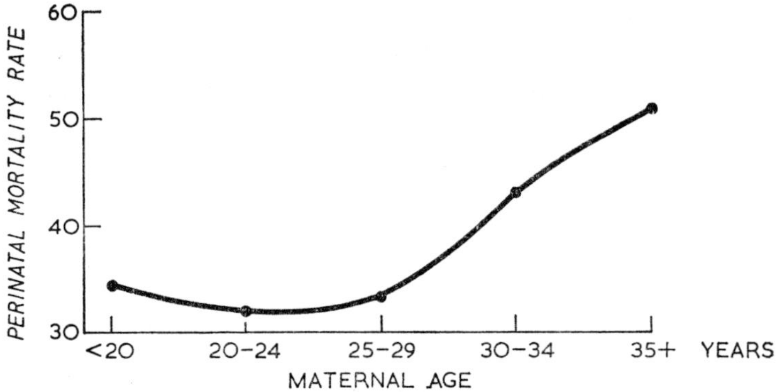

Figure **15/4** The perinatal mortality rate related to maternal age, Britain 1956.
Source: Butler, N. R., and Bonham, D. G. *Perinatal Mortality*, Livingstone, Edinburgh, 1963.

Individual hospitals rarely care for sufficient patients to obtain clear data, but in the British Perinatal Mortality Survey of 16,285 singleton babies born to married primigravidae, the perinatal mortality ratio rose from 32 per 1,000 in the age-group 20–29, to 43 per 1,000 in the age-group 30–34 and increased to 51 per 1,000 when the patient was aged 35 or more (Figure **15/4**). In a smaller series personally observed in Malaysia, the perinatal mortality of infants born to primigravidae aged 20–29 who had attended for pre-natal care at least twice was 20 per 1,000, but it rose to 48 per 1,000 amongst primigravidae aged 35 or more (Table **15/7**).

Table 15/7

Perinatal mortality in infants born to primigravidae in Malaysia (1958–62) related to the age of the mother

	Age of mother		
	10–19	20–29	30–45
Number of patients	2182	5341	376
Perinatal Mortality	21·1	20·2	47·9

One factor, although a minor one, is that congenital malformations, especially Down's syndrome, increase in frequency with advancing maternal age. The likelihood of the patient carrying an affected baby rises from 1 in 7,000 if the mother is under the age of 20, to 1 in 60 if she is over the age of 45.

As has been noted, the older primigravida has a slightly higher chance of delivering a low birth-weight baby (11·5 per cent as compared with 6·5 per cent amongst women aged 20 to 29).

These findings suggest that the older primigravida is best treated in a hospital staffed by obstetric specialists, equipped to perform Caesarean section safely and able to care for babies of low birth weight.

Psychological Problems

The psychological problems confronting the older primigravida are fears that pregnancy may be life-threatening to herself or to her fetus because of her age; fear that her fetus may be deformed; anxiety that she may be an inefficient mother; and concern about her ability to rear a child. These anxieties are compounded if the patient has had a period of involuntary infertility and has required investigations over a period of time before she became pregnant. She is also likely to have discussed pregnancy with parous neighbours, and to have obtained a considerable quantity of misinformation and mythology about pregnancy and the birth process.

The ability of the obstetrician to communicate readily and easily with the patient from early in pregnancy is essential and he must set aside time so that she may ask questions about matters which trouble her and receive clear answers. She should also be advised to obtain and read a book on matters connected with pregnancy and childbirth. One such book is *Everywoman*.

SIXTEEN

Social Factors in Reproductive Efficiency — II

In this chapter the effect of previous pregnancies, the age and the socio-economic status of the expectant mother on her reproductive efficiency will be discussed. In a way, the division into these three parts is rather arbitrary, as the three tend to be interconnected; but for a clearer appreciation of the problems, they will be dealt with separately.

The Effect of Parity on Reproductive Efficiency

In recent years, and particularly since the development of modern contraceptive technology, the proportion of first pregnancies to all other pregnancies is increasing, or, to put it another way, the average size of the family is diminishing. In Britain the average family size has dropped from above 6·25 in 1860 to 2·3 in 1970 (Figure **16/1**), although during the same period the proportion of women marrying by the age of 25 has increased from 32 to 57 per cent of all marriages (Figure **16/2**).

This reduction in natality has beneficial consequences, for statistical evidence shows that the complications of pregnancy and labour are fewest and the perinatal mortality is lowest in the second to fourth viable pregnancies. Both indices are slightly higher in the first viable pregnancy and increase considerably with the fifth and subsequent pregnancies. These data indicate that parity exercises a considerable influence on reproductive efficiency. Since the hazards of the second to fourth pregnancy are less than those associated with the first viable pregnancy (which was discussed in Chapter 15), only high parity, that is a woman having her fifth or subsequent baby, will be considered. Such women are also termed 'grande multiparae'.

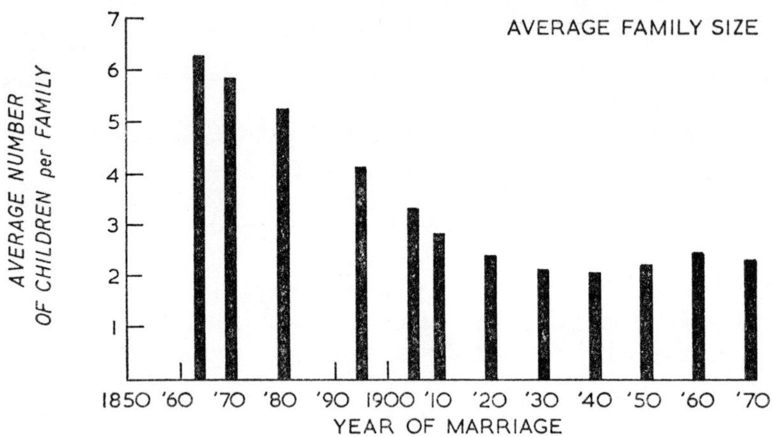

Figure **16/1** The secular change in average family size, England and Wales.
Source: Thompson, J. H.

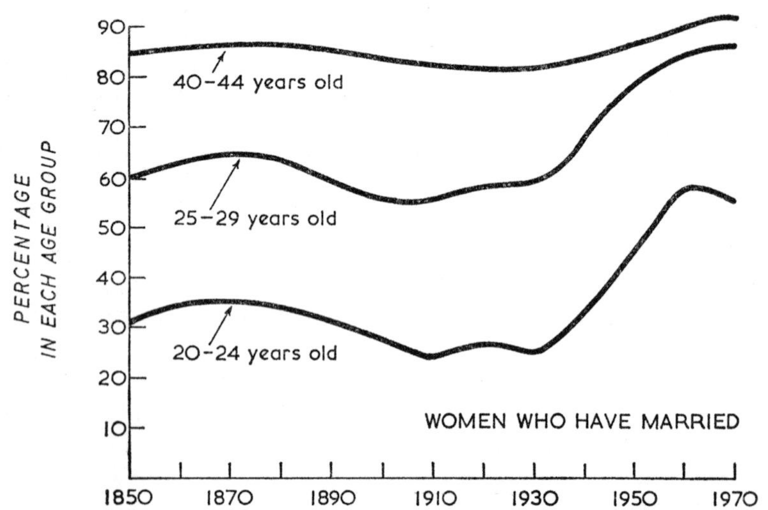

Figure **16/2** The secular changes in the proportion of married women in specified age groups, England and Wales.
Source: Thompson, J. H.

THE GRANDE MULTIPARA

The 'grande multipara' is generally considered to be a woman, irrespective of her age, who has previously had four pregnancies of over 20 weeks' duration. The term was originally introduced by Solomons, who studied a number of such patients in Ireland. In the past 20 years at least 15 reports have appeared in the literature in the English language, and the largest series was reported from London in 1967.

The number of grande multiparae per 100 pregnancies depends on cultural attitudes to large families, on the availability of contraceptives, and on the level of education of the population. An investigation in the U.S.A. in 1965 confirmed this hypothesis. Amongst white Americans, 13·2 per cent of the women aged 15 to 44 giving birth were grande multigravidae, whilst amongst black Americans, the percentage of grande multigravidae rose to 37·2. Black Americans, in general, married earlier, had a larger number of extramarital pregnancies, were of lower economic status and had a lower educational level than white Americans.

The same trend towards higher natality was found amongst white Americans when their age at marriage, educational attainment, socio-economic level (as measured by income and occupation of the husband) and place of residence were related to the parity of the wife. This analysis was made by the U.S. Bureau of the Census on the 1960 census. Those white Americans who had married early and had large families tended to have left school early with a low educational attainment, to be married to husbands whose income and social status were low, and to live in rural areas. Of the various factors analysed, age at marriage was the most important. The other factors had a lesser influence on natality, but when associated with early marriage of the girl increased the likelihood of high parity.

Since 1960, information and advice about contraception has been spread more widely and the differentials may be less marked when the 1970 census is studied.

In the United Kingdom, a survey was made by Law of grande multigravidae in the N.W. Metropolitan (London) Region of the National Health Service. Between October, 1962 and September 1963, 4,225 grande multiparae were delivered in the region, representing 5·9 per cent of all deliveries. But it is anticipated that with the increasing knowledge of contraception and the increasing availability of contraceptives the numbers of grande multigravidae will diminish over the next decade. Analysis of the series gave considerable information about the risk of pregnancy to grande multiparae in a developed nation, with a prepaid health service and a high standard of obstetric care. The survey forms the basis of the remainder of this section, although information from an Australian study has been added.

Obstetric complications

Since complications in pregnancy and labour are related to age as well as to parity, it is of interest to note that complications rose with age when only grande multigravidae were considered (Table **16/1**). It is also of interest that 26·3 per cent of the mothers were under the age of 30 and 60·8 per cent under the age of 35.

Hypertensive states occurred in pregnancy in 6·1 per cent of

Table 16/1

The effect of maternal age on the incidence of complications of pregnancy and labour amongst grande multiparae

Maternal age	20–24	25–29	30–34	35–39	40+
Percentage in age group	3·8	22·5	34·0	26·7	12·9
			Numbers		
No complications	125	735	1,072	800	365
Complications present	14	93	179	183	110
All	139	828	1,251	983	475
			Percentage		
No complications	90·0	88·8	85·5	81·9	76·9
Complications present	10·0	11·2	14·2	18·1	23·1
All	100	100	100	100	100

Source: North-West Regional Survey, 1962–63, London.

the patients. Fifty-three per cent of the hypertensive states were considered to be due to pre-eclampsia, 40 per cent to essential hypertension complicating pregnancy, and the remaining 7 per cent were not completely classified. The incidence of hypertensive states complicating pregnancy amongst grande multiparae in the British series is lower than the mean of 10 per cent recorded in most previous studies, and is probably a function of better pre-natal care. However, the incidence is twice that of women pregnant for the second to the fourth time, but lower than the incidence amongst primigravidae. Hypertensive disorders in pregnancy, therefore, have a U-shaped curve of incidence. Ante-partum haemorrhage occurred in 2·7 per cent of cases, which is double that found in women of lower parity. Of medical conditions complicating pregnancy none was found more frequently amongst grande multigravidae, and although anaemia is usually considered to be a frequent complication in these patients, in this series only 1·8 per cent of patients were anaemic. Unstable presentation has also been considered a sinister hazard to the grande multigravida, and Irish reports gave an incidence of 10 per cent. In the London series, unstable presentation was found in 1·8 per cent of all cases, and although this is higher than amongst women of lower parity, it does not constitute a significant hazard.

It can be seen that provided the grande multigravida seeks pre-natal care early in pregnancy, the dangers of complications of pregnancy are not increased.

Complications of labour

In most reports labour is considered to be a particularly dangerous time for the grande multigravida. In the London series, labour lasted more than 24 hours in 3·3 per cent of patients, the forceps rate was 1 per cent, the Caesarean section rate was 3·6 per cent. None of these rates are higher than those found amongst women of lower parity, but it was noted that the Caesarean section rate rose with the patient's age. Of the Caesarean sections, the indication was ante-partum haemorrhage in 32 per cent, failed induction of labour in 14 per cent, unstable presentation in 13 per cent, and previous Caesarean section in 11 per cent. Post-partum haemorrhage occurred in 5 per cent of patients, a rate more than twice that expected, so that this is a potential hazard, particularly if the patient has been delivered in unsuitable surroundings.

The infant of the grande multigravida

Several authors have observed that the infant of the grande multigravida tended to be above average in birth weight. This was confirmed by the British Perinatal Survey and by the London study. In the London series, 18·8 per cent of the babies

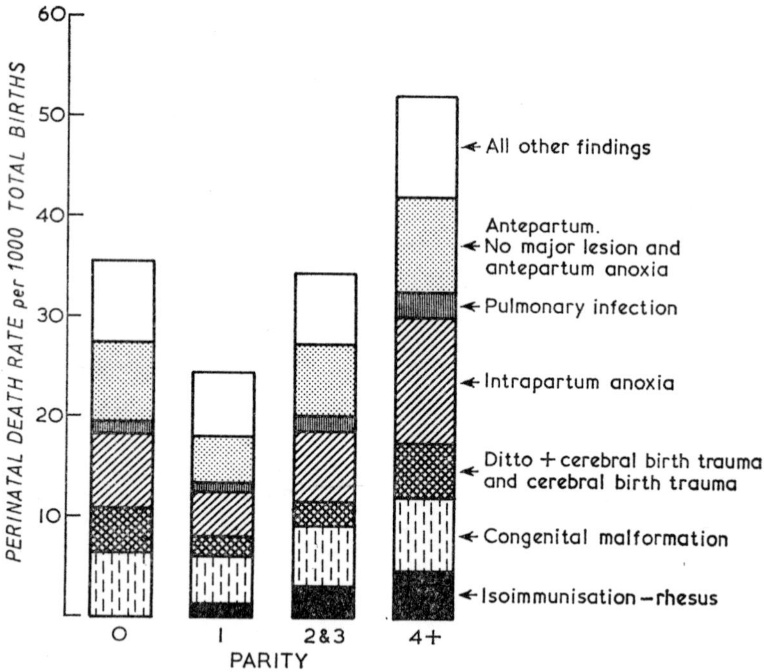

Figure **16/3** Necropsy findings of perinatal deaths related to maternal parity group.
Source: Butler, N. R., and Bonham, D. G.

exceeded 4,000 g (nearly 9 lb) at birth. The perinatal mortality of infants of grande multigravidae was 50·5 per 1,000; which is 50 per cent higher than the perinatal mortality of the infants of women para 2 to 3 as disclosed in the Perinatal Mortality Survey in Britain. One factor of importance is that congenital defects of the neural tube, particularly anencephaly, show a rising incidence in grande multigravidae, particularly the older grande multigravida.

In Figure **16/3**, which is reproduced from the British Perinatal Mortality Survey, the necropsy findings of the perinatal deaths occurring to women of various parities are shown. It can be seen that in each of the major groups, an increasing incidence of perinatal deaths occurred.

Conclusions

Since the majority of grande multigravidae tend to be of a lower intellectual level, to have a poorer economic status and less occupational and residential mobility than women of lower parity, they tend to avoid pre-natal care, and in many countries to seek home delivery. The patient is more likely to develop hypertension in pregnancy, to be anaemic, to have an antepartum haemorrhage and to have an unstable presentation. Labour is not likely to last longer, but postpartum haemorrhage is more likely to occur. The perinatal mortality of her infant is likely to be 50 per cent higher than that of a woman of lower parity. These hazards can be reduced considerably in countries where there is good pre-natal care which is readily available to patients, and where patients seek the care from early pregnancy. This means that a network of pre-natal clinics needs to be provided which are reasonably near the patient's home. In addition, the patient requires to be informed and educated about the need to seek the available pre-natal care from early in pregnancy, and to understand that if complications arise, she may require to be referred to a well-equipped obstetric hospital for treatment or confinement. The grande multipara who fails to seek pre-natal care is at risk. Not only are the complications of hypertension in pregnancy and anaemia likely, but malpresentations may remain undetected and lead to an obstructed labour. These patients have particular risk of postpartum haemorrhage, and if the patient is delivered in her home preventive measures (such as the injection of 'Syntometrine' at the time of delivery) should be taken, and transport be available to take the patient to hospital should this be necessary.

Grande multigravidae constitute a high risk group of patients. The risk will only be reduced by preventing the condition from arising by better dissemination of contraceptive advice, and by providing a good obstetric service to those who do not accept the advice.

Maternal Age and Reproductive Efficiency

In Chapter 15 the effect of age on reproductive efficiency was studied by examining the performance of the teenage primigravida and the older primigravida. This analysis indicated that the effect of age varied with the social status of the expectant mother and with her acceptance of adequate pre-natal care. Before considering social status it would be appropriate to summarize the findings regarding age, and to add some additional information.

Several studies, notably that carried out in Britain in 1946 by the Royal Commission on Population, have shown that the incidence of childlessness rises with age at marriage. In the British survey women who had married between 1900 and 1909 and who had been married for at least 10 years, were studied. During the period reviewed it was considered that fewer than 5 per cent of women practised voluntary conception control, and analysis of the data showed that there was no increase in the incidence of childlessness after 10 years of marriage. For these reasons the results were considered to be representative of involuntary sterility amongst British women. In Table **16/2**, it can be seen that the proportion of childless women increased with late age at marriage. Under the age of 30 this factor was not significant, but it became increasingly important if the age of the woman at marriage was 30 or more.

The effect of age on reproductive performance has been examined in Aberdeen, Scotland and in Kuala Lumpur, Malaysia. In these studies only primiparae who had attended pre-natal clinics on at least two occasions were included in the analysis, so that the variable of parity might be eliminated as far as possible.

In the Aberdeen study, the records of 5,339 married primiparae delivered between 1949 and 1954 in a single hospital were analysed. Aberdeen is an industrial city which had a population of 186,000 during the period under review. It is the commercial centre of an extensive and isolated agricultural region. The medical services of the region are highly organized, with good

Table 16/2

The age at marriage related to the percentage of women who had no children after 10 years of marriage

Age at marriage	*Per cent childless after* 10 *years of marriage*
15–19	6·2
20–24	8·4
25–29	14·3
30–34	22·7
35–39	39·4
40+	68·4
All ages	11·7

Source: *Report of Family Census 1946*, Royal Com. Pop., H.M.S.O., 1954.

transport facilities and good communication between family doctors at the periphery and the obstetric hospital at the centre. At the time of the study over 85 per cent of primiparae in the area received pre-natal care and gave birth in the hospital.

Kuala Lumpur is the capital of the State of Selangor, and of Malaysia. The city at the time of the study, between 1958 and 1962, had about 350,000 inhabitants and served an area of about 800,000 people. Two hospitals, the Government General Hospital and the Chinese Maternity Hospital, delivered 8,000 and 4,000 patients per year respectively, or about 80 per cent of all deliveries in the city. Between 1958 and 1962, 8,555 primiparous women who had attended the pre-natal clinic at least twice were delivered in the General Hospital. These formed the study group.

The social classification used in both investigations was that recommended by the Registrar-General in Britain in 1951. In this classification the population was divided into five classes:

Class I Professional, managerial and administrative
Class II Supervisory, non-manual blue- and white-collar workers, shopkeepers

Table 16/3

Reproductive efficiency related to maternal age in Scotland (Aberdeen) and Malaysia (Kuala Lumpur)

AGE	*Mild toxaemia* %		*Severe toxaemia/Eclampsia* %		*Prolonged labour* %
	Aberdeen	*Kuala Lumpur*	*Aberdeen*	*Kuala Lumpur*	*Kuala Lumpur*
10–19	13·4	3·6	4·4	2·2	2·1
20–24	15·4	4·0	4·2	2·3	4·1
25–29	15·3	4·0	5·4	1·7	5·1
30–34	23·6	8·5	5·2	4·2	9·7
35+	28·2	11·6	4·9	9·1	22·7
All	16·2	4·2	4·6	2·3	4·1

AGE	*Caesarean section* %		*Forceps delivery* %		*Perinatal mortality (per 1,000)* %	
	Aberdeen	*Kuala Lumpur*	*Kuala Lumpur*		*Aberdeen*	*Kuala Lumpur*
			Mid	*Low*		
10–19	2·1	1·6	1·7	2·9	39	21·1
20–24	3·1	2·0	4·9	4·9	25	19·2
25–29	5·8	4·2	5·7	6·0	25	21·3
30–34	11·6	9·0	8·7	9·7	34	48·4
35+	33·7	21·2	18·2	7·5	43	45·5
All	5·1	3·0	4·0	4·8	28	21·4

Class III Skilled workers
Class IV Semi-skilled workers
Class V Unskilled workers

In this Chapter only those factors which showed a significant variation with maternal age have been chosen (Table **16/3**). It can be seen that in both studies the incidence of mild pre-eclampsia rose after the age of 30. Severe pre-eclampsia and eclampsia only increased with age in the Malaysian study. The cause of pre-eclampsia is unknown, so that the reason for the increasing incidence with increasing age is unknown, although Nelson, who reported the Aberdeen figures, considers that it may be due to the unmasking of latent essential hypertension.

Statistics from the British Perinatal Mortality Survey suggest that this is not so and the good Aberdeen results may have been due to the excellent pre-natal care available. When all patients with essential hypertension were excluded, it was found in the British Perinatal Survey that the incidence of pre-eclampsia rose with age both in primigravidae and in multigravidae (Table **16/4**). The higher proportion of women with signs of pre-eclampsia is probably due to less stringent criteria for diagnosis

Table 16/4

The incidence of pre-eclampsia related to maternal age and parity

Maternal age	*Incidence of pre-eclampsia (per cent)*	
	Mild	*Severe*
Primiparae		
<25	21·6	8·2
25–34	24·5	9·4
35+	34·1	15·5
Multiparae		
<25	13·6	3·4
25–34	18·1	3·4
35+	22·3	5·7

Source: *British Perinatal Mortality Survey.*

used in the survey, which covered all deliveries occurring in Britain in one week.

In both the Scottish and Malaysian series the length of labour tended to increase with increasing maternal age. As has been mentioned in Chapter 15, Stewart and Bernard considered that the increased length of labour was due to an increasing incidence of uterine dysfunction rather than to a rising incidence of cephalopelvic disproportion. This was substantiated by the observation that there was no increase in the mean birth weight of the babies with increasing maternal age. The incidence of forceps delivery also rose, although this was not analysed in Aberdeen. In Kuala Lumpur, mid-forceps was differentiated from low forceps, as it was considered that the latter was often done for non-obstetric reasons, such as to save time after an episiotomy. The incidence of Caesarean section also rose with increasing maternal age both in Aberdeen and in Kuala Lumpur. The perinatal mortality shows a U-shaped curve, being higher in primigravidae aged 10–19, then falling until the age of 29, after which a rise occurred to reach a peak in the 35 and older age-group. The British Perinatal Mortality Survey confirmed this trend and showed that it related to all parities (Figure **16/4**).

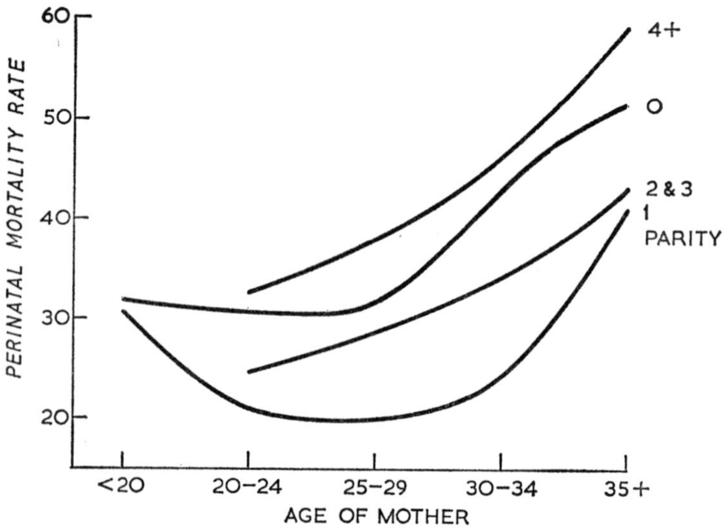

Figure **16/4** Perinatal deaths by maternal age and parity. Source: Butler, N. R., and Bonham, D. G.

One of the factors leading to a higher perinatal mortality is the increasing incidence of congenital defects, mainly of the central nervous system, which rise with maternal age. The most obvious defect is Down's syndrome. The incidence of this disorder is five times higher in infants of women more than 30 years old, compared with women under the age of 30. One per cent of pregnancies to women aged 40 or more results in a child with Down's syndrome, and this rises to one in 60 pregnancies if the mother is 45 or older (Table **16/5**).

Table 16/5

The risk of Down's syndrome in the child, related to the mother's age

Age of mother	*Risk of occurrence*	*Risk of recurrence*
30	1 : 1500	1 : 500
30–34	1 : 750	1 : 250
35–39	1 : 600	1 : 200
40–44	1 : 300	1 : 100
45+	1 : 60	1 : 20

Source: Redding and Hirshborn in *March of Dimes Articles*, Series Vol. 4, 4, 1968.

It is interesting to note that congenital malformations of a major nature occurred in 17·0 per 1,000 of all births in England and Wales, whilst the rate in Sweden was 11·2 per 1,000. In the Perinatal Mortality Survey of 1958, the social aspects of congenital defects were investigated. The survey confirmed earlier reports that advanced maternal age is an important factor in Down's disease, and in several other central nervous system tube defects. A strong association between the incidence of neural tube defects and Social Class IV and V was noted. There is also strong evidence that the incidence of the major neural tube defect, anencephalus, is higher in older multigravidae (Table **16/6**). If the lower incidence of congenital defects in Sweden is due to better social conditions, and to smaller families, completed before the age of 30, a reduction in congenital malformations may be expected as social conditions and contraceptive usage increases in other nations.

Table 16/6

Congenital defects. The risk of development related to maternal age
(*women aged* 35 *or more compared with women under the age of* 35)

Congenital defects	*Age*	
	<35	⩾35
Down's syndrome	1	7·7
Cerebral palsy	1	1·8
Anencephalus	1	1·9
Defects of circulatory system	1	1·7
CNS birth injury	1	1·6

Sources:
Newcombe, H. B., and Tavendale, O. G. *Mutat Res.*, **1,** 446, 1964, quoted by Day.
Fedrick, J. *Ann. Human Genetics*, **34,** 31, 1970.

Conclusion

The conclusion to be derived from these data is that with increasing maternal age, fertility decreases whilst complications of pregnancy and labour increase. The study of the rate of increase confirms that reproductive efficiency is at its peak between the age of 18 and 25, becoming less efficient below the age of 15 and after the age of 30.

The Effect of Social Status on Reproductive Efficiency

Evidence has been given in Chapter 6 and in Chapter 15 that socio-economic status has a considerable influence on reproductive efficiency. This influence operates from early childhood, and probably from intra-uterine life. The physique and health of the expectant mother greatly affect her reproductive performance and are themselves dependent on her genetic inheritance and the type of environment in which she has been reared. They also depend on the availability of a balanced diet in infancy and childhood, and on proper feeding habits.

Those women with the poorest physical health tend to come from the lower socio-economic groups, to have the largest number of siblings, to live in the worst environment, to have the highest rate of teenage extra-marital pregnancies and pre-nuptial conceptions, to have the highest total parity and to be the most reluctant to seek pre-natal care. On the other hand, women of superior health and physique tend to marry later, or to postpone conception for longer after marriage. As has been noted, the older the primigravida, the less efficient is her obstetric performance.

The problem in any analysis is that the factors of age, parity and socio-economic status are so interrelated, that it is difficult to determine the effect of any single factor. Possibly because of this, the literature is not very extensive and the problem is compounded by the fact that most reports have been based on collected hospital series and consequently include patients dealt with by a large number of obstetricians who have a wide spectrum of philosophies for conducting their practice. This has the effect of reducing the valid comparison of certain indices of obstetric efficiency. For example, examination of hospital reports from many countries show that the Caesarean section rate amongst paying patients is twice to three times as high as that amongst the 'higher-risk' patients in public wards. Clearly the reason for the higher rate cannot be obstetric, for as will be seen, obstetric problems are greater amongst the poorer section of the community. An analysis of the problem in Sydney revealed that the Caesarean section rate of different obstetricians attending paying patients in a certain hospital had a mean of 14 per cent, and varied from 9·5 to 25·0 per cent; whilst the mean rate amongst public patients was 5·5 per cent. Clearly subjective individual preference was the reason for the difference rather than objective obstetric criteria.

Because of this, the analysis will be confined to the series of primigravidae studied in Aberdeen and in Kuala Lumpur because in both centres there was agreement by the medical staff on procedures, and personal supervision was possible to clarify certain points. The British Perinatal Survey of 1958 will also be mentioned.

Table 16/7

Age at first viable pregnancy (>28 weeks gestation) related to husband's socio-economic status
(*Percentage of women in each age group*)

Year 1958–1962

Age at first viable pregnancy	*Kuala Lumpur*		*Aberdeen*	
	Husband's social class		*Husband's social class*	
	I *and* II	III *to* V	I *and* II	III *to* V
10–19	4·0	27·6	2·1	15·3
20–24	42·0	45·5	34·0	50·2
25–29	40·4	22·1	39·0	25·5
30–34	10·4	4·0	19·3	6·1
35+	2·2	0·8	5·6	2·9
n =	657	7,898	238	1,003

Year 1970

Age at first viable pregnancy	*Aberdeen*	
	Husband's social class	
	I *and* II	III *to* V
10–19	12·6	26·6
20–24	42·2	52·8
25–29	35·6	14·7
30–34	6·5	3·9
35+	3·2	2·0
n =	278	939

Source: for Aberdeen data, Prof. Ian MacGillivray.

Age at first pregnancy

Information from Scotland and Malaysia confirm the view that women in the higher socio-economic groups tend to postpone conception. The investigation made in Kuala Lumpur showed that 54 per cent of women, whose husband was in Social Class I or II, were aged 25 or more when carrying the first viable pregnancy, as opposed to only 27 per cent of women in Social Classes IV to V (Table **16/7**). Statistics from Aberdeen show a similar pattern, but it is to be noted that a secular change is occurring; when the data obtained in 1960 are compared with those of 1970, in the latter year more women of the upper socio-economic groups are becoming pregnant at an earlier age. Nevertheless, in two different types of society, women of higher socio-economic groups tend to delay childbearing.

Social class and pregnancy complications: Scotland

It would not be unreasonable to assume that the healthier the expectant mother, the less is she likely to develop complications in pregnancy, or to have difficulties in labour. It is easier to make the statement than to prove it, for the assessment of physical health is not exact and the indices are ill-defined. Investigations in Britain in the last 40 years have suggested that the reproductive performance amongst the upper socio-economic groups is superior to that of the lower groups, but until the Aberdeen workers investigated a well-defined population in the 1950s and 1960s, there was no proof of the hypothesis. Realizing that physical health was difficult to define objectively, the Aberdeen group related their assessment of physical health to that of body height, as the latter could be measured easily and accurately. Their findings indicated a positive correlation; 71 per cent of women with good health and physique were 163 cm (5 ft 4 in) or more, compared with only 30 per cent of short women (less than 155 cm (5 ft 1 in). It was also found that the proportion of short women increased steeply when the assessment of health and physique was graded fair or poor (Table **16/8**).

Body height is determined by the interplay of genetic inheritance and environmental factors, of which an important item is a good diet in childhood. The exact influence of

Table 16/8

Health and physique of Aberdeen primigravidae
related to body height
(*Percentage of women in each height group*)

Maternal height	*Health and physique*			
	Very good	*Good*	*Fair*	*Poor or very poor*
⩾ 163 cm	42	29	18	13
⩽ 155 cm	10	20	30	48

Source: Baird, D. 'Fertility and Health Status' in *Public Health and Population Change*. Ed. Sheps, M. C. and Ridley, J. C.

inheritance and environment remains in dispute, and the difficulty of separating the factors appears almost insuperable. Although genetic inheritance controls racial differences, in the rate and degree of growth, in all races studied the higher socio-economic groups had a higher proportion of tall people, who had a better physique. It could result from a pattern of social mobility which leads to an average movement of tall people upwards and short people downwards, as Tanner suggests. This assumes that taller men of the upper socio-economic groups tend to marry taller women. Although this syndrome of social mobility applies to developed nations, it cannot explain the findings in more traditional societies where marriages are generally arranged. It is more likely that the better growth, and physique, of the more affluent are due to a better home environment and better childhood nutrition. Evidence from several nations has shown that malnutrition delays growth, and increases the likelihood of infectious disease, which itself may delay growth. There is also a difference in the height, weight and general physique of the children according to the number of living siblings. The larger the family, the slower is the growth of each member during childhood and adolescence. As further evidence of the effect of good infant and childhood nutrition on growth, it has been observed that amongst European children there has been a steady increase in body height over the past 100 years. The magnitude of the increase has been about

0·3 cm (about a tenth of an inch) a decade from 1830 to 1880 and about 0·6 cm (about a fifth of an inch) a decade from 1880. This secular trend coincides with improvement of environmental sanitation, better childhood nutrition and a reduction in family size. This evidence supports the use by the Aberdeen workers of the readily measured and reproducible index of height as a measure of physique and health.

As a general rule, in Britain at least, those born and reared in an upper socio-economic environment tend to marry a partner from a similar social background. Illsley has shown that women who move upwards in the social scale on marriage,

Table 16/9

Maternal height and social class
(*Primigravidae* 1948–57, *Aberdeen by social class of husband*)

	Social Class		
	I + II	III	IV–V
	Percentage		
Tall (163 cm and over)	47	27	21
Medium	43	51	50
Small (155 cm and less)	10	22	29

Source: Baird, D. *J. Obst. Gynaec. Brit. Cwlth.*, **70,** 204, 1963.

tend to be taller than average. It is likely then that women in the upper social classes will be taller than those in the lower social classes. Investigations in Aberdeen have confirmed this observation (Table **16/9**). It was, therefore, possible for the Aberdeen workers to use body height and social class as indices against which they could measure reproductive performance. Statistical investigations in many centres have shown that the incidence of difficult labour due to cephalopelvic disproportion increases as body height diminishes. Since patients with disproportion tend to have longer labours and to require an operative delivery more frequently, the incidence of prolonged labour, forceps and Caesarean section will tend to rise. As might be expected, difficult labour is associated with a higher perinatal mortality, but it was found that the perinatal death rate from all other causes also increased as the patient's height and social status diminished. In Britain, the Aberdeen findings were extended and confirmed by the Perinatal Mortality Survey in 1958. The results are shown in Figure **16/5**. This figure shows that within the same socio-economic group, taller

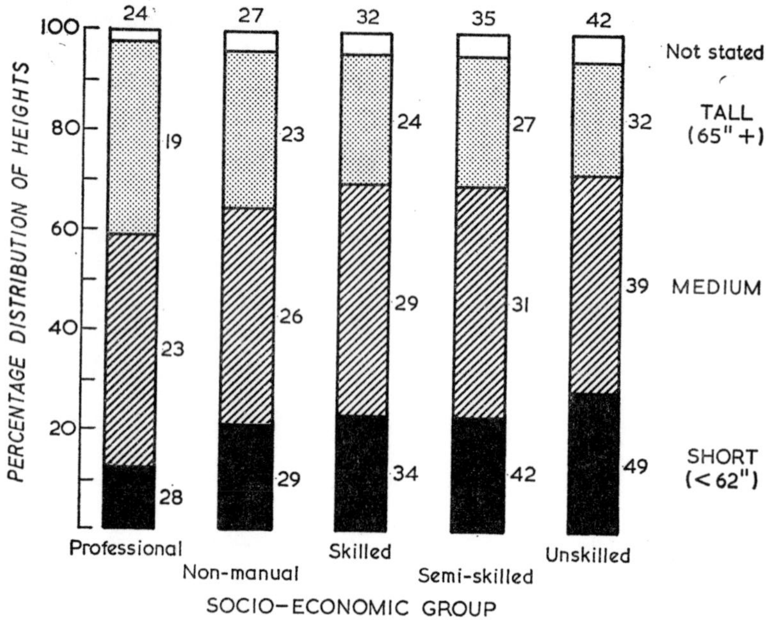

Figure 16/5 Perinatal mortality related to the height of the mother and the socio-economic status of the father, U.K. 1956. Source: Butler, N. R., and Bonham, D. G.

women have a lower perinatal loss than shorter women, and that as the socio-economic status of the patient diminishes the perinatal mortality in each height group is increased.

Social class and pregnancy complications: Malaysia

The effect of social class on reproductive efficiency is not so marked in the developing nations, if the model of Malaysia may be taken as giving valid information. Part of the problem is that the index of height was not found to be helpful in the Malaysian study. The findings of the Malaysian study are shown in Table **16/10**. Contrary to the Scottish study it can be seen that the overall incidence of pre-eclampsia was higher in the upper socio-economic groups, although that of severe pre-eclampsia and eclampsia was lower. Prolonged labour, Caesarean section and forceps delivery were all more frequent amongst

Table 16/10

The effect of social status on reproductive efficiency
(*Malaysian primiparae*, 1958–62)

	Class I *and* II $n = 657$		*Class* III, IV, V $n = 7,898$	
	Per cent			
Pre-eclampsia				
Mild	3·0		4·0	
Severe	0·8		2·3	
Total		3·8		6·3
Prolonged labour	6·6		4·1	
Caesarean section		4·7		3·0
Forceps				
Mid	13·0		4·0	
Low	18·7		4·8	
Total		31·7		8·8
Perinatal mortality (per 1,000)	16·7		21·4	

the higher socio-economic groups. In the analysis mid-forceps was separated from low forceps for the latter is often only performed for the convenience of the obstetrician, when an episiotomy alone would be sufficient to effect delivery. However, despite the increased incidence of obstetric interference, the perinatal mortality amongst the upper socio-economic group was lower than that of the lower socio-economic group.

Reasons for the difference between Scotland and Malaysia

Two factors require consideration in an attempt to explain the divergent findings of the two studies. The first is the influence of the age of the woman. In the Malaysian study, 54 per cent of the primiparae in Social Class I and II were aged 25 or more, and 13·6 per cent were aged 30 or more, compared with 63·9 per cent and 24·9 per cent of the Scottish primiparae of the same social classes.

The second factor is that obstetric efficiency is related to the nutrition of the mother during her own infancy and childhood as much as to her nutrition in pregnancy. It is true that a proper diet in pregnancy will eliminate anaemia, reduce the incidence of low birth-weight babies (although the factor of pre-pregnancy nutrition is important) and may alter the incidence of pre-eclampsia (although the evidence for this statement is conflicting).

If diet plays a part in the aetiology of pre-eclampsia, the higher incidence of mild pre-eclampsia amongst the Scottish primigravidae of the higher socio-economic groups could be due to overeating, particularly too much carbohydrate, whilst the higher incidence amongst the Malaysian primigravidae of the lower socio-economic groups could be due to under-nutrition.

However, as far as reproductive performance in labour is concerned, nutrition during infancy, childhood and adolescence is more important than diet in pregnancy. In 1946, a Scottish Scientific Advisory Committee reported that in pre-war Scotland, working mothers were underfed and their diets of poor quality. They stated that 'such diets are important causes of poor physique and maternal illhealth'. The children of such mothers formed the primigravidae studied 20 to 30 years later by the Aberdeen workers. The patients studied in Malaysia, between 1958 and 1962, had been born between 1928 and 1940, and had been children during the world economic depression and the Japanese occupation of Malaya. The parents of many had been of a lower socio-economic group than their children, who had achieved a higher status through education and subsequent employment in Government service. Such variables would reduce the difference between the obstetric performance of women in different socio-economic groups.

Birth Weight and Social Class

In the British Perinatal Mortality Survey it was noted that the birth weight for week of gestation rose with social class, but the differences between birth-weight curves were not always consistent. They were influenced by the parity of the mother, and once allowance had been made for associated effects showed no significant difference between social classes. This would suggest that given the diets obtainable in Britain, diet in pregnancy had a minimal effect on birth weight. However, in

Table 16/11

The birth weight of the baby related to the social class of the mother in Aberdeen, Scotland
(*Female infants only, weight in g*)

Pregnancy number	*Social class*		
	I, II	III	IV, V
1	3,250	3,200	3,120
2–4	3,370	3,340	3,240
5+	3,360	3,370	3,270

Source: Thomson et al. *J. Obst. Gynaec. Brit. Cwlth.*, **75**, 903, 1968.

Table 16/12

Mean birth weights of Malaysian babies related to the social class of the mothers (booked primiparae only) $n = 8,555$

Race	*Social class*	
	I *and* II	III–V
	Birth weight in g	
Chinese	3,100	2,950
Malay	3,010	2,840
Indian	3,015	2,265

the careful study in Aberdeen, the influence of social class on birth weight was seen and was most marked amongst women of lower parities (Table **16/11**). In Malaysia, the difference between the birth weight of the babies of primigravidae varied with social class and within each social class between the three races (Table **16/12**).

Three main ethnic groups live in Malaysia—the Malays, the Chinese and the Indians. Amongst the poorer women, the Indian diet was the least nutritious, and had the lowest protein content, whilst the Chinese diet had the highest protein content. Once the woman became wealthier, her diet improved, the birth weight of her infant rose, and the difference in birth weights of infants of different racial groups diminished.

Similar observations have been made in several other developing nations. For example, in South India, Ventatachalam found that the mean birth weight was much higher in the upper than in the lower socio-economic groups. He also found that if the poorest patients were taken into hospital from the 36th week of pregnancy and given an adequate, protein-rich, well-balanced diet, the mean birth weight of the infant was 200 g (about half a pound) greater than that of the infants of a woman not admitted. This observation emphasizes the need for good nutrition in pregnancy amongst the poorer sections of a community, as well as good nutrition in infancy, childhood and adolescence.

Perinatal Mortality and Social Class

In the Aberdeen study, the Kuala Lumpur study and the British Perinatal Mortality study, a positive correlation between perinatal mortality and social class was observed. In the British Perinatal Mortality Survey the factor of maternal height also had an influence as has been noted and is shown in Figure **16/5**, p. 426. It was also shown in the Aberdeen study, which related only to primigravidae.

The reason for the higher perinatal mortality in the lower socio-economic groups is probably multifactorial. The influence of poor childhood environment and nutrition on reproductive efficiency has been mentioned. Those women who have the lowest reproductive efficiency are the ones who are more likely to receive the least efficient medical care in pregnancy and labour. It follows that when the physical condition of the mother is poor, a high standard of obstetrical and social care is of particular importance. The efforts to reduce the perinatal mortality must, therefore, be twofold. The first is socio-political and should seek to improve family welfare by improving the general health of the mother and more particularly the female children through good nutrition. This in turn implies education of the mother so that she may alter traditional feeding patterns. As well as this, living conditions require to be improved so that the children may grow healthily. One way of doing this is to encourage family planning in the context of improving family welfare. The second approach, which should be pursued concurrently, is to improve standards of obstetric and child health care. This largely depends on medical organization, communications and skills, and will inevitably rely on a well-organized, highly-motivated health team.

SEVENTEEN

Social Factors in Low Birth Weight

The birth weight of any baby depends on a complex relationship between its genetically inherited growth potential and the effectiveness of the support provided by the maternal organism via the uterine blood vessels and the placenta. The growth potential of the individual fetus is unalterable, but its actual growth is modified by the growth support, which in practical terms means the quantity of nutrients and oxygen, made available to it. For the fetus to obtain maximal growth potential, the mother must be able to provide adequate amounts of protein and carbohydrate, and sufficient oxygen in the blood which bathes the placenta; the blood flow through the utero-placental area must be good; and the placenta must function sufficiently well to transfer the nutrients and oxygen to the fetal circulation, and to transfer waste products of metabolism from the fetus. So long as the maternal growth support exceeds that needed to achieve the fetal growth potential, the amount of growth of the fetus will depend on the latter; but when the growth support is inadequate, the growth potential will be limited, and growth retardation may occur.

Fetal growth potential is genetically determined, but except amongst the most healthy women *full* growth potential is rarely achieved. It is influenced by the sex of the fetus, male fetuses becoming heavier than females from the 30–35th week of gestation, so that at term the male infant weighs about 150 g (5 oz) more than the female. It is even more markedly affected by the presence of congenital defects. If the fetus is malformed, its growth potential is usually diminished, irrespective of the adequacy of the growth support, because of its inability to utilize the available nutrients.

Growth support is altered by a variety of factors, many being related to the socio-economic status of the mother, and to her nutrition and physical development from early childhood. It is also reduced in cases of multiple pregnancy, when it tends to become inadequate at an earlier gestational stage, because of the greater demands of the combined fetuses. For example, McKeown and Record have shown that the maternal organism is only able to supply sufficient growth support for about 3,000 g (6½ lb) of total fetal growth, without growth retardation occurring. However, except in cases of gross maternal disease, or extreme starvation, growth support is adequate to ensure

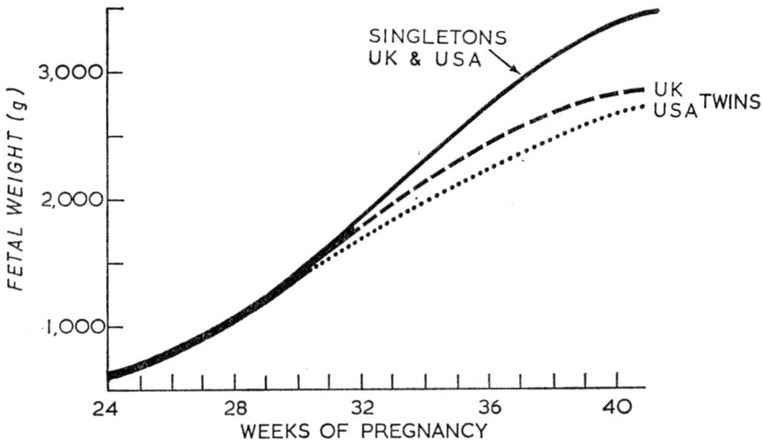

Figure **17/1** Growth retardation of the fetuses in multiple pregnancy.
Source: U.K.—McKeown, T., and Record, J. *J. Endocrin.* **8,** 386, 1953 and *Perinatal Mortality*, p. 126; USA—Hendricks C., *Obstet. and Gynec.*, **27,** 53, 1966.

maximal fetal growth (within the range of genetic growth potential) to about the 30th week of pregnancy, and differences will only become marked after the 35th week of gestation (Figure **17/1**).

Fetal growth in utero can be assessed by measuring the length of the fetus using radiology, or the biparietal diameter of its skull using ultrasonic echography (Figure **17/2**). Of the two methods ultrasound is the most useful and accurate in clinical obstetrics, but the apparatus is expensive and not generally available. An alternative method is to relate birth weight to

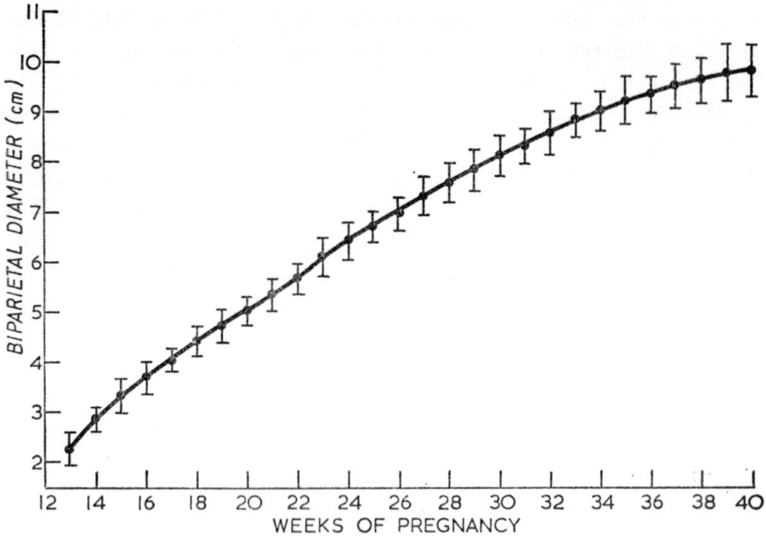

Figure **17/2** Fetal biparietal diameter measured by ultrasound related to gestational age.
Source: Campbell, S., *J. Obst. Gynaec. Brit. Cwlth.*, **75,** 568, 1968.

gestational age in cases where the mother's statement of the date of her last menstrual period is considered reliable. Although the reliability of this information has been disputed, studies by Yerushalmy in the U.S.A., by the Perinatal Mortality Survey in Britain, and personal observations in Australia, show that, in general, the information is both reliable and useful.

Using these indices it has been possible to make tables and charts in which the progress of fetal growth is plotted. This plot has been made in two U.S. studies; in two studies in Britain and in one in Australia. It is known that male fetuses tend to be heavier than female fetuses, at least after the 30th week of gestation, and that the infants of primiparous mothers tend to be lighter than those of multiparous mothers. Allowance has to be made for these factors. It has also been accepted that at each gestational age there will be a range of normality, because of the different genetic growth potential of different fetuses; and in research such factors must be allowed for. However, in clinical work these charts have great value in enabling the obstetrician to determine if a baby is growth-retarded at any given gestational age. In general, growth retardation is arbitrarily defined as occurring when the birth weight is below the mean minus 2 standard deviations for its week of gestation. A few workers take the 10th percentile (which approximately corresponds to minus 1 standard deviation) as the lower limit of normal. If the latter is used a rather large number of babies will be designated as growth-retarded, most of whom are not at risk. For this reason the lower limit of minus 2 standard deviations should be adopted, as it gives a more accurate evaluation of the problem of intra-uterine growth retardation.

Mean Birth Weight for Gestational Age

Currently the only statistics available of mean birth weight at different gestational ages are those obtained in Australia, Britain, the Netherlands, Sweden and the U.S.A. Comparison of the statistical data shows that in the four nations, which are all affluent and all predominantly Caucasian, growth of the fetus is linear up to about the end of the 35th week of gestation. At this time the mean fetal weight is about 2,500 g ($5\frac{1}{2}$ lb). In the last five weeks of pregnancy, variations occur. Swedish babies, whose parents are mainly tall and very well nourished, tend to be the heaviest, whilst American babies tend to be lightest at

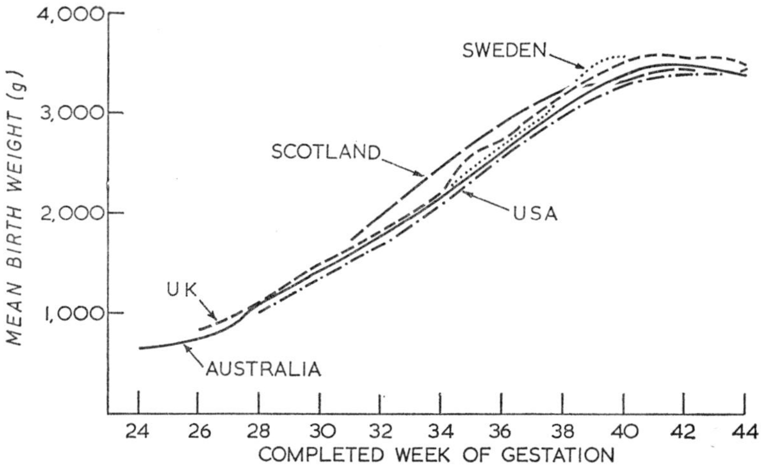

Figure **17/3** The mean birth weight at various gestational ages, several developed nations. Note that the mean birth weight at the end of the 35th gestational week is approximately 2,500 g.

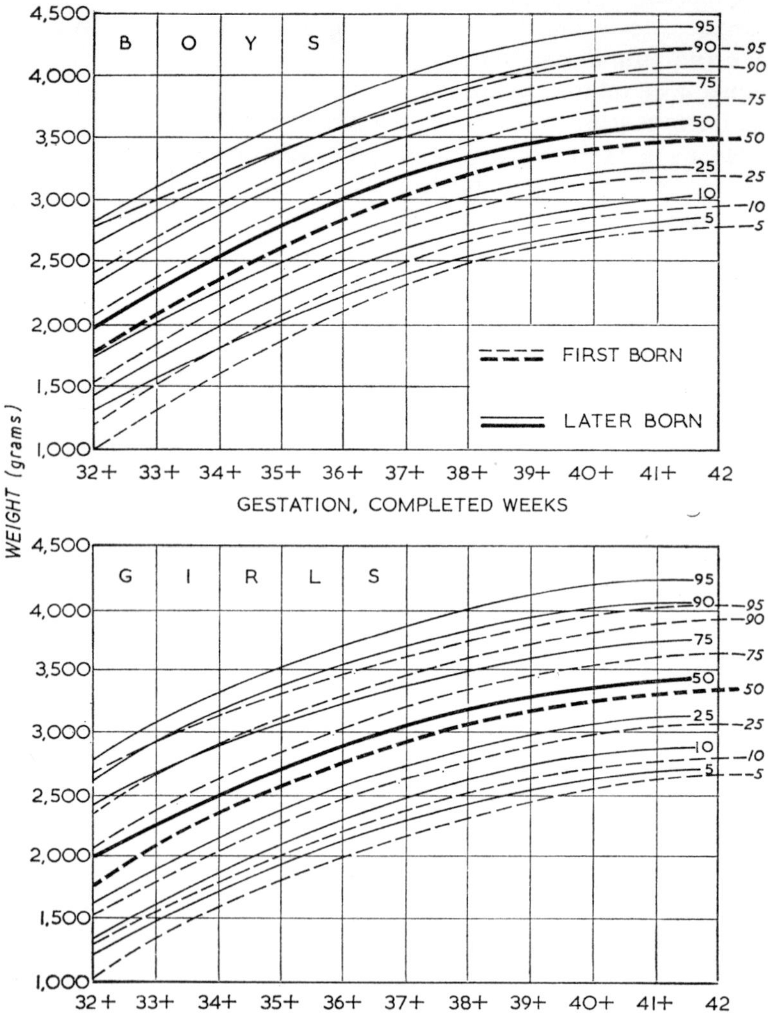

Figure **17/4** Weight charts prepared by Tanner and Whitehouse and based on information from Thomson *et al.* The centiles for first born are given by the interrupted lines and indicated by the italic figures; those for later born by the solid lines labelled in upright figures. Gestation is in completed weeks from the first day of the last menstrual period.

Source: Tanner, J. M., and Whitehouse, R. H.

each week of gestation, although the differences are not very marked (Figure **17/3**). The most sophisticated series of charts are those constructed in Aberdeen from the study of 5,200 singleton births to married women. These were drawn up by **Thomson** and his colleagues and make allowance for the increased weight of male fetuses over female fetuses from the 32nd week of pregnancy, and the effect of increasing parity on fetal weight (Figure **17/4**). Of particular relevance was their

Table 17/1

Mean birth weight of babies of various ethnic groups in selected nations

Ethnic group and nation	*Mean birth weight (g) Socio-economic group* *High*	*Low*	*Per cent less than* 2,500 g
Caucasian			
Australia, New Zealand	3,500	3,200	5–7
Scandinavia, U.K.	3,500	3,100	4–7
U.S.A.	3,400	3,200	6–8
South Africa	3,400		4–7
African			
U.S.A.	3,400	3,000	10–14
Nigeria	3,200	2,750	10–24
Congo	3,000	2,850	
South Africa	3,050		9–12
Chinese			
Malaysia	3,100	2,885	9–12
Hong Kong	—	3,030	7–10
Singapore	—	3,180	—
Malay			
Indonesia	3,020	2,815	—
Malaysia	2,905	2,750	18–20
Philippines	2,889		—
Singapore	3,170		—
Indian			
South India	2,950	2,750	25–36
Malaysia	2,915	2,645	18–24
South Africa	—	—	18–22
Singapore	3,020		—

finding that a gradient existed between mean birth weight and the social class of the husband, but that when the mean birth weights were standardized for length of gestation and maternal height, the gradient disappeared. This suggests that the mother's nutrition in infancy and childhood has an important bearing on the weight of her infant. If her socio-economic environment in childhood is inadequate, she will grow less tall than she should have, and is more likely to deliver a smaller infant.

The variation in the mean birth weight is more apparent when mean birth weights reported from the developed and developing nations are compared. In Table **17/1** data are given of mean birth weights of infants born to mothers of different racial groups in different countries. The Table shows the effect of social class on mean birth weight. Once again the importance of childhood nutrition, which in turn is related in some degree to family spacing and welfare, is emphasized.

Low Birth Weight

The definition of low birth weight resulted from the conclusions of an expert committee of the World Health Organization which met in 1948 and in 1950. This definition, which has been endorsed by most member nations, identifies a *low birth-weight infant as one with a birth weight of 2,500 g or less and/or a gestation period of less than 37 completed weeks.*

This definition was determined after obtaining birth weight data, mainly of white infants born to mothers living in the developed nations. It is not very accurate even in these nations, as it has been demonstrated by studies in Holland, Scotland, Sweden and the U.S.A. that the mean birth weight at the end of the 35th week of gestation is 2,500 g (about $5\frac{1}{2}$lb). That it is inappropriate in the developing nations was realized originally, and has been confirmed subsequently. In these nations, principally because of poor maternal growth support, mean birth weights tend to be lower, particularly if the mother is in the lower socio-economic group. This means if the criterion of low birth weight is taken as a weight of 2,500 g ($5\frac{1}{2}$ lb) or less, a larger proportion of infants in the developing nations will be found to be of low birth weight. In the developed nations between 5 and 10 per cent of all babies born are of low birth weight as defined by the WHO. By the same definition, 15 to 30 per cent of infants would be put in this category in many Asian, African and South American nations.

Studies in Malaysia have shown that the chances of survival and the vitality of Malay infants weighing 1,800 g (4½ lb) were comparable with those of European infants weighing 2,200 g (5 lb) at birth and delivered in the same hospital. Studies in other Asian countries have shown substantially similar findings. For example, low birth-weight infants born in New Guinea had a lower neonatal mortality than Australian children of the same weight groups, and the mortality of Indian low birth-weight infants born in Calcutta was less, when compared with infants of similar weight born in the U.S.A.

The WHO definition of low birth weight is not entirely acceptable for another reason. The examination of data from the British Perinatal Mortality Survey in 1958 showed that 33 per cent of infants who were of low birth weight were born *after* 37 completed weeks of pregnancy. A similar investigation of data collected between 1957 and 1959, in New York by Yerushalmy, showed that 45 per cent of low birth-weight infants were born after 36 completed weeks' gestation. These data indicate that two separate populations are included in the group of infants designated as of 'low birth weight'. In the larger group, pregnancy has been curtailed for one reason or another, with the result that a *premature baby* has been born, whose weight is appropriate for its gestational age. The smaller group, comprising between 20 and 35 per cent of all babies designated as being of low birth weight, are inappropriately underweight for the gestational age. These babies are either congenitally defective, or have suffered from inadequate maternal growth support during intra-uterine development. This has led to intra-uterine growth retardation and the birth of a *dysmature baby*. Combinations of the two types of low birth weight also occur. In these cases a premature baby is born which is also dysmature. Since the response of the two types of low birth-weight baby to survival is quite different, it is important to distinguish between them, although the aetiological factors leading to the births tend to be similar whether the infant is premature or dysmature.

It should also be clear from the discussion that the critical cut-off point of 2,500 g (5½ lb) and 37 completed weeks has been selected for clinical rather than biological reasons, and that there is a need for a revision to determine a more discriminating point of separation. It is suggested that a more appropriate definition would be:

Low birth weight

A low birth-weight infant is one which in the developed nations weighs less than 2,500 g ($5\frac{1}{2}$ lb); and in the developing nations, 2,000 g ($4\frac{1}{2}$ lb) or some other appropriate weight. This weight is normally attained at the end of the 35th completed week of gestation. In the developed nations, about 30 per cent of low birth-weight infants will have a greater gestation interval than 35 completed weeks. Such infants have been growth retarded in utero, and are *dysmature*. Babies whose weight is less than 2,500 g ($5\frac{1}{2}$ lb) at the end of the 35th week of gestation and whose weight is appropriate for age are considered *premature*.

The Diagnosis of Growth Retardation

The separation of true premature from dysmature infants prior to delivery is not always easy. The most useful single index is knowledge of the date of the last menstrual period and of the women's menstrual cycle. This information is most reliable if it was obtained prior to the 10th week of pregnancy, and particularly if a vaginal examination was performed at that time which confirmed uterine growth and related it to the period of gestation.

In many instances the patient is not seen until after the 30th week of pregnancy and often has forgotten the date of her last period, or has been disbelieved by the obstetrician when she has stated it. In such cases failure of fetal growth determined indirectly by estimating the fundal height is suggestive. If the height of the fundus of the uterus palpated per abdomen is less than that expected, fetal intra-uterine growth retardation may be suspected, but the measurement is rather inexact (Figure **17/5**). Another clinical finding of value is that the mother's weight is stationary, or that she is losing weight between visits. This is suggestive of dysmaturity rather than prematurity. In centres where ultrasonic equipment or facilities for measuring oestriol in blood or urine are available, the failure of observable fetal skull growth, or of persistently low oestriol levels on serial assay, may suggest dysmaturity, but neither method is consistently accurate nor exact.

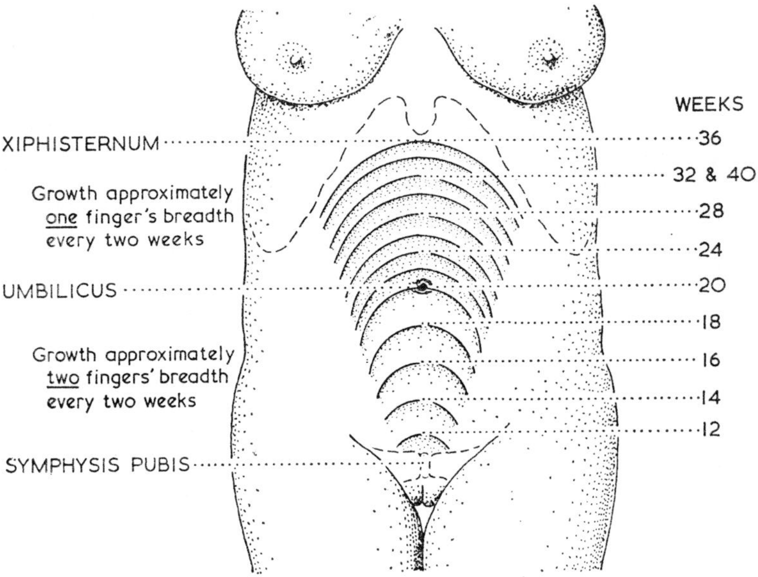

Figure **17/5** The abdominal markings of uterine growth related to the number of completed weeks after the last menstrual period.

The greatest diagnostic problems occur amongst mothers of the lower socio-economic groups, who have pre-eclampsia, anaemia or ante-partum haemorrhage, as the infants of these mothers may be both premature and dysmature.

Aetiological Factors in Low Birth Weight

SOCIO-ECONOMIC FACTORS

In studies from various parts of the world, which were reviewed by Day, it appears that adverse socio-economic conditions play a more important part in the aetiology of low birth weight than do obstetrical factors. Support for this opinion comes from the known fact that mean birth weights are lower amongst the poorer classes of affluent nations, and amongst the majority of pregnant women in the developing nations, when compared with the mean birth weights of infants in developed nations. In Scotland, Baird noted that the percentage of low birth-weight infants born to primiparae under the age of 20, whose husbands, or fathers, were of the lower socio-economic groups, was significantly higher than the percentage born to primiparae aged 20 to 29, of the same socio-economic groups, but this higher incidence disappeared if the woman was in Social Class I or II. Baird also analysed the effect of social status of the husband and of the woman's father on the incidence of low birth weight. In this analysis the age of the expectant mother was ignored,

Table 17/2

Incidence of low birth weight related to the social class of the parents
(*All Aberdeen primiparae 1951–59, single births only*)

Husband's social class	*Wife's father's occupation*			*All classes*
	I *and* II	III	IV *and* V	
Professional and managerial (I and II)	4·3	6·7	8·9	5·6
Skilled (III)	5·1	6·5	7·6	6·8
Semiskilled and unskilled (IV and V)	14·0	11·1	10·9	11·0
All classes	5·4	7·1	8·7	7·6

as was maternal height, although both might have influenced the findings. The results, which are shown in Table **17/2**, indicate that the lower the social class of husband or father, the higher the percentage of low birth-weight infants. A study in Edinburgh by Drillien suggested that the social class into which a woman married, had a minor influence on her chance of delivering a low birth-weight baby compared with the social class into which she had been born and in which she had been reared. The reconciliation of these two points was clearly stated by the Scottish sociologist Illsley: 'The use of the husband's social class in vital statistics tends automatically to focus attention on the conditions existing at the time of maternity . . .

(but it) has a much wider significance. Generally speaking, like marries like; for example, the wife of a professional man, irrespective of her father's social class, will normally possess before marriage the personal qualities, education and social habits that fit her for that role. "Husband's social class" is useful as a research tool, not only because it accounts for the immediate way of life of a mother, but because it reflects her life history, the conditions of her upbringing, and her personal qualities.'

The effect of socio-economic factors on the incidence of low birth weight is also shown in a study made in Chicago between 1963 and 1965 and quoted by Wallace. The percentage of babies, weighing 2,500 g ($5\frac{1}{2}$ lb) or less, born to mothers living in 'neighbourhoods in the national fourth quartile of the socio-economic index' was 14·5; whilst the percentage amongst mothers living in the rest of Chicago was 8·3, almost exactly the same as the overall U.S. rate of 8·2 per cent for the same period, and the differential was greater for black than it was for white underprivileged mothers.

Another factor of importance is that the frequency of low birth-weight infants increases when the birth interval is shorter than 2 years. This finding was obtained from a study by Douglas of 13,300 single births to married English women, and the effect was independent of age. It was confirmed in a study in the U.S.A. by Bishop. These investigations suggest that the effect of frequent pregnancy as a cause of low birth weight is only significant amongst women of the lower socio-economic groups. Since such women are brought up in a worse environment, tend to conceive at an earlier age, are less likely to obtain prenatal care early in pregnancy and are more likely to work in late pregnancy, the socio-economic findings also play a role.

As has been noted, maternal age has an effect on the incidence of low birth weight. Both the British Perinatal Mortality Survey, and surveys in the U.S.A., show that low birth-weight babies are more likely to be born if the mother is under the age of 20, is primiparous and has pre-eclampsia. The evidence is that many of these infants are dysmature rather than premature. On the other hand, an increasing incidence of low birth weight occurs amongst grande multiparae. This may be due to age, to reduced birth intervals or to parity, but the effect is that pregnancy is curtailed and a premature infant is born. In both instances the effect of maternal age cannot be separated from socio-economic status.

The effect of parity alone on the incidence of low birth weight is less clear. Douglas noted that low birth weight was more frequent amongst primiparae than in women pregnant for a second or third time. After this the frequency rose again, and exceeded the rate for primigravida after the fifth pregnancy, particularly if the interval between pregnancies was less than 2 years. In the British Perinatal Mortality Survey the same trend was noted, but the differences were not marked. The incidence of low birth-weight babies amongst primiparae was 7·6 per cent, amongst women pregnant for the second to fourth time it was 6·0 per cent, and amongst grande multiparae it rose to 7·4 per cent. It is likely that socio-economic factors are more important than parity per se in the aetiology of low birth weight.

It has been claimed that pre-natal care from early pregnancy reduces the incidence of low birth weight. How this operates is not clear, except that the factor of anaemia may be eliminated by treatment, pre-eclampsia may be detected early, and patients with multiple pregnancy, or with placenta praevia, may be admitted to hospital. Since these conditions account for 40 per cent of the obstetric complications associated with low birth weight, the claim has substance. However, the greatest impact of adequate pre-natal care is likely to be amongst the poorer women of the developed nations and most women in the developing nations. In the developed nations the overall incidence of low birth weight has not decreased in the past 40 years despite an increased acceptance of pre-natal care, which suggests that the influence of pre-natal care in reducing the incidence of low birth weight may be low in these nations, and other factors may operate.

OBSTETRIC FACTORS

This discussion would be incomplete if the obstetrical factors leading to low birth weight were ignored. In both developed and developing nations, *severe pre-eclampsia* and *severe essential hypertension* may lead to the birth of a low birth-weight baby. In some instances the baby becomes growth retarded because of insufficient maternal growth support, due to reduction of uterine blood flow. In other cases pregnancy has to be terminated early because of the increased hazard to the infant in utero, and this leads to the delivery of a premature baby. Severe pre-eclampsia is most common in first pregnancies, especially if the mother is aged less than 20 or more than 30, but even then it complicates less than 5 per cent of all pregnancies. However, pre-eclampsia is an important cause of low birth weight, and in several studies was a factor in between 15 and 35 per cent of pregnancies in which a baby of low birth weight was delivered (Table **17/3**).

Table 17/3

Factors associated with low birth-weight live births
(*Percentage incidence*)

Associated factor	*Aberdeen Scotland* (1954–58) $n = 540$	*Kuala Lumpur Malaysia* (1955–64) $n = 2{,}100$
No associated condition	48·0	40·0
Pre-eclampsia	34·7	19·3
Multiple pregnancy, uncomplicated	4·3	15·0
Ante-partum haemorrhage	7·4	8·4
Congenital malformations	1·3	1·0
Maternal disease	4·3	15·0*
Miscellaneous	—	1·3

* Mainly anaemia.

Multiple pregnancy occurs in about 1·2 per cent of all pregnancies, and has a three- to five-fold greater chance of being complicated by pre-eclampsia than a singleton pregnancy. As well as this, at any given gestation date, after the 30th week, the weight of each baby is less than that of a singleton of equivalent maturity. This indicates that the maternal growth support is inadequate to enable maximal growth to occur. The babies are growth retarded, although this is rarely severe, unless the pregnancy is also complicated by severe pre-eclampsia. Multiple pregnancy is complicated by hydramnios in about 5 per cent of cases, and the excessive distension of the uterus may lead to the onset of premature labour. About 50 per cent of infants born of a multiple pregnancy are of low birth weight, and are either premature or dysmature (small for dates or growth retarded). Dysmature babies have a lower perinatal mortality than premature babies. In a study of survival rates of twins, shown in Table **17/4**, the survival of an infant born of a multiple pregnancy was greater than that of a singleton at all weights of all low birth-weight babies, which would substantiate the claim that dysmaturity is a main factor in low birth weight amongst multiple pregnancies, although prematurity also occurs. There is suggestive evidence that the incidence of low birth

Table 17/4

Survival rates for single and multiple gestations (life births only)

Birth weight (g)	*Single*		*Multiple*	
	No.	*Per cent survival*	*No.*	*Per cent survival*
401–1,000	196	4·1	112	8·9
1,001–1,500	253	52·2	174	60·3
1,501–2,000	599	81·6	392	91·8
2,001–2,500	2,312	96·2	799	97·6
Over 2,500	35,736	99·5	1,049	99·5
Total	39,096	98·3	2,526	91·0

Source: Kohl. Obstetrical Statistical Cooperative, 1958.

weight will be reduced if the patient receives an improved diet (including folic acid from the 30th week of pregnancy) and adequate rest from the 30th to the 35th week. Multiple pregnancy accounts for only 1·2 per cent of all pregnancies, but 30 per cent of low birth-weight infants are products of a multiple pregnancy.

Ante-partum haemorrhage is also a factor in low birth weight, but since ante-partum haemorrhage is a complication of parity, and especially high parity, the influence of socio-economic factors may be considerable. In most series, ante-partum haemorrhage complicates 2 to 3 per cent of all pregnancies, but is a cause of the delivery of a low birth-weight baby in between 6 and 12 per cent of cases (Table **17/3**).

The effect of *maternal disease* on low birth weight cannot be separated from social factors. Cardiac disease, especially rheumatic heart disease, is more frequent in the lower socio-economic groups, as is pyelonephritis. Both conditions increase the likelihood of low birth weight. The incidence of anaemia, both iron deficient and megaloblastic, is more common amongst the poorer sections of the community in the developed nations and amongst many more women in the developing nations. Anaemia leads to retardation of intra-uterine growth of the fetus, and either to stillbirth or to the

Table 17/5

The effect of maternal anaemia on low birth weight (in Malaysian patients)

	Anaemic patients Hb ⩽ 6·5 g *n* = 2,250	*Non-anaemic patients* Hb > 6·5 g *n* = 70,798
Incidence low birth weight*	18·1%	5·7%
Perinatal loss		
Mature infants only	45 per 1,000	23 per 1,000
Low birth-weight infants	52 per 1,000	57 per 1,000
Stillbirth rate	91 per 1,000	16 per 1,000

* Indicates a birth weight of 500–1,999 g.

Source: Llewellyn-Jones, D. 'Severe Anaemia in Pregnancy'. *Aust. N.Z. J. Obst. Gyn.*, **5**, 191, 1965.

birth of a dysmature baby (Table **17/5**). In the developing nations and particularly amongst the lower socio-economic groups, this preventible disease is a significant cause of low birth weight. *Uterine malformations*, which complicate less than 3 per cent of pregnancies, are often associated with the onset of premature labour and the birth of a low birth-weight, premature infant. Uterine malformations have no association with any socio-economic group, but the incidence of premature labour appears to be higher amongst women of the lower socio-economic groups. However, this may be due to socio-economic variables.

FETAL FACTORS

Genetically determined *fetal defects* appear to have a higher incidence amongst the infants of older women of the lower socio-economic groups who are of high parity. This applies particularly to malformations of the central nervous system. Chromosomal defects are found in association with 25 to 35 per cent of spontaneous abortions (also called early fetal deaths) and, as Yerushalmy has shown, the incidence of abortions increases with age and decreased pregnancy interval. Fetal defects may also be caused by the transplacental passage of virus in cases of maternal viral infection, particularly if this occurs in early pregnancy. Although viral infections occur in all social classes, the chance of infection is greater amongst women living in more crowded conditions, in a poor environment. Fetal defects are found in about 2 per cent of all births and about half of these infants are of low birth weight.

OTHER FACTORS

Because of the increasing habit of *cigarette smoking* amongst women in developed nations, the effect of cigarette smoking has been studied. In surveys in Britain and the U.S.A., the greater the number of cigarettes smoked, at least in the second half of pregnancy, the greater was the difference in birth weights of infants born to smokers and non-smokers. When the statistics were analysed it was found that the excess of low birth-weight babies was due to intra-uterine growth retardation rather than to curtailed pregnancy (Figure **17/6**). The effect of social status complicates the issue. In Britain it was found that whilst only 20 per cent of mothers in Social Classes I and II were smokers, 35 per cent of mothers in Social Class IV and V smoked. Smoking was also found to increase with maternal age. However, scrutiny of the data indicated that the effect of smoking on reduced birth weight was independent of maternal age, parity or social class, although these factors together with pre-eclampsia, ante-partum haemorrhage and anaemia would increase the incidence of low birth weight amongst smokers. In a study of a large number of women, Butler et al. concluded that cigarette smoking in pregnancy reduced the mean birth weight of the infant by 170 g (6 oz), and increased the perinatal

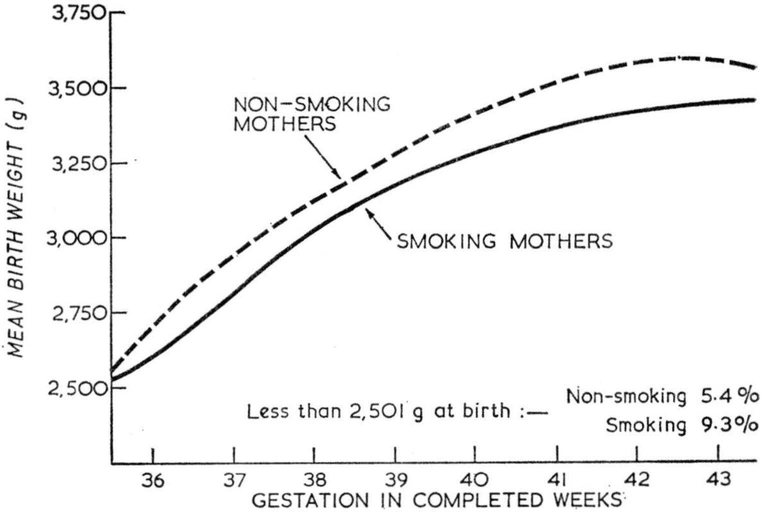

Figure **17/6** The effect of maternal cigarette smoking on mean birth weight.
Source: Butler, N. R., and Alberman, E. D., *Perinatal Problems*, p. 72, Livingstone, Edinburgh, 1969.

mortality by 28 per cent (from 32 to 41 per 1,000). However, if a woman ceased to smoke cigarettes by the 20th week of pregnancy, the adverse effect on infant birth weight and on perinatal mortality disappeared. For this reason every effort should be made to discourage cigarette smoking in pregnancy.

The relation between *nutrition* in pregnancy and low birth weight remains confused, and a well-designed experimental model is almost impossible to devise. One measure of maternal nutrition in pregnancy can be made by determining weight gain in pregnancy. The problem in such a study is to subtract the weight gain due to fluid retention. Thomson and his colleagues in Aberdeen have studied this problem and concluded that women who were more than 20 per cent underweight for height at 20 weeks' gestation, and who gained less than 10 kg (22 lb) in pregnancy, were likely to have a higher proportion of low birth-weight babies than other women. This finding suggests that poor nutrition during pregnancy in a woman who herself had suffered nutritional deprivation throughout her own childhood leads to the birth of a low birth-weight baby.

Table 17/6

Low birth weight related to the altitude of the mother's place of residence in the U.S.A.

Altitudes in metres	*Low birth-weight babies (per cent)*
0–999	6·7
1,000–1,500	8·5
2,000–2,500	10·7
2,500 or more	23·7

Source: Lichty et al. *Amer. J. Dis. Child.* **93,** 666, 1957.

The *altitude of the mother's place of residence* also plays a factor in the incidence of birth weight. The most complete study of this factor was made in the U.S.A. by Lichty and his colleagues, and the correlation between altitude and the low birth weight is shown in Table **17/6.** Why high altitude is associated with low birth weight is unclear. It is unlikely to be due to increased cosmic radiation, as there is no increase in congenital defects, and current opinion is that the lowered partial pressure of oxygen and reduced erthyrocyte saturation may be the main factors involved.

The Mortality of Low Birth Weight

It is evident that the less mature the infant the less is its chance of survival. In as far as birth weight can be related to maturity, the less the birth weight of the baby the greater its mortality. In Britain for example, over 95 per cent of babies weighing less than 1,000 g (2¼ lb) died, but when the birth weight exceeded 2,500 g (5½ lb) the mortality was less than 3 per cent (Figure **17/7**). Improved neonatal care given in special units can save more very small babies, but 40 per cent of infants weighing 1,500 g (3¼ lb) or less at birth have moderate or severe handicaps, either mental, neurological or physical when assessed at the age of 5 to 7.

The more premature the baby, the greater are its difficulties in adjusting to extra-uterine life and the higher the neonatal

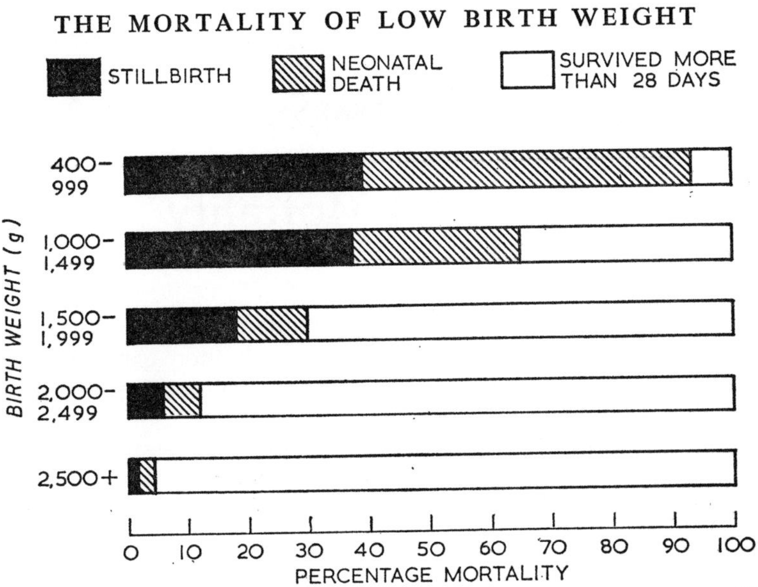

Figure 17/7 Perinatal mortality by weight at birth, U.K. 1967.

mortality. In contrast, the greater the degree of pre-natal nutritional deprivation the greater is the likelihood of intra-uterine death. Thus dysmature babies are more likely to die in utero, and consequently become fetal deaths, whilst premature babies are more likely to die in the neonatal period. The combination of prematurity and dysmaturity is particularly lethal.

It is clear that the incidence of low birth weight, with its high mortality, can be reduced if more women will accept family spacing and seek pre-natal care, secure in the knowledge that any pregnancy which they have is likely to terminate with a live, healthy baby of normal birth weight.

EIGHTEEN

Perinatal Mortality

In recent years, with the increasing availability, acceptance and sophistication of pre-natal care, and with increasing medical care for high risk cases in well-equipped, well-staffed hospitals, the maternal mortality has been reduced considerably. The reduction has been particularly marked in the developed nations, but the maternal death rate is falling in the developing nations. The effect of this, in many nations, is that the maternal mortality is now computed as a ratio per 10,000 or even per 100,000 births (see Chapter 19). The relative infrequency of maternal death has reduced the importance of this measure as an index of the quality of health care available within a nation.

Because of this, increasing attention has been paid recently to perinatal deaths; that is deaths of the fetus or child occurring around the time of birth. The concept of perinatal mortality has replaced the older computation of stillbirth and neonatal death rates, as it has been realized that identical factors may affect the fetus in late pregnancy or in the early neonatal period, leading in the former case to death in utero, and in the latter to neonatal death. To separate the two events is not only artificial, but gives incomplete information, so that avoidable factors which might be identified are overlooked and corrective action not taken.

Many nations now accept that the number of perinatal deaths may be an appropriate index of the quality of maternity care available, since maternity care is increasingly concerned in improving the welfare of the fetus, and in ensuring the birth of a healthy living child. Thus good fetal care necessarily implies good maternal care.

The Components of Perinatal Mortality

Without clear definition, the components of perinatal loss cannot be clearly identified, and inaccurate data will be recorded. This has been a concern of the World Health Organization, who have appointed sub-committees and expert committees at intervals since 1950. These committees have reviewed the international situation concerning the great diversity of definitions of live births and fetal deaths (that is abortions and stillbirths) in use in different countries, and have sought to obtain agreement in setting up uniform definitions, which might command general acceptance.

Over the years these concepts have evolved, and currently accepted definitions may be subject to change.

Live birth

The following definition of live birth was adopted by the WHO Assembly in 1951:

'Live birth is the complete expulsion or extraction from its mother of a product of conception, irrespective of the duration of the pregnancy, which, after such separation, breathes or shows any evidence of life, defined as beating of the heart, pulsation of the umbilical cord, or definite movement of the voluntary muscles, whether or not the umbilical cord has been cut or the placenta is attached; each product of such a birth is considered live born.'

The definition is not entirely satisfactory, particularly as some fetuses delivered by therapeutic termination of pregnancy, at an early stage of gestation, may show signs of life as defined. An Expert Committee appointed in 1970 to consider the 'Prevention of Perinatal Mortality and Morbidity' noted this, and so that very immature fetuses which could only survive for short periods even though they showed transitory signs of life might be excluded, recommended that a viability criterion should be added to the definition. The words 'irrespective of the duration of gestation' were replaced by the words 'weighing 500 g (1 lb 2 oz) or more, or if less than this surviving for at least one hour'.

Fetal deaths

The definition of fetal death must obviously be the converse of that of live birth, and the 1950 definition of the WHO states:

'Fetal death is death prior to the complete expulsion or extraction from its mother of a product of conception, irrespective of the duration of pregnancy; the death is indicated by the fact that after such separation the fetus does not breathe or show other evidence of life, such as beating of the heart, pulsation of the umbilical cord, or definite movement of voluntary muscles.'

In 1950 the WHO recommended that fetal deaths should be divided into four groups.

Group I	Less than 20 completed weeks of gestation
Group II	20 completed weeks but less than 28
Group III	28 completed weeks of gestation and over
Group IV	Gestation period not classifiable in Groups I, II or III.

It was also recommended that fetal deaths in Group I were described as *early fetal deaths*, and that this term should replace the term abortion as applied to a product of conception. Fetal deaths in Group II should be called *intermediate fetal deaths*, whilst fetal deaths in Group III should be termed *late fetal deaths*. The term stillbirth should be discontinued as it was synonymous with late fetal death, and the latter had no connotation with breathing. It may be recalled that in 1925, a special committee of the League of Nations defined stillbirth as 'the birth of a fetus after at least 28 weeks of pregnancy in which pulmonary respiration does not occur; such fetus may die either before, during or after birth, but before it has breathed'.

The definitions of 1950 have proved to have considerable disadvantages, particularly as in many cases the gestation period has been unknown or inaccurately recorded. Some nations, for example the U.S.A. and Australia, have attempted to overcome this by adding a weight criterion. Thus in the U.S.A. an intermediate fetal death is one in which the gestation period is 20 completed weeks but less than 28 completed weeks and/or the fetus weighs between 400 and 999 g (14 oz and 2¼ lb). Analysis of birth weight and gestation period statistics in Australia and Malaysia suggests that this criterion is inaccurate, and a birthweight of 500 g (1 lb 2 oz) is much more closely related to 20 weeks' gestation in both developed and developing nations. Moreover, a weight criterion is much more likely to be recorded accurately than is a gestation period criterion.

It is therefore suggested that live births and fetal deaths are classified as follows:

PERINATAL MORTALITY RATIOS

GROUP	LIVE BIRTH	FETAL DEATH
I	Up to 499 g	Up to 499 g (early fetal deaths)
II	500 g, up to and including 999 g	500 g, up to and including 999 g (intermediate fetal deaths).
III	1,000 g and over	1,000 g and over (late fetal deaths)

In the above classification the weight division of 500 g corresponds to a gestational age of 20 completed weeks; and the weight division of 1,000 g to one of 28 completed weeks, so that late fetal deaths continue to correspond to 'stillbirths' as defined by the League of Nations in 1925.

Neonatal deaths

Conventionally, neonatal deaths are those deaths which occur in the first 28 days of life. Because over 65 per cent of the deaths occur within the first 24 hours of birth, and over 90 per cent within the first week, neonatal deaths may be conveniently divided into two categories.

1. *Early neonatal deaths*, that is deaths occurring between birth and the end of the 7th day of life, or, more accurately, up to, but not including, the moment the infant becomes 168 hours of age.
2. *Late neonatal deaths*, that is deaths occurring from the beginning of the 8th day (the 168th hour of life) up to, but not including, the moment the child reaches the 29th day of life.

Perinatal Mortality Ratios

The definitions presented are necessary so that perinatal mortality may be defined. The Eighth Revision Conference of the International Classification of Diseases of the WHO held in 1965, defined the perinatal period as extending from the 28th week of gestation to the 7th day of life. However, the Conference encouraged nations to collect pertinent data from the 20th week of pregnancy up to the 28th day of life. About half the nations in the European Region of the WHO, and a few in other Regions, have adopted the recommendation and report fetal deaths occurring at 28 weeks, or more, of gestation, and deaths of live-born infants occurring in the first week after birth. A total of 41 out of 132 nations report perinatal mortality ratios. A very few nations, or parts of nations, notably the U.S.A., some Canadian provinces, and the State of New South Wales in Australia, report perinatal mortality ratios which include fetal deaths of at least 20 completed weeks' gestation, or at least 400 g weight (in some cases 500 g weight), and infant deaths occurring within a period of 28 days after birth. It can be seen that two definitions of perinatal mortality are current.

1. *The extended perinatal mortality ratio*, which is defined as:

   Fetal deaths of infants weighing 500 g or more at birth, and all neonatal deaths occurring from the day of birth up to the end of the 28th day of life, expressed as a ratio per 1,000 total births. This can be more briefly expressed as intermediate and late fetal deaths plus neonatal deaths per 1,000 births.

The use of the extended perinatal mortality ratio increases the proportion of deaths for the following reasons: (1) Although 0·5 to 1·5 per cent of all births fall into Group I (500–999 g), only 5 to 15 per cent of live-born infants in this Group survive; (2) 20 to 40 per cent of all perinatal deaths are of babies in Group I, and (3) although late neonatal deaths in the developed nations only form about 5 to 10 per cent of all neonatal deaths, they form a much larger proportion in the developing nations. As an example of the increase, the standard perinatal mortality in the State of New South Wales, Australia, in 1970 was 19·5 per 1,000; whilst the extended perinatal mortality was 27·5 per 1,000, an increase of 42 per cent.

2. *The standard perinatal mortality ratio*, which is defined as: Late fetal deaths plus early neonatal deaths per 1,000 total births.

It is recognized that most nations will prefer to use the standard perinatal mortality period in calculating their statistics.

The Purpose of Reporting Perinatal Mortality Ratios

The problems involved in collecting perinatal mortality statistics, particularly if the extended period is chosen, are great and the expense involved is considerable. The procedure must be shown to have value if a nation is to embark on collecting and evaluating the information. Data collection involves: (1) the registration of all births, and (2) the registration of all perinatal deaths. If the information is to be of value, additional data are required. These include: (3) information about the birth weight of all registered births, (4) the establishment of a perinatal death certificate, which gives birth weight, demographic information, autopsy data and information about the course and complications of pregnancy, (5) similar data to be collected for all births. Obviously the last three steps are costly, and currently impractical to establish in most nations. Although the first two steps could be established with relative ease, less than one-third of the nations of the world have done so. Despite this, statistics of perinatal mortality have considerable value both at the national or regional level and at city or hospital level.

At a national or regional level the data are valuable as: (1) They permit health planners to identify avoidable factors and to suggest corrective action which may be taken. (2) They permit the annual assessment of the extent of perinatal mortality and morbidity, and the changes which occur in response to the development of new services. (3) The information obtained provides those concerned with administering health services, including teaching and research, with means to measure the effectiveness of the services in meeting stated objectives. (4) It enables health planners to direct investigation to explain why certain areas of the nation have a rate different from the mean. (5) With accurate data (i.e. when steps 3 to 5 have been introduced) the information can be used as a longitudinal research tool for multiple cause correlations and analysis.

Although the statistics can be very misleading when limited to data collected from a single hospital or from a single city, the study of perinatal mortality by committees is a stimulating method of education, leading to the closer co-operation between administrators, obstetricians, paediatricians and resident staff to improve obstetric and neonatal care. It also permits the identification and correction of potentially dangerous procedures, in the pre-natal period, during labour and in the neonatal period.

Table 18/1

Perinatal and infant mortality statistics, crude birth rate, and total population in various nations, 1965

Country or territory	*Perinatal mortality per 1,000 total births*	*Late fetal deaths per 1,000 births*	*Deaths under 7 days per 1,000 live births*	*Infant mortality per 1,000 live births*	*Live births per 1,000 population*
Guatemala	48·7	29·5	19·2	92·6	45·3
Chile	48·3	24·2	24·1	107·1	31·5
Philippines	42·9	18·2	24·7	72·9	24·6
Ecuador	40·3	23·8	16·5	93·0	44·0
Western Malaysia	40·2	23·2	17·0	50·0	36·7
Argentina	39·9	23·9	16·0	56·9	21·4
Portugal	39·5	23·7	15·7	64·9	22·8
Colombia	38·6	17·7	20·9	82·4	36·8
Italy	36·2	19·2	17·1	36·0	19·2
Mexico	35·6	21·4	14·3	60·7	44·2
Venezuela	35·6	19·9	15·7	47·7	43·5
Hungary	35·0	11·4	23·6	38·8	13·1
Scotland	32·0	18·2	13·8	23·1	19·3
Japan	30·1	21·9	8·2	18·5	18·6
Greece	29·9	15·7	14·2	34·3	17·7
Austria	29·8	12·0	17·8	28·3	17·9
Fed. Republic of Germany	29·0	12·4	16·6	23·9	17·7
France	28·2	15·4	12·8	21·9	17·8
Yugoslavia	28·1	10·1	18·0	71·8	20·9
Belgium	27·6	13·7	13·9	23·7	16·4
England & Wales	27·3	16·0	11·3	19·0	18·1
U.S.A.	26·5	10·7	15·9	24·7	19·4
Canada	26·3	11·6	14·7	23·6	21·4
Poland	25·1	11·3	13·8	41·7	17·3
Australia	23·6	11·9	11·7	18·5	19·7
Netherlands	23·4	13·3	10·1	14·4	19·9
Switzerland	23·1	10·6	12·5	17·8	18·8
Czechoslovakia	22·8	8·2	14·6	25·5	16·4
Sweden	19·9	10·3	9·6	13·3	15·9
Bulgaria	18·3	9·9	8·4	30·8	15·3

Source: *Demographic Yearbooks,* U.N., New York.

International Perinatal Mortality Statistics

Comparison of perinatal mortality ratios between nations is not particularly informative at this stage of registration, as so few nations record accurate data, although a study in 1970 by a WHO Expert Committee did show certain trends. The statistics in Table **18/1** relate to this study, but in this particular table only nations with populations exceeding 5 million have been chosen. It should also be noted that the standard perinatal mortality ratio has been recorded (i.e. late fetal and early neonatal deaths per 1,000 total births).

It can be seen that the perinatal mortality ratio in 1965 varied from 18·3 to 48·7 per 1,000 total births, and that the more developed the nation, in general, the lower was the perinatal mortality ratio. In many nations which currently do not record perinatal mortality data, sample surveys have shown that the perinatal mortality ratios are higher than those shown in Table **18/1**, so that the problem of perinatal mortality is considerable. The influence of socio-economic factors such as poor diet, frequent childbearing and inadequate pre-natal care are factors leading to the higher ratios, and these factors, together with infectious disease, operate to produce high late neonatal mortality ratios, and high postneonatal mortality ratios (children aged 1 month to 1 year). In some nations between 200 and 300 children of every 1,000 born fail to survive to the age of 5.

Secular Trends in Perinatal Mortality Ratios

In most advanced nations for which statistics are available, the perinatal mortality ratios have fallen since recording was first instituted in about 1935. Samples of these statistics are shown in Figure **18/1**. Because of different registration practices in different nations, problems arise in obtaining comparable statistics, but as far as possible allowance has been made for these, and the statistics are the best currently available.

The Causes of Perinatal Mortality

Since a main function of perinatal mortality data collection is to enable health planners to identify avoidable factors and to suggest remedies, it is necessary to subdivide gross perinatal mortality ratios into separate groups. Originally perinatal deaths were recorded on the International Form of Medical

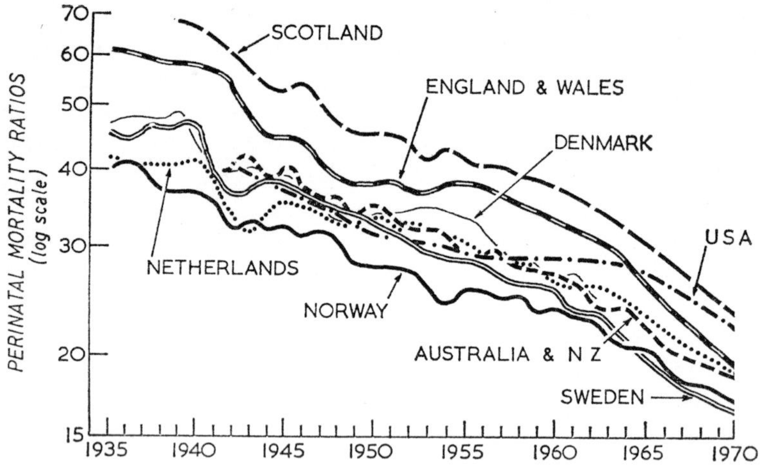

Figure **18/1** The secular trend in perinatal mortality ratios in some developed countries.
Source: U.N. *Demographic Yearbooks.*

Certification of Cause of Death. This Certificate was designed to allow the certifying practitioner to indicate what, in his opinion, was the underlying cause of death. By this was meant what was the disease or injury which initiated the train of events leading directly to death. In the death certificate the sequence of events was entered in Part I of the form, with the underlying cause stated on the lowest line. A second part, Part II, was also provided to enable the certifier to report any other conditions which may have contributed to the death but which were not related to the sequence entered in Part I.

This certificate has proved very useful in collecting data for single cause mortality statistics; but it has certain limitations when two or more disease processes have contributed more or less equally to the death. In this case the certifier has to make a choice. The situation is even more complex with late fetal deaths and early neonatal deaths, as three factors are frequently involved: conditions in the fetus or child itself; conditions in the mother affecting the fetus or child; and conditions arising from the process of birth.

In 1963 a sub-committee of the Expert Committee on Health Statistics of the WHO considered this problem and came to the conclusion that if fetal and maternal conditions were recorded independently, in different sections of the certificate the relationship between the two would not be known. 'It seemed preferable, therefore, to use a sequential arrangement allowing the certifier to indicate the relationship and to record what, in his opinion, was the underlying cause whether in the child or the mother.'

This opinion was endorsed by the International Conference for the Eighth Revision of International Classification of Disease, and most countries have accepted this opinion, and record perinatal mortality data in this manner (Figure **18/2**).

Examples of how data is recorded in this way is shown in Figure **18/3**, which is reproduced by permission of the Government of New South Wales, Australia.

For the analysis of single-condition mortality statistics, this certificate has proved useful, but recently there has been a growing awareness of the need for multiple-condition analysis in order to present a truer picture at ages of death where multiple causation is common. This is particularly so in the perinatal period, as there is often an interplay of several causes, or circumstances, not necessarily attributed to mother or child. A difference of opinion has arisen between various experts since 1963, and in consequence a new form is under trial in selected centres.

In this form the certifier lists separately 'maternal diseases and conditions affecting the fetus' and 'fetal conditions' and has to select one from each group as the main disease or condition. Until multiple cause analysis can be performed, statistical departments are recommended to make separate tabulations of the main fetal and the main maternal cause, and a cross-tabulation of a condensed list of each. Since the International Classification of Disease lists over 160 causes, the lists may become too complex for study by people other than health statisticians.

The Clinico-pathological Classification of Perinatal Deaths

Because of this, Baird and his colleagues have suggested a clinico-pathological classification, as they felt that the pathological

Medical Certificate of Cause of Perinatal Death

To be completed—

(a) in respect of a still-born child of at least 20 weeks gestation or 400 grammes weight at delivery—by a legally qualified medical practitioner who attended the mother during the confinement or who has viewed the body of the child after the still-birth.

(b) in respect of a live-born child dying on the day of his birth or within 28 days thereafter—by a legally qualified medical practitioner who attended the child before death or who has viewed the body of the child after death.

NOTE—Please tick in relevant boxes thus ☑

A. Particulars relating to Mother

1. Full name ....
2. Address of usual residence ....
3. Age last birthday .... years. 4. Number of previous pregnancies ....

B. Particulars relating to Child

5. Name, if given .... 6. Sex ....
7. Date of death, if live-born ...., 19..... 8. Age at death .... (minutes, hours, or days)
9. Place of death or still-birth ....
10. Time and date of birth: .... *a.m./p.m. on ...., 19.....
11. This birth was: Single ☐ Twins ☐ Triplets ☐ .... ☐
12. Weight at birth .... grammes, or alternatively .... lb .... oz.
13. Period of gestation .... completed weeks from first day of last menstrual period to date of delivery.
14. Did child breathe after complete expulsion or extraction from the mother? Yes ☐ No ☐.
15. Did heart beat cease—
    - (a) Before labour commenced .. .. ☐
    - (b) During labour but before delivery .. .. ☐
    - (c) Before delivery but not known whether before or during labour ☐
    - (d) After delivery .. .. ☐
    - (e) Not known whether before or after delivery .. .. .. ☐
16. If heart beat ceased before labour commenced, please estimate how long before: .... hours, or .... days.
17. If heart beat ceased after delivery, please state time .... *a.m./p.m., and date ....

18. **CAUSE OF DEATH** (in BLOCK LETTERS)

PART I

State approximate interval between onset and death, if known

A. Causes in Child or Foetus—

Disease or condition directly leading to death ....

due to } † ....

due to } ....

† Morbid conditions, if any, giving rise to the above cause, stating the underlying condition last.

B. Maternal Conditions or Other Causes giving rise to the underlying cause in the child or foetus—

....

due to ....

PART II

Other significant conditions in child, foetus, or mother contributing to the death but not related to the disease or condition causing it ....

....

---

19. Post mortem was held ☐ is to be held ☐ is not to be held ☐

I hearby certify that
- * I attended the mother of the still-born child during confinement
- * I attended the child before death
- * I viewed the body of the child after death

and that the particulars stated above are true to the best of my knowledge and belief.

Signature .... *Date* ....

Residence ....

Full name of medical practitioner: ....
(in BLOCK LETTERS)

* Strike out whichever is inapplicable.

Figure **18/2** The form of perinatal death certificate used in New South Wales, Australia.

EXAMPLES OF REPORTING CAUSE OF DEATH

Example 1—Placenta praevia causing severe haemorrhage at 31 weeks gestation. Caesarian section performed, complicated by undiagnosed twins. Weight of this child (second twin) 1,532 grammes, condition poor at birth, died aged 7 hours. Post mortem examination showed hyaline membrane disease. Item 18 (Cause of Death) on medical certificate should be completed as follows:

18. **CAUSE OF DEATH** (in BLOCK LETTERS)	**PART I**	State approximate interval between onset and death, if known
A. Causes in Child or Foetus—		
Disease or condition directly leading to death	*HYALINE MEMBRANE*	*7 HOURS*
due to †	*PREMATURITY*	
due to †		
† Morbid conditions, if any, giving rise to the above cause, stating the underlying condition last.		
B. Maternal Conditions or Other Causes giving rise to the underlying cause in the child or foetus—		
	ANTE-PARTUM HAEMORRHAGE	
due to	*PLACENTA PRAEVIA*	
	PART II	
Other significant conditions in child, foetus, or mother contributing to the death but not related to the disease or condition causing it	*CAESAREAN SECTION*	
	UNDIAGNOSED TWINS	

Example 2—Pregnancy normal. Baby born at 40 weeks gestation, weight at birth 3,380 grammes. condition good. **Cyanosis appeared 2 days** after birth and child died on fifth day. Postmortem showed death to be due to pulmonary atresia.

Part I	A.	Pulmonary atresia.	4 days.
	B.	—	
Part II		—	

Example 3—Admitted at 37 weeks gestation, membranes not ruptured, foetal heart sounds not heard, spontaneous normal delivery of a macerated foetus. Large retroplacental haematoma. Postmortem showed cause of death to be anoxia.

Part I	A.	Intra-uterine anoxia	
	B.	Concealed accidental antepartum haemorrhage.	
Part II		—	

Example 4—Mother Rh negative, Rh antibodies present at 28 weeks. Evidence of mild pre-eclamptic toxaemia from 34 weeks. Spontaneous labour at 36 weeks, foetal heart sounds ceased 1 day before labour commenced. Foetus hydropic.

Part I	A.	Haemolytic disease.	
	B.	Rh iso-immunisation.	
Part II		Mild pre-eclamptic toxaemia.	

Example 5—Baby born at 41 weeks. Condition at delivery poor, cyanosed from birth, tracheo-oesophageal fistula diagnosed and ligated but baby developed broncho-pneumonia on fourth day and died on the fifth day.

Part I	A.	Broncho-pneumonia.	1 day.
		Tracheo-oesophageal fistula.	
	B.	—	
Part II		—	

Example 6—Mother had a history of hypertension and developed pre-eclamptic toxaemia. A severe haemorrhage occurred at 32 weeks and mother was delivered of 1,400 gramme infant which died aged 2 hours. Postmortem finding was death due to atelectasis.

Part I	A.	Atelectasis.	2 hours
		Prematurity.	
	B.	Premature separation of placenta.	
		Pre-eclamptic toxaemia.	
Part II		Chronic hypertension.	

Figure **18/3** Examples of perinatal mortality recording.
Source: Department of Health, New South Wales, Australia.

classification, which was based on *how* the baby died, not *why* it died, was important, but not particularly helpful in meeting the objectives of perinatal mortality surveys. For example, the autopsy of a 2,500 g ($5\frac{1}{2}$ lb) late fetal death might

Table 18/2

Summary of clinico-pathological causes of perinatal death

A. MAINLY ENVIRONMENTAL OR SOCIO-ECONOMIC CAUSES	
1. Unexplained, low birth weight	Infant weighs 2,500 g or less at birth
2. Antepartum haemorrhage (without toxaemia of pregnancy)	*a*) Abruptio placentae *b*) Placenta praevia *c*) Origin uncertain
3. Malformations	*a*) Anencephalus and other malformations of the CNS *b*) Cardiac, multiple or other congenital malformations
4. Maternal disease	Diabetes; cardiac disease etc. Essential hypertension
B. MAINLY OBSTETRIC CAUSES	
5. 'Toxaemia'	*a*) without antepartum haemorrhage *b*) with antepartum haemorrhage
6. Mechanical/Trauma	*a*) Difficult labour *b*) Malpresentation of the fetus *c*) Cord complications
7. Unexplained, normal birth weight	Infant weighs more than 2,500 g
8. Serological incompatibility	*a*) Rhesus *b*) Other
9. Infection of fetus or infant	
10. Miscellaneous	

NOTE:

The mainly environmental causes are those in which it was considered that the cause related mostly to unfavourable factors in the mother's environment, her socio-economic background, or to diseases which she had acquired.

The mainly obstetrical causes were cases in which it was thought that a higher standard of obstetric care might have influenced the outcome.

It is accepted that there will inevitably be considerable overlap between the two main groups; and some difficulty may occur in deciding in which subgroup the death is to be entered.

only show anoxia, but the important matter was how this arose. Was it due to a preventible factor, or not? The classification divides perinatal deaths into ten main groups, and is shown in Table **18/2**. The following information is derived from Sir Dugald Baird's article in *Perinatal Problems*.

MAINLY ENVIRONMENTAL CAUSES

Unexplained, low birth weight

Deaths of babies weighing 2,500 g ($5\frac{1}{2}$ lb) or less in developed nations and 2,000 g ($4\frac{1}{2}$ lb) (or some other nationally determined weight) in developing nations, where no other obvious cause of the death has been found, are entered in this category. Pregnancy has been normal apart from being curtailed, and labour has been substantially normal. There is no obvious cause for the low birth weight. Autopsy findings, when this has been performed, reveal only the *mode* of death, e.g. anoxia, but do not indicate how the anoxia occurred. An autopsy finding of atelectasis, hyaline membrane disease or of massive pulmonary haemorrhage is consistent with placing the death in this category. Cases in which placental dysfunction, or dysmaturity, is thought to have occurred, are currently best included in this category if no other condition (e.g. pre-eclampsia, congenital defect or maternal disease) is present.

Antepartum haemorrhage

All cases in which the cause of death was obviously, or probably, the result of antepartum haemorrhage, are placed in this category except when the haemorrhage was associated with 'toxaemia', in which case the death is included in that category.

Malformation

In many cases the congenital defect is obvious, without autopsy (e.g. anencephalus), but autopsy is desirable in all cases as additional malformations may be discovered. In the classification *severe congenital defect* takes precedence over all other potential causes of death in a particular case; but great reliance is placed on the pathologist's report.

Maternal disease

Cases in which the mother suffered during pregnancy from an incidental medical or surgical condition, such as diabetes, heart disease or infection which apparently led to the fetal or early neonatal death are placed in this section. If hypertension is not complicated by proteinuria, and was present in the first half of pregnancy or persisted when the patient was seen at the post-natal visit, the case is entered in this category; in all other cases hypertension is entered under 'toxaemia'.

MAINLY OBSTETRIC CAUSES

'Toxaemia' (pre-eclampsia)

Cases in which the maternal diastolic blood pressure exceeded 90 mm of mercury or more on two successive days after the 20th week of pregnancy, after being below that level in early pregnancy, are placed in this category. The presence of proteinuria adds to the accuracy of the diagnosis and if it is present the condition is categorized as severe pre-eclampsia. If there is any doubt whether the hypertension preceded pregnancy or occurred in late pregnancy, the case is put in this category.

Mechanical/trauma

Cases in which the death was due, or apparently due, to mechanical obstruction, damage during labour, or difficulty in delivery are entered under mechanical causes. In deciding whether to enter the death in this group a careful study of the history of the labour may be crucial. All deaths associated with breech delivery or shoulder presentation are considered to be due to mechanical causes unless a severe congenital malformation is present, or the child weighs less than 1,500 g ($3\frac{1}{4}$ lb) and some other cause of curtailed pregnancy (e.g. severe pre-eclampsia or antepartum haemorrhage) is associated. Such infants are placed in the appropriate category on the grounds that any remedial action would be better directed to controlling or preventing the cause of the immaturity rather than in the better conduct of the labour. A second group of cases included in the group are those due to cord complications. If it is desired these can be classified separately.

Unexplained, normal birth weight

Babies which weigh more than 2,500 g (5½ lb) (or 2000 g, (4½ lb) in some nations) and either die in utero without any warning and in the absence of any maternal disease, or, after a normal labour, fail to establish respiration, are entered in this category. Deaths in which placental dysfunction is diagnosed on clinical or laboratory evidence are included in this group at present, provided the child weighs more than 2,500 g (5½ lb).

Serological incompatibility

Amongst Caucasians, rhesus isoimmunization is the main problem, but this is less common in Dravidians and Malayans, and is almost unknown amongst Chinese. Amongst these ethnic groups, and amongst Africans, other blood incompatibilities may cause death. Except where there is a gross congenital malformation, this cause is given priority in entering a death.

Infection of the fetus or infant

In these cases there is evidence of overwhelming intra-uterine infection (i.e. after prolonged rupture of the membranes), or the baby's condition is satisfactory at birth but death from infection occurs in the neonatal period. Neonatal tetanus, which is all too common in some countries, would be included in this category.

Arguing in support of the clinico-pathological classification as opposed to a purely pathological classification, Baird points out that although the two classifications have a fair measure of agreement in cases of congenital malformation and in serological incompatibility, in all other groups 'there is a wide scatter' when a cross compilation is made. He notes that 'post-mortem evidence of cerebral birth trauma and of infection was often unreliable as an indication of why the baby died, in the light of the sequence of clinical events which culminated in death'. In his study he considered that the need to evaluate the clinical story was important as 'no pathological lesion was found in 15·7 per cent of all deaths, and in over 30 per cent deaths were classified clinically by us as prematurity of uncertain origin' (*unexplained, low birth weight* in this book). A study of perinatal mortality in a hospital in Australia endorses Baird's view. In the study no pathological lesion was found to indicate why death occurred in 18 per cent of cases.

Two examples will show the difficulties of classification more clearly:

1. The patient was aged 35, and it was her sixth pregnancy, her largest baby having weighed 4,000 g (9 lb). She received pre-natal care and was normal throughout, going into labour spontaneously at the 37th week of gestation. After an 8-hour labour and a second stage lasting 30 minutes, she delivered a male child weighing 3,200 g (7 lb). The baby's Apgar score was 8–9. Half an hour after birth the child became cyanosed and dyspnoeic. It improved after resuscitation, but further episodes recurred with death at 15 hours after birth. An autopsy indicated the cause of death as 'cerebral haemorrhage—due to birth trauma: subdural haemorrhage and tentorial tear, with evidence of pulmonary infection.' The clinico-pathological classification was 'unexplained, normal birth weight'. This was decided after reviewing the history of the labour which did not explain how cerebral trauma could have occurred, nor did it explain the presence of pneumonia.

2. The patient was a known hypertensive, and was aged 26. This was her third pregnancy. She received pre-natal care at sporadic intervals, and her blood pressure levels were reported not to exceed 160-170/100-105. No significant rise occurred, but this may have been due to the fact that she was taking methyl-dopa. When 32 weeks pregnant, the membranes ruptured spontaneously, and labour started 12 hours later. Labour lasted 6 hours, and a 1,500 g (1 lb 12 oz) female child was born which developed the respiratory distress syndrome and died 28 hours after birth. Autopsy stated that death was due to hyaline membrane disease. The clinico-pathological classification placed the death in the category 'maternal disease', because of the pre-existing hypertension. This would alert the physician to the problem of curtailed pregnancy and premature birth in a subsequent pregnancy, and would suggest that increased pre-natal attention be given.

The Application of the Clinico-Pathological Classification

In Table **18/3**, information from the British Perinatal Mortality Survey and the New South Wales (Australia) perinatal mortality statistics have been classified using the clinico-pathological method. It can be seen that in those two nations the proportion of cases falling into each group is not dissimilar. The exception is toxaemia, and part of the reason is that in Britain most cases of hypertension complicating pregnancy have been included in this section, whilst in New South Wales greater care was taken to establish whether the patient had pre-eclampsia or essential hypertension complicating pregnancy.

Table 18/3

Standard perinatal mortality classified by clinico-pathological method

	NSW 1970 % *of total*	*U.K.* 1958 % *of total*
Environmental		
1. Unexplained, low birth weight	23·3	17·4
2. Ante-partum haemorrhage	14·2	13·1
3. Malformations	14·4	18·0
4. Maternal disease	5·9	2·4
Obstetric		
5. Toxaemia	6·1	13·1
6. Mechanical/Trauma	14·0	13·0
7. Unexplained, normal birth weight	10·5	15·1
8. Serological incompatibility	4·2	4·8
9. Infection	3·4	1·1
10. Miscellaneous	4·0	2·0
	100·0	100·0
	n = 1,684 Rate 19·4	n = 2,210 Rate 30·5

The division of the deaths into the two main groups of *mainly environmental causes* and *mainly obstetric causes* enables health planners to identify problems which require further investigation and the differential allocation of resources. This analysis is particularly valuable when different regions within a nation are compared. For example, in Figure **18/4**, the United Kingdom has been divided into three zones, North, Central and

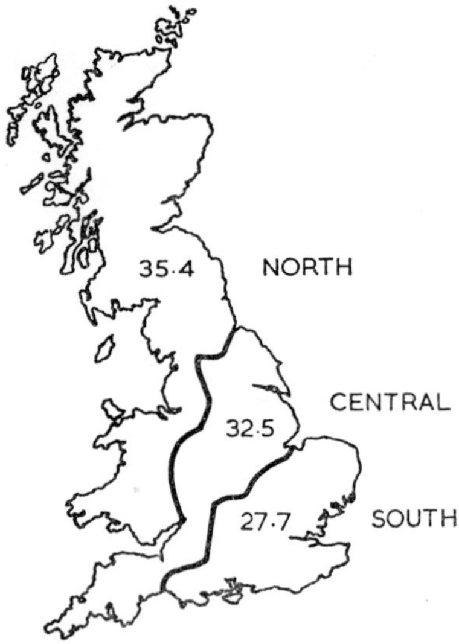

Figure **18/4** Perinatal mortality ratios in the geographical zones of the United Kingdom.
Source: Butler, N. R., and Alberman, E. D.

South. The Northern Zone includes North and North-West England, Scotland and Wales. This zone is characterized by dependence on heavy industry and coal mining. It is an area which is particularly affected during economic recession, when rates of unemployment tend to be higher than in the other two zones. Nutrition tends to be poorest within this zone, and this is reflected by the lower average height of the women (25 per cent of women are under 62 inches tall), by the higher proportion of women of the lower socio-economic groups (37 per cent are in socio-economic groups III to V), and by the higher parity of the mothers.

The Central Zone includes the East and West Ridings of Yorkshire and the Midlands, North Midland and South Western Regions. This zone depends mainly on light industry and continues to attract people from the less prosperous Northern Zone.

The Southern Zone is dominated by Greater London and includes the South-Eastern, Eastern and Southern regions. It is the most prosperous part of the United Kingdom, has the highest standard of living, the lowest unemployment rate, and the

Table 18/4

Perinatal death rates by clinico-pathological cause in geographical zones of Britain: single legitimate deaths. March to May 1958

	North			*Central*			*South*		
	Urban	*Rural*	*Total*	*Urban*	*Rural*	*Total*	*Urban*	*Rural*	*Total*
Mainly environmental									
Unexplained, low birth weight	7·4	5·6	6·5	6·1	5·1	5·6	5·8	4·5	5·0
Antepartum haemorrhage	5·3	5·1	5·1	4·6	4·7	4·7	3·7	3·7	3·7
Malformations	7·2	6·1	6·7	6·7	6·2	6·5	5·4	4·4	4·8
Maternal disease	Unable to compute: included in miscellaneous								
Mainly obstetric									
Toxaemia	4·3	4·3	4·3	3·6	4·5	4·2	3·7	3·5	3·6
Mechanical/trauma	4·6	4·8	4·7	3·5	4·8	4·3	3·3	3·5	3·6
Unexplained, normal birth weight	4·9	4·8	4·8	4·7	4·5	4·6	4·4	3·8	4·1
Serological incompatibility	1·4	1·5	1·4	1·2	1·4	1·3	1·2	1·4	1·3
Infection	Unable to compute: included in miscellaneous								
Miscellaneous	1·9	1·5	1·8	2·1	1·1	1·5	1·6	1·3	1·5
Perinatal mortality rate	37·1	33·7	35·4	32·6	32·4	32·5	29·0	26·6	27·7

Adapted from Table 13/1 of *Perinatal Problems* by kind permission.

lowest proportion of people in the lower socio-economic groups (30 per cent are in Groups III–V). The average maternal height is the highest in Britain and the average parity the lowest.

The three zones have been further subdivided into urban and rural areas.

In Table **18/4** it can be seen that the overall perinatal death ratio fell from the Northern Zone to the Southern Zone. *Mainly environmental causes* showed falls in the three main sections, suggesting that the better physique and nutrition of women in the South Zone was a factor. When malformations are further subdivided into central nervous system malformations, and all other malformations, the former had a high incidence in the North, but there was no difference in the rates for all other malformations. Amongst *mainly obstetrical causes* the lower rate associated with toxaemia and mechanical causes is noticeable in the Southern Zone.

It was also noted that the ratios in the rural areas of both the Northern and Central Zones were higher. When further information was sought, a factor was found which may be important. This was that in the Northern Zone, only 47·5 per cent of all mothers delivering had been under the supervision of obstetrical specialists or their staff, compared with 61·6 per cent in the Southern Zone; and in each zone fewer patients living in rural areas received specialist supervision. This suggests that the higher ratios were due to less adequate pre-natal and hospital facilities and a lower standard of obstetric care.

The 'High Risk' Mother

Use of the clinico-pathological classification of the standard perinatal mortality in Australia, Scotland and England and Wales, has enabled the investigators to identify mothers who have the greatest risk of losing their baby either in the late fetal period or the early neonatal period. This information is shown in Table **18/5**. Study of the various subgroups indicates that of the environmental causes, low socio-economic status (which frequently implies poor nutrition and inadequate obstetric care) is the major factor; whilst of the obstetric causes, high parity, increasing age, and inadequate obstetric care are important factors. It is clear from this analysis that peri-

Table 18/5

Standard perinatal mortality by clinico-pathological classification showing mothers likely to have the highest risk

Cause of death	*High risk mothers*
1. Unexplained, low birth weight (15–25 per cent of all)	Low socio-economic status Reduced height In all social classes, highest in women under 20 and over 35 Para 4 or more Cigarette smoking
2. Antepartum haemorrhage (12–16 per cent of all)	Para 4 or more Low socio-economic status
3. Malformations (15–20 per cent of all)	
a) CNS	Increase with diminishing socio-economic status Primiparity Increased rate in primiparae under the age of 20
b) Other	Increase with increasing parity, and age
4. Maternal disease (3–7 per cent of all)	Increase with increasing maternal age: no effect from parity
5. 'Toxaemia' (6–12 per cent of all)	Primiparae Women over 30 History of toxaemia in a previous pregnancy
6. Mechanical/Trauma (12 to 16 per cent of all)	Primiparity, especially if aged 30 or more Short stature Para 4 or more (inadequate obstetric care)
7. Unexplained, normal birth weight (10 to 15 per cent of all)	Primiparae, especially aged 30 or more Para 4 or more Post term (i.e. 42 weeks' gestation) especially in older primigravidae
8. Serological incompatibility (3–5 per cent of all)	Increasing parity
9. Infections (1–4 per cent of all)	None discerned apart from ? increasing age

Information from *Perinatal Problems*, Chapter 12, by Sir Dugald Baird and A. M. Thompson; *Perinatal Mortality Committee reports*, The Women's Hospital, Crown Street, Sydney.

natal mortality ratios will be reduced if increased attention is given to maternity and child health services, including family planning programmes. These matters are considered at greater length in the next section.

Factors Influencing Perinatal Mortality

Factors which influence perinatal mortality adversely may be socio-economic or environmental, due to maternal disease or due to fetal defects. This is rather an artificial division for it is obvious that there will be a considerable interplay between the groups. For example, women of the lower socio-economic groups tend to marry and have children at an earlier age, to have a shorter interval between pregnancies, and to have more pregnancies, than women in the higher socio-economic groups. They are, in addition, liable to be less well nourished, more subject to anaemia, to have less knowledge of hygiene, to be less adaptable to modern methods of child care and more likely to continue to use potentially dangerous traditional methods. They have less ready access to skilled obstetrical attention, both in the pre-natal period and during labour.

AGE AND PARITY

Studies in Britain and the U.S.A. confirm the direct relationship between age and parity and a rising perinatal mortality ratio. This is shown in Table **18/6** and in Figure **18/5**, which is derived from the careful study made in Britain in 1958. The adverse effect of increasing age, and at all ages, of high parity is obvious. At all ages and parities, cigarette smoking increases the perinatal mortality. But this is a peculiarly Western habit, particularly in Atlantic seaboard nations.

SOCIO-ECONOMIC STATUS

In Britain, the socio-economic status of the couple was defined in terms of the husband's occupation, because of the tendency of men to marry women of their own socio-economic group, or if of a lower group, women who had shown special qualities of beauty, intelligence or personality. It can be assumed that higher socio-economic status is associated with more favourable physical, educational and social opportunities during childhood

Table 18/6

Effect of maternal age on perinatal mortality
(*Age-specific perinatal mortality ratios*)

Maternal age	*U.S.A.*	*U.K.*
Under 20	59	33
20–24	37	27
25–29	40	27
30–34	42	35
35–39	54	49
40+	102	

Sources:
U.S.A. Yerushalmy, J. et al. *Amer. J. Obst. Gynec.* **71,** 80, 1966.
U.K. Butler, N. R., and Alberman, Ed. *Perinatal Problems,* Table 2.6, 1969.

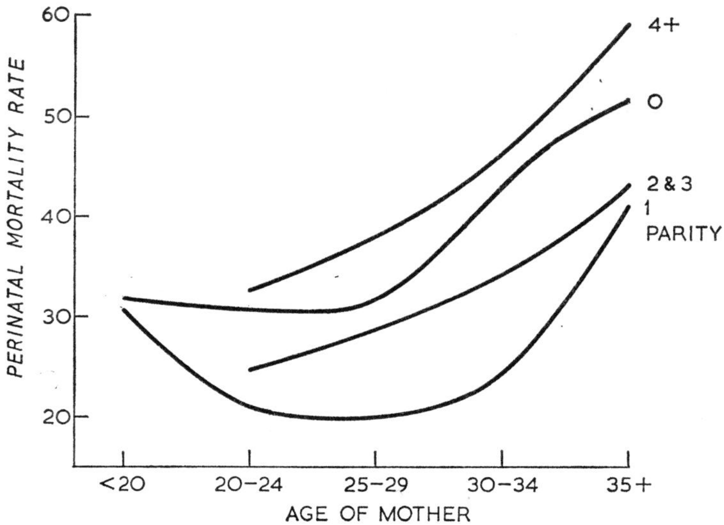

Figure **18/5** Perinatal deaths by maternal age and parity.
Source: Butler, N. R., and Bonham, D. G.

and adolescence. Socio-economic status influences age at marriage, but the effect of this factor is diminishing. One study by Daly and his colleagues in Britain in 1955 has shown that standardization for age and parity in each social class scarcely affects perinatal mortality as (1) the trends are similar in all socio-economic groups and (2) the relatively higher perinatal mortality amongst the older primiparae (aged 30 or more) who

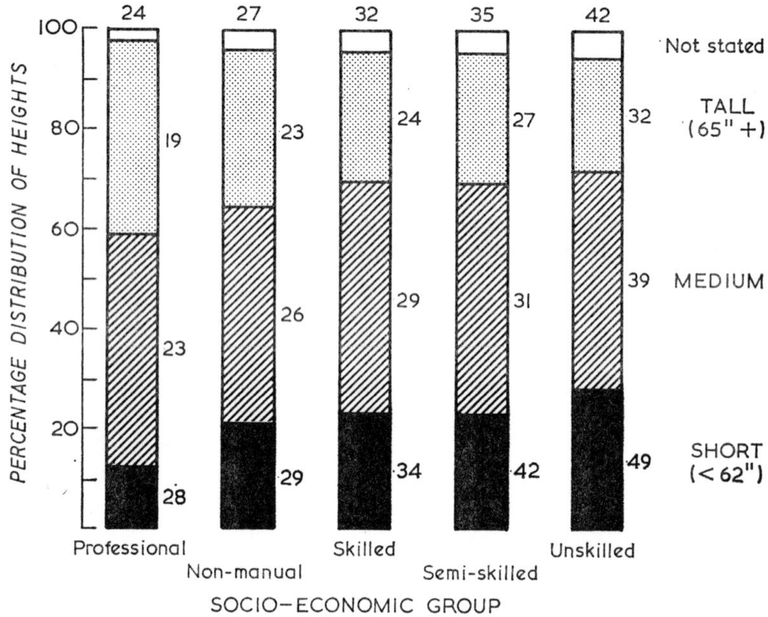

Figure 18/6 Perinatal mortality related to the socio-economic status of the father and the height of the mother, U.K. 1956. Source: Butler, N. R., and Bonham, D. G.

are mainly found in the higher socio-economic groups, is offset by the higher perinatal mortality in grande multigravidae (gravida 5 or more) who are found mainly in the lower socio-economic groups. In the British study the effect of maternal height was found to influence the mortality in each socio-economic group. Height is considered an indicator more of nutrition during infancy and childhood than due to a genetically operating factor.

In Figure **18/6**, it can be seen that the overall perinatal mortality ratio rose from 24 per 1,000 in the highest socio-economic group to 42 per 1,000 in the lowest socio-economic group.

Similar findings are reported from the State of Indiana, U.S.A., where higher perinatal mortality rates were found in areas of urban overcrowding lived in by people of the lower socio-economic groups. These areas also had the highest percentage of low birth-weight babies. The converse is found in the thinly populated rural areas of Indiana. Here both the incidence of low birth-weight babies and the perinatal mortality ratios were lower than the average for the State (Thompson).

BIRTH INTERVAL

It has long been suspected that a reduced interval between births leads to an increased perinatal mortality ratio. That this is so has been shown by Yerushalmy. The extended perinatal mortality ratio has been calculated and related to the interval between the end of one pregnancy and the conception of the next child (judged by the date of the last menstrual period) (Table **18/7**). The shorter the birth interval (at least up to three years), the higher is the perinatal mortality of the next child.

Table 18/7

Birth interval related to perinatal mortality ratios

Interval between birth and conception	*Fetal death (20 weeks or more) per 1,000 total births*	*Neonatal death (up to 28 days) per 1,000 live births*	*Extended perinatal mortality*
Less than 4 months	40·2	37·9	78
4–11 months	24·2	20·2	44
12–23 months	19·6	10·7	30
24–35 months	19·1	7·6	27
36 or more months	27·0	11·4	38

The significance of a short birth interval extends beyond an increase of perinatal mortality, for if the child survives, it tends to replace its immediately older sibling on the breast, which may lead to the death of that sibling from infection enhanced by malnutrition, or to the protein-calorie deficiency disease of marasmus and kwashiorkor.

The reasons for the raised perinatal mortality with reduced birth interval are not fully understood. In Britain, Douglas studied over 13,000 single legitimate births and concluded that regardless of maternal age and parity, the frequency of low birth-weight infants increased with birth intervals shorter than 24 months, which means a birth-conception interval of 15 months or less. Since low birth weight is a significant factor in raised perinatal mortality, this could be a major reason for the increase.

GEOGRAPHICAL DOMICILE WITHIN A NATION

This factor has been examined in the U.S.A. by Hunt and Huyuk, and in Britain by the Perinatal Mortality Survey. In the U.S.A., the perinatal mortality ratio was highest in the larger urban aggregations (over 500,000 population); lowest in smaller urban aggregations, and intermediate in rural areas. This difference is due to the poorer socio-economic status of the mothers living in the urban slums and the provision of a poorer quality of obstetric care; factors which apply to rural areas, but with less force. In Britain the differences are small, but once again the urban perinatal mortality ratio exceeds that of the rural areas by a small margin. Similar findings were made in New South Wales, Australia (Table **18/8**).

Table 18/8

Effect of urban or rural domicile on perinatal mortality

	Australia 1969–70[1]	*U.K.* 1958[2]	*U.S.A.* 1962[1]
Urban			
Aggregations of 50,000 or more	27	37 (Urban combined)	41
Other Urban	25		34
Rural	30	34	32

1. Extended perinatal mortality = intermediate and late fetal deaths + neonatal deaths.
2. Standard perinatal mortality = late fetal + early neonatal deaths.

FACTORS INFLUENCING PERINATAL MORTALITY

THE EFFECT OF PRE-NATAL CARE

The consistency of the trend in the three countries examined suggests that a major factor in lowering perinatal mortality is the availability of high quality obstetric care. This is supported when the relationship between pre-natal care and perinatal mortality is examined. In a study by Kohl in New York in 1958, amongst the 28,000 parturients, the perinatal mortality fell from 166 per 1,000, when no pre-natal care was sought, to 130 per 1,000 when the patient attended 8 or more times. Similar findings were obtained in an investigation in Australia.

THE EFFECT OF 'HIGH RISK' MOTHERS ON PERINATAL MORTALITY

The effect of socio-biological-economic factors on perinatal mortality cannot be fully analysed without a study of their relationship to adverse factors which may be present in the mother before pregnancy or may arise during pregnancy. These mothers constitute a 'high-risk', and their identification would aid the reduction of the perinatal mortality rate. The clinico-pathological classification, or preferably multiple-cause analysis, when this is available, will permit the more ready identification of the problem cases.

Pre-eclampsia (or the specific hypertensive disease of late pregnancy) is diagnosed by examination of the patient's blood pressure and her urine for the presence of protein. The condition only occurs after the 20th week of pregnancy, and affects twice as many primiparae as multiparae. The diagnosis is made if a patient develops hypertension for the first time after the 20th week of pregnancy. If the maximum diastolic blood pressure is between 90 to 99 mm of mercury, present on two successive days, the condition is classified as *mild* pre-eclampsia; if the diastolic blood pressure is 100–109 mm it is classified as *moderate pre-eclampsia*; and if the diastolic blood pressure is 110 or more it is classified as *severe pre-eclampsia*. The presence of protein in the urine, not due to infection, associated with any diastolic blood pressure exceeding 90 mm also is classified as *severe pre-eclampsia*. In several studies, the perinatal mortality has been shown to rise from 40 per 1,000 in mild pre-eclampsia, to 80 per 1,000 in moderate pre-eclampsia, reaching 120 per 1,000 in severe pre-eclampsia. Pre-eclampsia is the main cause leading to the perinatal death of the infant in 6 to 12 per cent of all cases.

Although pre-eclampsia currently is not preventible as its aetiology is unknown, early detection and adequate treatment of mild pre-eclampsia prevents the disease becoming severe. If this is to be achieved, freely available pre-natal care and facilities for hospital admission if ambulant treatment seems insufficient must be provided.

Antepartum haemorrhage

The studies reported earlier indicate that antepartum haemorrhage is the main cause of perinatal loss in 12 to 16 per cent of

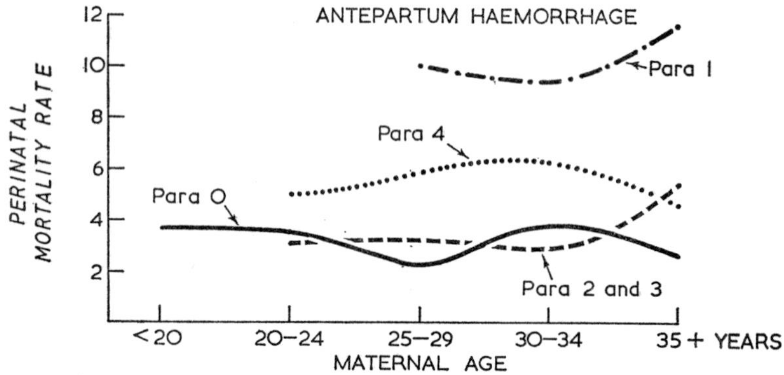

Figure **18/7** Perinatal mortality related to antepartum haemorrhage—various parities.

Source: Baird, D., and Thomson, A. M., in Butler, N. R., and Alberman, E. D., editors: *Perinatal Problems*, p. 211.

all cases. Antepartum haemorrhage can be subdivided into abruptio placentae (which accounts for 25 to 65 per cent of all cases); placenta praevia (15 to 35 per cent); and antepartum haemorrhage of uncertain origin (5 to 25 per cent). The incidence of the disorder in pregnancy increases with increasing maternal parity (Figure **18/7**). The obstetrician can do little to prevent perinatal deaths from abruptio placentae, apart from making family planning measures available to prevent conception in women who already have three or more children. However, with skilled obstetric care, available blood for transfusion, and adequate hospital accommodation, the perinatal mortality due to placenta praevia can be reduced from over 250 per 1000 to under 100 per 1000.

Serological incompatibility

This accounts for 4 to 8 per cent of all perinatal deaths in predominantly Caucasian nations, but is less frequent in Indo-Malay races, and rare amongst Chinese. In typical Caucasian communities, one fetus in every 200 is affected to some extent. Prophylactic injections are now available, which given within 72 hours of birth in a non-sensitized woman will offer over 98 per cent protection to becoming rhesus iso-immunized.

Haemoglobinopathies are of importance, particularly in Africa, and are associated with an increased perinatal risk, which can be much reduced by careful screening and good prenatal care of affected pregnant women.

Anaemia

In the British study severe maternal anaemia was rarely found. However, in many developing nations, maternal anaemia is both common and a significant cause of perinatal death. In one study in Malaysia by Llewellyn-Jones, amongst a population with a mean haemoglobin level of 10·1 g in early pregnancy, haemoglobin levels of 6·5 g or less were detected in 3 per cent of the women. Severe maternal anaemia was associated with a perinatal mortality of 134 per 1,000, three times higher than that amongst non-anaemic women. The main effect of anaemia is to reduce fetal oxygenation and possibly amino-acid transfer, with resulting intra-uterine growth retardation and the occurrence of an intermediate or late fetal death, or the birth of a low birth-weight infant. If born alive the infant has no greater risk of dying than any other infant of similar birth weight. Anaemia in pregnancy is entirely preventible and any perinatal death due to this disease is the result of inadequate obstetric care.

Other maternal causes

With increasing age the incidence and severity of essential hypertension, chronic renal disease, and diabetes increases; and the effects of heart disease become more severe. The same is true for maternal infections, which also increase with increasing parity.

In tropical countries, malaria is a significant factor in causing low birth weight and an increased perinatal loss. Studies in Africa indicate that although the fetus is rarely affected by falciparum malaria, the placenta is infected in 15 to 30 per cent of cases. When this occurs, placental function is disturbed and fetal growth retardation is likely.

Untreated maternal syphilis is a hazard to the fetus in utero, leading either to fetal death or to congenital infection, whilst gonorrhoea is a hazard to the neonate.

The dangers to the fetus of maternal disease can be diminished by good pre-natal care with appropriate medical advice and therapy; whilst the dangers of many infections can be eliminated by prophylactic measures and by serological testing to detect non-clinically obvious syphilis.

Low birth weight as a factor

Many of the maternal conditions mentioned lead to the birth of a low birth-weight baby, either because of the disease process, or because pregnancy is terminated to rescue the infant from a hostile environment. In other cases congenital defects lead to the birth of a low birth-weight baby which is either born pre-term, or growth retarded in utero, or is of low birth weight because of a combination of the two conditions. However, in 15 to 25 per cent of cases of perinatal death, a baby of low birth weight is born, and the cause of the onset of premature labour cannot be determined. One factor which is of importance is the occurrence of multiple pregnancy. The low birth weight of twins is in part due to pre-term delivery, but more importantly is due to growth retardation in utero. This growth retardation is not placental in origin, but is due to inadequate maternal growth support. By this is meant that insufficient nutrients are made available by the maternal blood stream to enable the full fetal growth potential to take place. If this is the explanation, an improved uterine blood flow should reduce the frequency of curtailed pregnancy and pre-term labour. There is evidence that increased rest, particularly during the vulnerable gestation period from the 30th to 35th week, has this effect. The increased attention to mothers with a multiple pregnancy should also reduce the incidence of moderate and severe pre-eclampsia which is three times as common as in women with single pregnancies. In the British survey the perinatal mortality of first born twins was 97 per 1,000, that of second born twins 121 per 1,000 compared with a rate of 33 per 1,000 for singletons. The reason for the higher perinatal mortality amongst second twins may be that they have a lower birth weight, but in all probability other factors are present.

Obstetric factors

In the clinico-pathological classification, 12 to 16 per cent of the deaths were considered due to mechanical or traumatic conditions arising during parturition. Although this group included cord complications, some of which are impossible to detect, it is sufficiently large even in a nation with good communications and an efficient medical service to cause concern. It is interesting to note that when the perinatal death ratio from this cause in the British Perinatal Survey was compared with that of the Aberdeen district in Scotland, the ratio in Aberdeen was significantly lower. Aberdeen has a highly organized obstetric service, with good two-way communication between midwives, general practitioners and the specialist staff of the obstetric hospital. The perinatal mortality ratio in Aberdeen was 40 per cent lower than that of the rest of the country.

The importance of good communications between all types of health worker caring for the expectant mother, of an efficient medical service and of a well-organised web network of obstetric care in reducing perinatal mortality is emphasized by Aberdeen's example.

FACTORS IN THE CHILD

It is known that increasing maternal age is associated with a higher incidence of certain neurological congenital defects, but this is a minor factor in perinatal mortality ratios, although *congenital defects* themselves account for from 15 to 20 per cent of all perinatal deaths. Factors in the child causing perinatal death are difficult, if not impossible, to separate from the maternal factors which led to the birth, particularly the pre-term birth of the child. For example, the fact that the child died of *hyaline membrane disease*, is mainly due to the fact that it was born prematurely, as the disorder increases steadily with gestation periods below 35 weeks. In the British Perinatal Mortality Survey, hyaline membrane disease was found in 22 per cent of autopsies on neonatal deaths. When the infant was more than 38 weeks gestation at birth, hyaline membrane disease was found in only 8 per cent of all neonatal deaths; between 35 and 37 weeks it rose to 14 per cent; between 32 and 34 weeks to 34 per cent; and if the gestation period was 31 weeks or less, to over 40 per cent. Sex is also involved and several investigations show the disease is more likely to affect male infants of low birth weight. Low birth weight is not the only association of hyaline membrane disease. The method of delivery is an important factor, as Caesarean section, particularly when performed before the onset of labour, is associated with a higher incidence of hyaline membrane disease in the infant, even when gestation age is taken into account (Usher). The current management of hyaline membrane disease is complex and only moderately successful, but it would appear desirable, when possible, that infants at particular risk of developing the condition are treated in special units able to give intensive neonatal care.

Pulmonary infection

This was even more commonly found in the British study, being present in 31 per cent of the autopsies on neonates. It was considered the primary cause of death in 36 per cent, and was associated with congenital malformations in 19 per cent, hyaline membrane disease in 12 per cent, cerebral trauma in 14 per cent and evidence of intrapartum anoxia in 12 per cent.

Apart from pulmonary infection, infections are uncommon amongst neonates in the developed nations, although occasionally meningitis develops. The situation is different in the developing nations, where the neonate is much more likely to be infected from the environment to which it is exposed. Low birth-weight infants are particularly likely to become infected. A serious, and common, infection in some developing nations is due to the custom of smearing the cut umbilical cord with cow dung. This leads to neonatal tetanus, which is entirely preventible.

Intraventricular haemorrhage

This occurred in 10 per cent of neonatal deaths, often in association with other pathology, usually hyaline membrane disease or pulmonary infection. The main aetiological factor was extreme immaturity; the baby usually weighed less than 1,800 g (4 lb), often being small for dates.

Massive pulmonary haemorrhage

This was found in 8 per cent of neonatal deaths, and in two-thirds of these it was the only pathological finding. The condition was unduly common after severe pre-eclampsia, and in dysmature (growth-retarded) babies.

The Reaction of the Mother to Perinatal Death

In contrast to the small psychological reaction to induced abortion, perinatal deaths produce a marked sense of maternal bereavement. The usual initial reaction is one of emptiness, restlessness and physical exhaustion. In addition, many women feel that the fetal or neonatal death occurred because of something they have done in pregnancy, or because of divine retribution for errors or transgressions. Finally, a feeling of failure exists; the mother feels she has failed her husband or her family. Psychiatrists are of the opinion that the proper management of bereavement plays an important part in preventive psychiatry, and that grief at the loss of a fetus or neonate is no less strong than grief following the death of an older child or a spouse. It has also been observed that the psychological recovery is slower in women who suppress their grief.

These women need support, reassurance, explanation and help. A leading article in the *British Medical Journal* in 1967 entitled 'Broken Hearts' which discussed grief, suggested that 'a willing ear tolerant of confusion and anger, is probably more important than tonics or sedatives'. The doctor needs to be sympathetic and factual and he should not delay in telling the mother that her child is dead. He may encounter hostility or resentment but must accept these, and give the parents a simple, rational explanation of the cause of the death. Later, when the initial impact has diminished, he should reinforce his explanation and answer often unformulated questions about the prognosis for a subsequent pregnancy. Unfortunately, few doctors are prepared to do this, most relying on the treatment of physical symptoms by prescribing sedatives liberally, whilst avoiding all communication about the death (Giles). But, Giles concludes, 'To have relieved a patient's anxiety, loneliness and guilt, and to have established her trust and confidence for the future are the rewards of a doctor's readiness to talk with a woman who has lost her baby in the perinatal period.'

The Reduction of Perinatal Mortality

The analysis of the causes of perinatal mortality in this Chapter indicates that the rate is influenced by two main, but inter-related factors. These are (1) the physique, health and reproductive habits of the mothers, and (2) the quality and availability of obstetric and neonatal care offered them.

In certain developed nations the standard perinatal mortality is between 14 and 20 per 1,000. With present knowledge this is about as great a reduction as can be achieved. To achieve it, a multi-pronged long-term approach is required, which starts with education of children and continues through the reproductive years.

1. Preparation for Childbearing and Child Health

Education in the school years should include preparation for family life. In this course, which should be taken by both sexes, the physiology of human reproduction, human sexuality, family planning and the impact of nutrition and hygiene on health should be stressed. The development of good nutritional habits is of importance in developed and developing nations, as the evidence given in this Chapter indicates that nutrition in infancy and childhood is as important to successful childbearing as is nutrition in pregnancy. There is much merit in the view that the course should form part of the course in human biology, which would replace the biology currently taught in many schools. Since in many nations only primary education is compulsory, the education should start at this level, and for those who then cease formal education, continuing health education should be made available, including information on family planning and nutrition, by the mass media and through health and community services. As a complement to this education, school health programmes should seek to identify physical and mental disorders in childhood and adolescence and to remedy these before childbearing begins. Where funds are available, supplementary instruction should be given in the period prior to marriage, when advice on family planning, child care and responsible parenthood should be made available.

2. CARE IN PREGNANCY AND PARTURITION

The principle of optimal care in pregnancy and childbirth, is that a web-network of services should be established so that prenatal care is readily accessible to every pregnant woman. In the majority of nations, it is envisaged that the key person in this web-network will be the midwife. It is envisaged she will make first contact with the patient in most cases. Her personality in motivating pregnant women to seek pre-natal care, as early as possible in pregnancy, will be crucial to the success of the campaign. In her care of the pregnant woman, she will emphasize nutrition, hygiene, childbearing, breast feeding and family spacing, in addition to screening the expectant mother for abnormalities. If any are discovered, she will refer the patient to the next level of the network. In the developed nations the first contact of the pregnant woman may be shared by midwife, general practitioner and obstetrician, but the principles of care and referral remain the same. The only way in which the network will operate most efficiently is if the expectant mother can be referred from the periphery to the centre with administrative ease and the minimal distress or anxiety to the patient. For this to occur demands a unified service with good communications, co-operation and co-ordination between personnel at all levels and between the health personnel and the community.

During pregnancy, the patients at higher risk need to be identified. The first selection is made at the initial visit on the basis of age, parity, past medical disorders and obstetric history. A secondary selection is made should abnormalities arise during pregnancy. Ideally, at all levels in the web-network the patient's blood should be examined for anaemia and ABO blood group. In appropriate circumstances the examination should include

Rhesus group and serological evidence of syphilis. There is an urgent need for a sturdy efficient haemoglobinometer to be devised for use by midwives. Routine testing of the urine, particularly for protein, is mandatory; and all personnel should be able to record the patient's weight and blood pressure accurately. If sufficient doctors are available, it is desirable that each pregnant woman be seen by a physician, who has received additional obstetric training after graduation, between the 30th and 35th week of pregnancy, although supervisory midwives could well replace doctors in this task. The object of this assessment is to ensure that no higher-risk mother has been missed, and to reassess the procedures done by less trained staff. In developed nations, where most pre-natal care is conducted by doctors, it is hoped that the referral would be to a specialist obstetrician, if he is not already caring for the patient.

Throughout pregnancy, by means of discussion and demonstration, the importance of nutrition, child hygiene and welfare and family planning are stressed, and expectant mothers are educated and motivated in these matters.

3. CARE IN LABOUR

For the foreseeable future the vast majority of pregnant women, probably over 85 per cent of the 100 million women giving birth annually, will be attended in pregnancy and childbirth by traditional midwives or by trained midwives. Less than 5 per cent, mainly in the U.S.A., Canada, Australia, New Zealand and parts of Europe, will be attended by doctors. Because of this, facilities must be made available, and guidelines established, to ensure the abnormalities of labour are detected early, that patients at 'high risk' are only cared for in the best available environment, and that patients can be readily and easily transferred from the periphery to the central hospital of the web-network. Such a service will only be effective if two-way communications and visits occur between the various levels. The key to success is motivated personnel. This means that the specialists from the centre must visit the periphery and must engage in informal discussions of problems with doctors and midwives. Personal contact is invaluable.

4. CHILD HEALTH AND HYGIENE

Throughout pregnancy the opportunity should be taken to educate mothers in child health and hygiene. One particular matter to stress is the value of breast feeding in the control of infant mortality, since there is strong evidence, particularly in the developing nations, that failure of lactation in the mother is followed by a raised infant mortality. In addition to this, instruction on child nutrition should be given, cultural taboos on foodstuffs explained, and the mothers informed about the value of prophylactic inoculations against smallpox, tuberculosis (BCG vaccination), tetanus, diphtheria, poliomyelitis and typhoid.

In many developing nations neonatal tetanus is a problem, because of traditional beliefs in managing the divided umbilical cord. Expectant mothers should be shown ways of dealing with the cord hygienically, and additionally, the mother should be actively immunized against tetanus with tetanus toxoid in the last months of pregnancy (preferable before the 35th week) as this has been shown to protect the fetus.

ORGANIZATION OF THE WEB-NETWORK

In both the developed and in the developing nations, the *regional hospital* should be the centre of the web-network. The size of the region will depend on local circumstances, and can only be determined after studying local conditions. If the region is too large, communication problems are magnified; if it is too small the service tends to be inadequate. In addition to having well-equipped and staffed obstetrical and paediatric departments, the senior obstetrician and senior paediatrician should be specialist advisers to the regional MCH services. In all regional hospitals, and in selected district hospitals, a well-equipped and well-staffed fetal and neonatal intensive care department should be established.

The regional hospital should be linked with *district hospitals*, which should be sufficiently equipped to provide appropriate laboratory services, to have adequate ward accommodation for pre-natal patients, and to provide facilities for midforceps deliveries, Caesarean section and neonatal care. The aim should be that the district hospital will be closely related to the community it serves. In general it should deliver more than 1,000 patients a year and should have a doctor with postgraduate gynaecological training in charge of the obstetric section. In the developed nations, the district hospital would co-ordinate the MCH work of general practitioners and midwives in the area. In the developing nations, a third level in the web-network is envisaged. This is the *health centre* which serves between 15,000 and 30,000 people. The health centre would have obstetric beds and would be under the care of a doctor and/or supervisory midwife. The doctor would have been trained to perform assisted vaginal delivery, manual removal of the placenta, vasectomy and the insertion of the IUD. He would have a knowledge of neonatology, and would be skilled in health education, including family planning. Each health centre would supervise between 3 and 7 subcentres which would be situated so that no patient needed to travel more than 5 to 10 km (3–6 miles) to receive attention. The subcentre would be staffed by midwives who would co-operate with traditional midwives in the domiciliary care of the expectant and parturient mother.

Efficient transport services should be available so that a patient requiring special attention may readily be transferred from her home to the appropriate level in the network. Similarly, when possible, a 'flying obstetric squad' should be provided by the centre to bring skilled attention to seriously ill patients at the periphery, so that treatment may be given before referral.

NINETEEN

Maternal Mortality

The death of a mother in pregnancy, in labour, or after childbirth, is one of the greatest tragedies which can befall a family, for the entire family structure is temporarily, or permanently, disorganized.

The quality of the obstetric care offered to women in a country or a region can be measured, to some extent, by studying the maternal mortality rate—the lower the rate the better the implied quality of medical care. In most developed countries maternal deaths are studied on a State or Regional basis by properly appointed Maternal Mortality Committees whose function is to analyse the factors causing each death, and to recommend measures to prevent future deaths. Unfortunately, in most of the developing countries the available vital statistics are highly inaccurate, and analysis of maternal deaths can only be made on the basis of experience in individual hospitals. This does not necessarily reflect the conditions in the area. Despite these limitations, the study of maternal mortality trends is of great importance to all health workers who care for pregnant women. The method of establishing and conducting maternal mortality studies differs in different nations. Because of this diversity, three examples are given to show how the studies have evolved, and what their impact has been on the maternal mortality rate. The nations chosen as examples are the U.S.A., Britain and Australia. In addition, the activities of the World Health Organization will be mentioned.

The United States of America

In the U.S.A., the National Committee on Maternal Welfare was established in 1920. Its aim was 'to encourage the analysis of maternal deaths in every State, county and community and to try, if possible, to prevent maternal deaths by education of the laity, the hospital members, the community and also the medical profession'. Progress was slow, however, and 13 years elapsed before the first analysis of maternal deaths in New York State during 1930–32 was published. Subsequently, most other States have followed New York's lead. The main impetus for this change in the late 1920s was the realization that the maternal mortality in the U.S.A. compared unfavourably with that of other countries. Obstetricians felt that this would only be remedied if maternal deaths were analysed, and decisions were made to determine if the cause of death was obstetric or non-obstetric. If the cause of death was obstetric, investigations would be made to see if factors were present, which, if avoided, would have prevented the death. The analysis tried to determine whether the doctor, the patient or the family had been at fault. However, the purpose of the enquiries was educative, not punitive.

Unfortunately, not all States used the same definitions for maternal deaths and consequently comparison of statistics was impossible. To remedy this, the American Medical Association established a Committee on Maternal and Child Care which began its work in 1950, and in 1955 called a national conference to develop guidelines for State maternal mortality committees. The result of this meeting was the publication of the *Guide for Maternal Death Studies*, published in 1957 and revised in 1964. The guide recommended that as an initial step the co-operation of all the medical societies, and of the doctors in the area under study was obtained, and that the co-operation of the appropriate health department was sought. The health department was asked to inform the Maternal Mortality Committee when a maternal death occurred. The committee then obtained as much information regarding the death, by questionnaire and personal interview, as was possible. In particular, information was sought from the patient's doctor, and from hospital records. All identification was removed and the case, identified by a number, was analysed by the committee, who issued an annual report.

The *Guide for Maternal Death Studies* further defined maternal death as 'the death of any woman dying of any cause whatsoever while pregnant or within 90 days of the termination of the pregnancy, irrespective of the duration of the pregnancy at the time of the termination or the method by which it was terminated'. By 1968, 30 States had agreed to this definition and 31 issued reports on maternal deaths.

BRITAIN

In 1928, the maternal death rate was 4·4 per 1,000 live births, a level little changed since 1900. Because of public concern, a departmental committee of the Ministry of Health was appointed in that year to advise upon maternal mortality and morbidity. Two years later, in 1930, the committee issued its report and recommended amongst other things, that the concept of a 'primary avoidable factor' be introduced. This was defined as a 'departure from accepted standards of satisfactory care from which ensued the chain of events resulting in death'. As well, it was recommended that the enquiry be strictly confidential and neither the name of the patient, the attending doctor, or the hospital (if the patient had died in hospital) would be disclosed. However, little further action was taken until 1949 when the Royal College of Obstetricians and Gynaecologists suggested to the Ministry of Health that maternal deaths might be investigated more usefully if the technique adopted in the U.S.A. was followed. After two years of consultation, a new system was introduced, the original confidential nature of the enquiry being maintained. As in the U.S.A., information was sought from all those who could provide it, from the midwives or doctors who had been associated with the maternal death being investigated. It was determined that the information would be entered on a standard form, marked '*Strictly Confidential*, for medical use only' and issued by the Ministry of Health.

Maternal mortality was defined as 'the death of a woman within one year of pregnancy and childbirth'. The deaths were classified under two headings: maternal deaths and associated deaths. *Maternal deaths* were further defined as those 'due to complications of pregnancy, labour and the puerperium'. This definition included deaths due to abortion or ectopic gestation, which since 1952 have accounted for between 15 and 20 per cent of all deaths. Maternal deaths accounted for about 80 per cent of all deaths of pregnant women. The *associated deaths* were defined as those due to disease, violence or accident involving the death of a pregnant or parturient woman, but which were not the result of pregnancy, labour or the puerperium.

This classification is not without its problems. The first is that it may be difficult to decide whether a death should be classified as maternal or associated. An example would be if a diabetic patient, whose diabetes is out of control, dies during Caesarean section. The second problem is that, as in the U.S.A., the definition gives a time following delivery after which the death ceases to be classified as a maternal death. One example is a death from malignant trophoblastic disease occurring more than 12 months after the expulsion of a hydatidiform mole. How should such a death be classified? Luckily these complicated cases are relatively few.

The success of the British confidential enquiry depends on having one person responsible in each area of the country for obtaining the information accurately. This in turn depends on accurate recording of data in hospital and other case records. One side-effect of the enquiry has been to improve the quality of the record-keeping, which is of importance for the future when computers will be used increasingly. A positive feature of the confidential enquiries is that the information obtained by the enquiry has led to much more accurate information about maternal mortality. For example, Stallworthy and Bourne quote that in the years 1958 to 1960 the statistics of the Registrar General for England and Wales attributed 61 of the maternal deaths to puerperal phlebitis and thrombosis, whilst the more detailed investigations of the enquiry revealed that in only two of the cases was this the real cause. Conversely, the Registrar General attributed pulmonary embolism as the cause of death in only 36 cases, whilst the enquiry considered that this was the cause of death in 101 women.

Each region has a designated regional assessor, who has the authority to seek additional information, and who submits the documents to the Ministry of Health, where two senior obstetrical advisers co-ordinate the records, make further assessments, and draft the report. Since 1952, five reports have been issued, each covering maternal deaths in a 3-year period. The Reports on Confidential Enquiries into Maternal Deaths have recorded a progressive reduction in the number of deaths over the period

1952–67, and after analysis of the avoidable factors have indicated ways in which improvements might be made.

Australia

Confidential enquiries into maternal death have been conducted since 1939, when the State of New South Wales set up a Committee, under the Department of Health, for this purpose; and other States followed this example. Because of the small, relatively affluent population of each State, and a fairly high standard of health care, the numbers of deaths available for analysis were few, which limited the value of any recommendations made. It was therefore decided, in 1962, to seek the agreement of all States to publish a report on all maternal deaths in Australia. This task was given to a subcommittee of the National Medical and Health Research Council, and the first reports were published in 1969 and 1972. These reports dealt with the maternal deaths occurring in the years 1964 to 1966 and 1967 to 1969 respectively. The method for obtaining information was similar to that used in Britain.

International

The problems connected with the American and British definitions have led to further consideration of the problem by an especially appointed Committee on Maternal Mortality of the Federation Internationale de Gynaecologists et Obstetricians (FIGO). This committee has developed a definition of maternal mortality which has been approved by the World Health Organization.

In the FIGO definition, maternal death is defined as 'the death of any woman dying of any cause while pregnant or within 42 days of termination of pregnancy, irrespective of the duration and the site of the pregnancy'. The FIGO Committee also recommended that the maternal mortality rate was calculated per 10,000 live births. Live births were further defined as 'the birth of a live-born infant that weighs 500 g or more and in the absence of known birth weight has an estimated duration of 20 weeks or more, calculated from the first day of the last menstrual period'. Finally, the numerator in this rate was to include *all* maternal deaths, whether due to direct obstetric causes, indirect obstetric causes, or non-obstetric causes.

Direct causes of maternal death include such conditions as abortion, ectopic gestation, pre-eclampsia and eclampsia, ante-partum and post-partum haemorrhage and puerperal sepsis. Indirect causes include conditions which, although present

Table 19/1

Main causes of maternal death

International classification number	*Cause of death*	*Percentage of all deaths*		
		U.K. 1955–66* *national statistics*	*Australia* 1964–69† *national statistics*	*Malaysia* 1953–62‡ *hospital statistics*
642, 685, 686	Toxaemia of pregnancy	12	11	11
643, 644, 760	Haemorrhage, ante-partum	7	5·5	9
671, 672	,, post-partum	5	5·5	13
647, 673–5, 677	Difficult or traumatic labour	9	6	10
640, 641, 680–3, 689	Infection (excluding septic abortion)	5	5	4
684, 687	Vascular accidents	13	15	3
645, 650–2	Abortion and ectopic gestation	18	16	18
648, 660, 676, 678, 688	Other direct causes (including deaths due to complications of anaesthesia)	8	7	7
VII, VIII	Cardiac or respiratory conditions	8	12	4
646, IV	Diseases of blood (including anaemia)	1	—	8
I	Infectious disease	2	2	3
II	Neoplastic disease	3	4	0·5
III, V, VI, IX–XVI	Other indirect conditions	9	11	9·5
		100	100	100
	Total deaths	3,887	512	360

* *Confidential Enquiry into Maternal Deaths in England and Wales*, 1955–57, 1958–60, 1961–63 and 1964–66, H.M.S.O., London.

† *Maternal Deaths in the Commonwealth of Australia*, N.H.M.R.C., Canberra, 1969 and 1972.

‡ *Maternity Hospital, Kuala Lumpur: Annual Clinical Reports*. (The Hospital is the main hospital for 1,000,000 people.)

before 'pregnancy, are aggravated by pregnancy: examples are cardiac disease, anaemia, thyroid disease, diabetes and certain malignancies'. Non-obstetric causes include car accidents, malaria, typhoid fever and some other infectious diseases.

These examples have been given to demonstrate the variety of ways in which maternal mortality survey committees can be established and operate. In summary, the efficiency of the surveys depends on the input of accurate detailed information obtained either voluntarily, or as a statutory duty, from the records of those who have attended the dead woman, from hospital protocols and from all other sources. For this to be obtained the information must be strictly confidential, so that no person is at risk of litigation, and in the published report all identification must be removed. The information received must be carefully evaluated so that avoidable factors may be identified. The purpose of the report is educative, rather than juridical, and to be effective it requires to be circulated widely and discussed by all health workers who deal with maternity. Evidence from several nations shows that the knowledge that a committee is investigating maternal deaths improves the standard of case-histories, which is highly desirable. Finally, the full value of the enquiries will only be obtained if the avoidable factors are remedied. This means that state and county health officers, hospital administrators and individual doctors must be prepared to act on the information derived from the confidential enquiries, to improve the quality of maternity care in their region.

In Table **19/1**, a short tabulation of maternal deaths using the international classification of disease is shown, and statistics from Britain, Australia and Malaysia are given.

The Impact of Studies on Maternal Mortality

The value of maternal mortality committees in reducing maternal mortality is difficult to determine because of other measures which have occurred over the same period. However, the studies have made general practitioners and obstetric specialists aware of the problems; they appear to have encouraged consultation; and within health services and in hospitals have identified areas for improvement of maternity care, for example, the need for blood banks, the dangers of inhalational anaesthesia and the inadequacy of obstetric emergency services. That the enquiry itself has value is shown in Britain where the maternal mortality fell from 8·7 per 10,000 in 1950 to 2·5 in 1965. During this time there were no obvious pharmaceutical or obstetric advances, so that the drop must at least in part be due to the greater awareness by medical attendants of the problems described in the analysis of the deaths. The impact of the studies would be greater if their published work received wider publicity, for ultimately the best ways to reduce maternal mortality are to improve the coverage of pre-natal care to a hundred per cent of the population and to ensure that all medical attendants of whatever degree of skill, know their limitations as well as their abilities, and are not afraid to seek consultation or to refer the patient. The importance of education is shown by an American study in Ohio of maternal deaths over 10 years, in which 65 per cent of them were found to have been avoidable. Similar analyses in Britain, between 1952 and 1966, showed that over 43 per cent of the deaths directly due to pregnancy and childbirth (including abortion) were thought to have been avoidable.

Secular Changes in Maternal Mortality

In all developed nations, and in many developing nations, the maternal death rate has dropped considerably since about 1935. Britain is an example of a developed nation where vital statistics are very accurate. Since 1934, the maternal mortality rate in Britain has been falling. In 1934 it was 52 per 10,000 live births, a rate similar to that which had existed for the previous 30 years (Figure **19/1**). The most striking fall, initially, was of the deaths caused by sepsis, and this was due to Colebrook's work on cross infection by droplets, and to the discovery of the sulphonamides and penicillin. But other factors have played a major part. The wartime food policy provided extra rations for pregnant women if they attended for antenatal care, and this led to the increasing use of antenatal clinics in early pregnancy and to the early detection of abnormalities. Hospital beds were made available so that patients requiring hospital attention could be easily admitted. Simultaneously, the blood transfusion services made blood readily available, and the spectre of death from haemorrhage receded. In medical schools greater emphasis was laid on adequate obstetric training in the undergraduate period. The Royal College of Obstetricians and Gynaecologists played its part by recommending postgraduate experience for all those doctors who intended to care for pregnant women, and in suggesting improvements in the design of the maternity units of hospitals. The training of nurse-midwives was improved, as it was realized that their area of responsibility in obstetric care

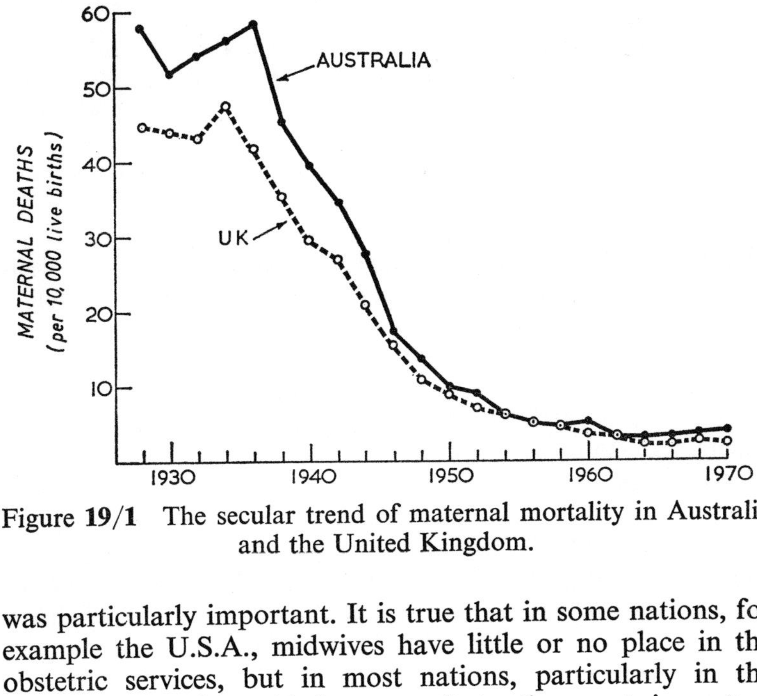

Figure **19/1** The secular trend of maternal mortality in Australia and the United Kingdom.

was particularly important. It is true that in some nations, for example the U.S.A., midwives have little or no place in the obstetric services, but in most nations, particularly in the developing world, midwives constitute the most important section of health workers offering maternity care, so that better training should reduce maternal mortality significantly. In the post-war years the rapidity of the decline in the mortality rate has decreased in developed nations, but statistics from several countries show that the rate is still falling slowly (Table **19/2**), towards what will probably be the minimum—less than one death per 10,000 births.

Table 19/2

The decline in the maternal mortality rate since 1939 in selected developed nations
(*Direct causes only*)

Country	*Year*			
	1939	1957	1965	1970
Australia	41·0	6·0	4·3	3·0
Canada	43·0	5·0	3·2	3·1
New Zealand	36·0	7·0	2·2	3·2
United Kingdom	32·0	4·8	2·5	1·8
U.S.A.	41·0	4·0	3·3	2·2

Factors Associated with Maternal Mortality

PARITY

The effect of increasing parity upon maternal mortality is considerable. In Britain, the pregnancies in which the rate is below average are the first, second and third, the first being slightly more at risk than the other two. The slightly higher risk in first pregnancies is due to the increased number of extramarital pregnancies occurring in that group. The problems of extramarital pregnancy are considered in Chapter 15. It was noted in that chapter that extramarital pregnancy was only a hazard if it was concealed and if pre-natal care was not sought early in pregnancy. From the fourth pregnancy onwards the risk rises considerably (Figure **19/2A**). If the parity-specific maternal mortality is calculated (i.e. the death rate per 10,000 births in each parity group) the increasing maternal mortality with higher parity is emphasized (Figure **19/2B**).

The effect of parity was strikingly apparent in a study of the mortality rates in a hospital in Malaysia which admitted all primigravidae and all women pregnant for the sixth or subsequent time, but which selected patients pregnant for the second to fifth time. In this last group only those women who had had an abnormal pregnancy or labour in the past, or whose present pregnancy was abnormal, or whose social conditions were unsuitable for home delivery, were accepted. Between 1953 and

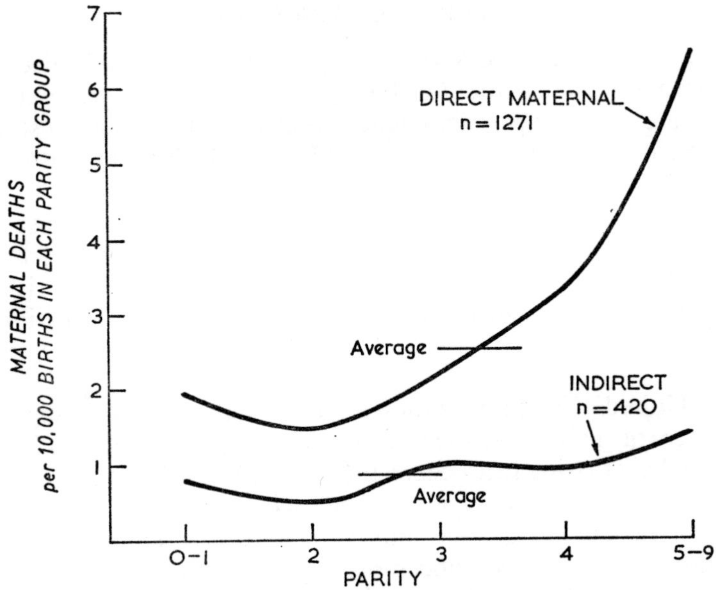

Figure **19/2A** The effect of parity on maternal mortality in the United Kingdom.

Source: *Confidential Enquiries into Maternal Deaths*, Ministry of Health.

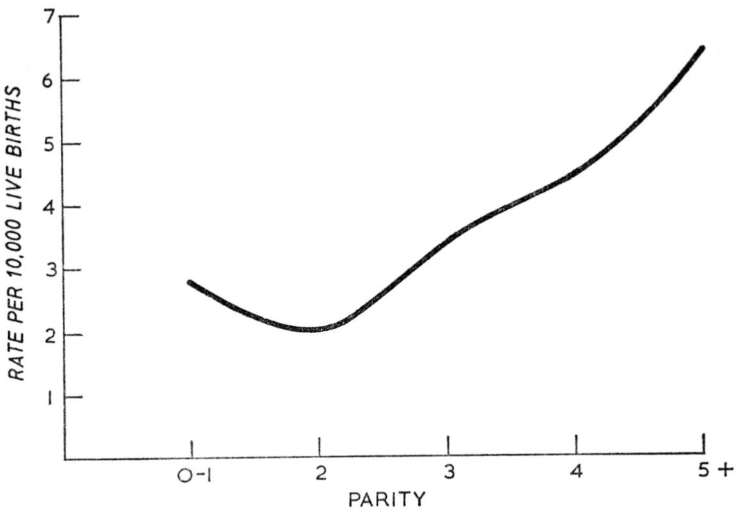

Figure **19/2B** Parity-specific maternal death rates in the United Kingdom.

Source: *Confidential Enquiries into Maternal Deaths.*

1962, 73,284 deliveries took place and 283 women died; a maternal mortality rate (excluding abortions) of 35 per 10,000. The rate amongst primigravidae was 28 per 10,000; amongst the selected gravidae two to five, 32 per 10,000; amongst the gravidae six or more, 51 per 10,000.

The increased risk to the grande multipara is quite clear. If women decided to reduce the number of pregnancies they had, a reduction in maternal mortality would follow this decision alone. This is currently taking place in most developed nations.

AGE

The United Kingdom studies indicate that the risk is slightly greater for girls under the age of 20 than for women aged 20 to 24, and that rising rates occur thereafter; but it is probable that the important factor is not age but extramarital pregnancies in the under-20 age-group, and greater parity amongst older women. When age-specific mortality rates are calculated, the rising maternal mortality with increasing age is confirmed; but the risk to women under the age of 20 disappears (Figure **19/3A**). Similar findings are reported from the U.S.A., where the lowest maternal mortality is found amongst women aged 20 to 24. The rate is almost four times greater amongst women aged 35 to 39, and eight times greater in women aged 40 to 44.

In the Netherlands a longitudinal study of maternal mortality (including abortion)—direct causes only—confirms the increasing risk of death with increasing age. This is shown in Figure **19/3B**. It can be seen that the maternal mortality is much higher after the age of 30 than before. Any cultural change which reduces childbearing after this age, and leads to a shift in the mean age of childbirth to younger age-groups will effectively reduce maternal mortality.

AGE AND PARITY

In Britain, the fifth Confidential Report, 1969, includes an age-parity analysis. It was found that the risk of maternal death increased with age independent of parity. The analysis showed that the safest age for a mother to have her first baby was between 20 and 25, whereas the primigravida aged 40 years or more was at the greatest risk. At all ages the maternal death rate was considerably increased amongst women having their fifth,

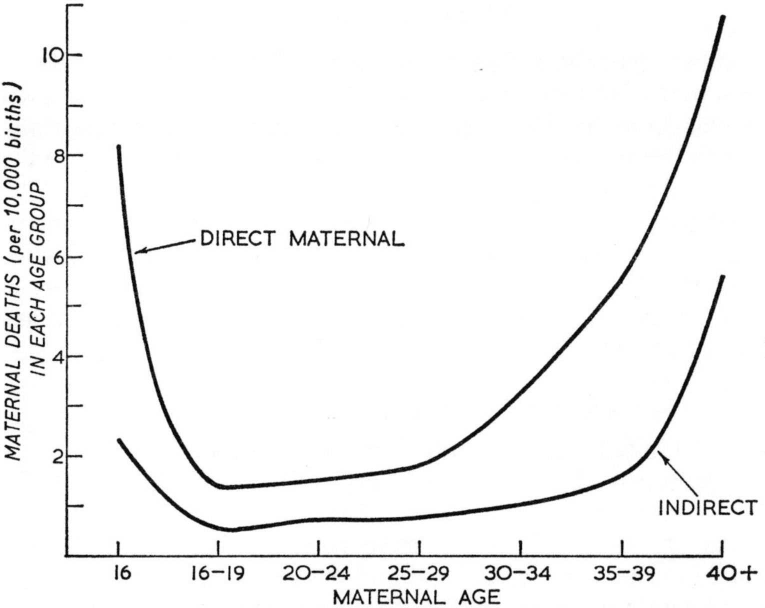

Figure **19/3A** Age-specific maternal death rates, U.K. 1961–66. Source: *Confidential Enquiries into Maternal Deaths.*

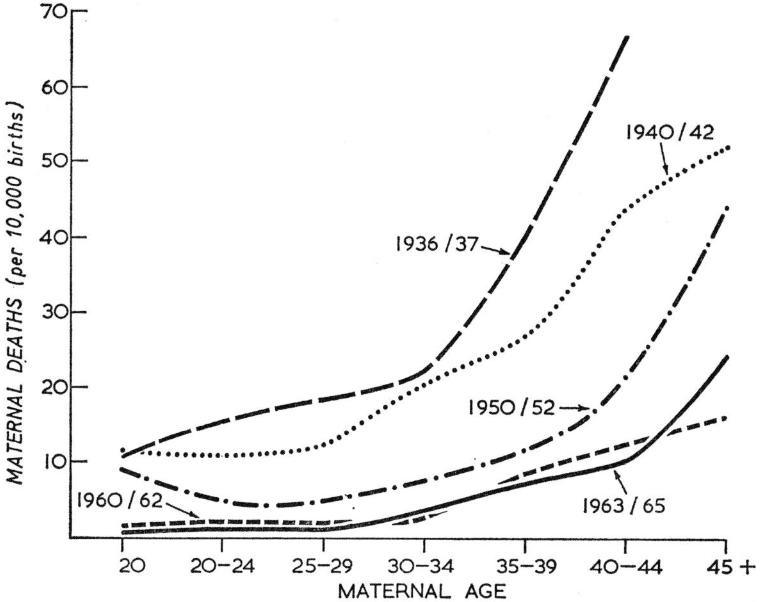

Figure **19/3B** Age-specific maternal death rates, the Netherlands 1936–65. Source: Bronte, J. T. P., and Verbrugge, H. P.

or subsequent child. The authors concluded that the reduction in maternal mortality in England and Wales in the period 1964 to 1966, compared with the previous 3-year period, was partially due to the fact that fewer babies were born to women over the age of 29 and fewer women had five or more children. The importance of this observation to the concept of family planning cannot be over-emphasized, as the fragmentary evidence from developing nations confirms the British findings, and in these nations the overall maternal mortality is ten times that of England and Wales.

SOCIAL CLASS AND ECONOMIC STATUS

In the United Kingdom the maternal mortality rate increases as the social class of the husband falls. The effect of social class cannot be considered in isolation, as women of the lower social classes are likely to have been the least privileged in nutrition, housing, education and social amenities from birth. In Malaysia a similar association was noted: the rate amongst

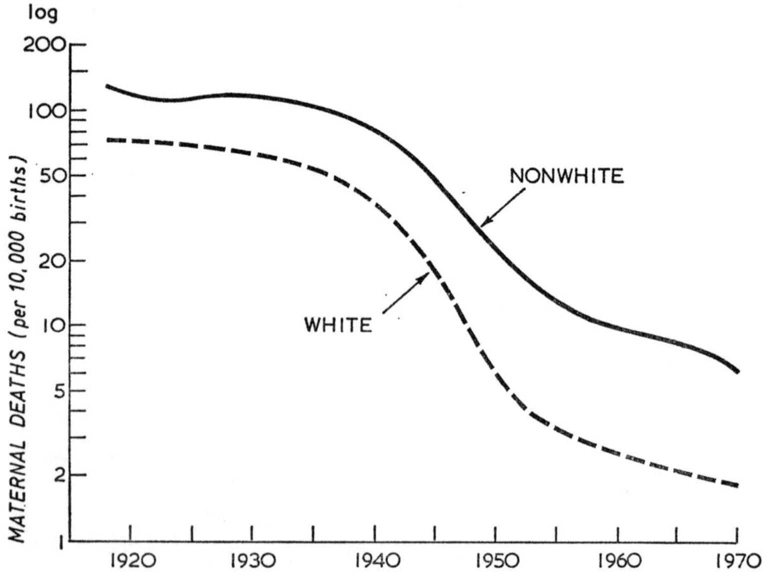

Figure **19/4** Maternal mortality by racial group, U.S.A. 1918–70. Source: National Center for Health Statistics. U.S. Department of Health, Education and Welfare.

wives of professional or managerial groups, upper echelon clerks and skilled workers being one-sixth that of the wives of unskilled workers. In the U.S.A. similar differences are noted when the rates amongst Black Americans are compared with the rates amongst White Americans (Figure **19/4**). This increase is related to poverty rather than racial origin as will be shown later (page 519).

ANTENATAL CARE

The most significant immediate factor affecting maternal mortality rates is the availability of antenatal care, and its acceptance by the community. Unfortunately, those very groups which have the highest mortality rate (the unmarried primigravidae, the high multigravidae, and those of the lower socio-economic groups) are those women who least often avail themselves of the facility. This is reflected by a tenfold increase in the mortality rate in Malaysia amongst those who did not attend antenatal clinics, as can be seen in Table **19/3**.

Table 19/3

Effect of antenatal care on the maternal mortality rate per 1,000 births (*Kuala Lumpur*, 1953–62)

	Numbers	*Deaths*	*Rate*
Antenatal care	59,449	77	1·3
No antenatal care	13,835	206	14·9
	73,284	283	3·8

ENVIRONMENTAL FACTORS

Information relating to the type of women at risk and the immediate cause of death is of little value unless further related to the environmental factors which permit them to operate. In the British *Confidential Enquiries into Maternal Deaths* for the years 1958 to 1967, it was considered that 40 per cent of the deaths directly due to pregnancy and childbirth had avoidable factors. In a further analysis of the cases, the fault lay primarily with the following persons: the general practitioner, in

33 per cent; the patient or relative, in 33 per cent; the hospital medical staff, in 24 per cent; the midwife (hospital or domiciliary), in 6 per cent; the ante-natal clinic doctor, in 2 per cent; other doctors, in 2 per cent.

A similar study in Malaysia showed that 75 per cent of 283 deaths (excluding abortion and ectopic gestation) were probably preventible (i.e. avoidable factors were present). The main fault lay with the patient or her relatives in 46 per cent; with inadequate obstetric care outside the hospital in 23 per cent; and with inadequate care in hospital in the remaining 31 per cent of deaths.

IDENTIFICATION OF POTENTIAL HIGH RISK MOTHERS

Several of the U.S. surveys have sought to identify women who would be at greater risk of death should they become pregnant. A recent study from the Collaborative Project on Cerebral Palsy, which involves hospitals in several States, analysed 40 maternal deaths which occurred amongst 40,360 pregnancies between 1959 and 1965. A previous investigation in New York had identified that potentially high risk mothers were those aged less than 17 or more than 40; those who were single; those who were grossly overweight ($>$ 90 kg or 14 stone) or underweight ($<$ 45 kg or 7 stone); those who had cardiovascular disease, renal disease, hypertensive disease or diabetes; grande multiparae; and women with a poor infant 'survival rate'. The last was considered to be present when the ratio between the number of children currently alive to the total number of pregnancies was 0·5 or less. It was noteworthy that of the 40 women dying, 28 fell into the high risk category and 20 had stated that they had not wished to become pregnant, so that the pregnancy was not only unwanted and unwelcome, but lethal.

THE MAIN CAUSES OF MATERNAL DEATH

In analysis of the reports of the Maternal Mortality Committees of Australia, England and Wales, and those of certain States in the U.S.A., it is of interest that the same main causes of death appear in almost the same order of frequency (Table **19/4**). In that table it can also be seen that in 20 to 60 per cent of each of the groups, avoidable factors were present which might

Table 19/4

Most common causes of maternal deaths (Australia, England and Wales, New York State)

Cause	*Percent of deaths*	*Proportion avoidable*
Abortion and ectopic gestation	15–25	70
Haemorrhage	10–25	60
Toxaemias of pregnancy	5–20	55
Trauma, difficult labour	5–15	50
Thrombo-embolism	5–15	20
Infection	5–10	50
Cardiorespiratory (including anaesthetic)	5–10	50

Table 19/5

The secular change in the main causes of maternal mortality (per 10,000 births) in England and Wales since 1931

Cause	1931	1952–54	1955–57	1958–60	1961–63	1964–66
Abortion (including septic abortion)	10·1	0·7	0·68	0·60	0·55	0·51
Sepsis (excluding septic abortion)	10·5	0·33	0·36	0·25	0·14	0·22
Toxaemia	7·5	1·19	0·89	0·60	0·42	0·26
Haemorrhage:						
Antepartum	2·1	0·52	0·32	0·30	0·18	0·17
Postpartum	2·0	0·55	0·33	0·27	0·17	0·09
Pulmonary embolism (excluding abortion deaths)	3·1	0·67	0·74	0·60	0·51	0·35
Trauma and difficult labour	6·0	0·48	0·42	0·41	0·31	0·30

have contributed to the death. For this reason these categories require further consideration. As an introduction to this discussion it should be observed that in England and Wales the mortality rate from each of these causes has been declining since 1931. In Table **19/5**, and Figure **19/5**, this is clearly shown.

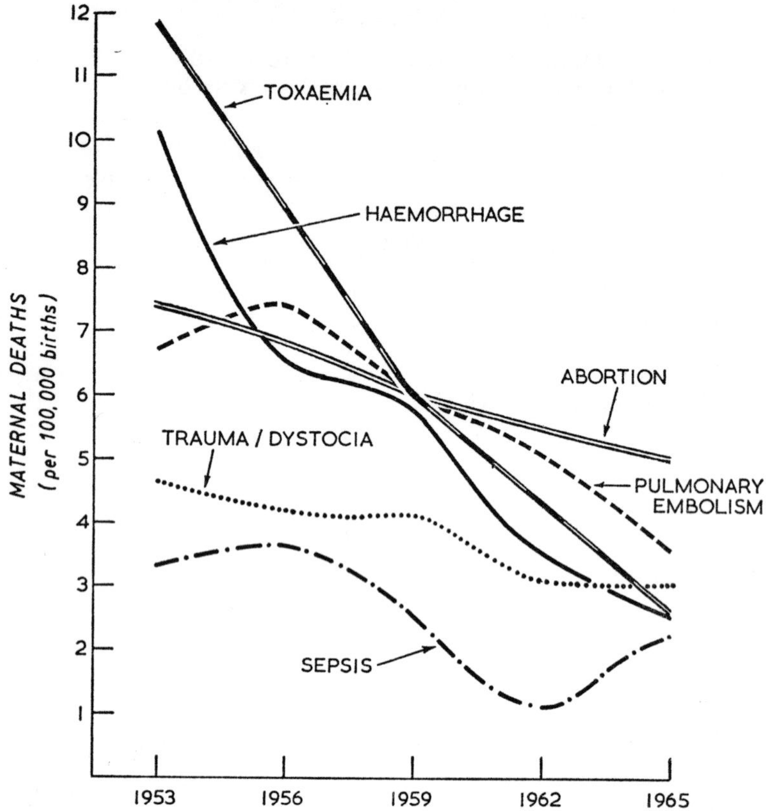

Figure **19/5** The secular change in the main causes of maternal death, U.K.

ABORTION

The grave consequences of unskilled, unhygienic, illegally induced abortion have been stressed in Chapter 13. It will be noted in Table **19/4** that between 15 and 25 per cent of all maternal deaths are due to abortion. Investigation of the reported case protocols indicates that there was evidence that the abortion was illegally induced in between 60 and 75 per cent of all deaths in this group. Since most of the deaths were due to haemorrhage, or, more usually, overwhelming infection, the cases could be placed in those categories, but this device would obscure the importance of induced abortion as a cause of maternal death. Such deaths will only be eliminated if illegal abortion is markedly reduced. Such a reduction could be effected by making contraceptive measures freely available; by letting all people, particularly women of the lower socio-economic groups, know that they may be obtained easily; and by legalising abortion to deal with unwanted pregnancies resulting from failure of contraception. These measures would do much to reduce the mortality due to abortion (see Chapters 12 and 13).

HAEMORRHAGE

This category includes two groups—antepartum haemorrhage and postpartum haemorrhage—which should be considered separately.

Antepartum haemorrhage

The incidence of both placenta praevia and abruptio placentae increases with increasing parity, but not with increasing maternal age. Since multiparous women tend to be more likely to be anaemic, this adds to the risk. There is much merit in recommending family limitation as a preventive measure, and ensuring that all pregnant women are screened for anaemia, and treated if it is found. The hazards of antepartum haemorrhage will be further reduced if all women who have a significant vaginal bleed after the 20th week of pregnancy are admitted to a well-staffed, well-equipped maternity hospital after the initial bleed, without delay and without vaginal examination. In all the reports studied, failure to take note of the bleeding episode, and the performance of a vaginal examination in inappropriate surroundings, led to further more severe haemorrhage. Within hospital the most important factor in preventing maternal death is that adequate supplies of blood are available. It is often not realised that in abruptio placentae considerably greater quantities of blood may be lost to the circulation than is indicated by the loss per vaginam, or by the clinical condition of the patient. As a clinical guide, Table **19/6**, which is reproduced from *Fundamentals of Obstetrics and Gynaecology: Volume I—Obstetrics*, is shown. The second major avoidable factor in the management of antepartum haemorrhage is surgery by insufficiently skilled doctors.

Table 19/6

Comparison of the clinical picture in the various grades of accidental haemorrhage

	Severity of bleeding		
	Mild	*Moderate*	*Severe*
Pulse	No change	Raised	Raised
Blood pressure	No change	Lowered	Lowered
Shock	None	Often	Always
Oliguria	Rare	Occasionally	Common
Hypofibrinogenaemia	Rare	Occasionally	Common
Uterus	Normal	Tender	Tender and tense
Fetus	Alive	Usually dead	Dead
Blood loss in ml	Less than 500	500–1,499	1,500–3,000

Postpartum haemorrhage

Although it is taught traditionally that postpartum haemorrhage occurs more frequently, and has a higher mortality with increasing parity, evidence from Australia and Britain suggests that hazardous postpartum haemorrhage can occur at all parities. It is especially dangerous in women who have failed to obtain pre-natal care and are anaemic. Correction of these two avoidable factors would be sufficient to reduce the mortality considerably. In domiciliary midwifery—and over 80 per cent of women delivering a baby in any year throughout the world are confined at home—postpartum haemorrhage is a particular hazard. In most instances the birth attendant is inadequately trained to cope with the problem; often the house is at some distance from more skilled help; and frequently the means of access—the roads, paths or rivers—are difficult to traverse. Deaths are therefore inevitable. However, by strategically placing hospitals and health centres, by recruiting 'bare-foot doctors', by making available stocks of blood substitutes, and eventually blood, many more deaths from postpartum haemorrhage will be avoided. Whilst such measures require organization, a simple measure would reduce postpartum haemorrhage. This is the use of oxytocics given prophylactically with the birth of the child by birth attendants who have been trained in the use of this regimen.

Conclusion

The high incidence of avoidable factors in this group of maternal deaths, both in the developed and more particularly in the developing nations of the world, emphasizes the importance of preventive obstetrics.

'TOXAEMIAS OF PREGNANCY'

The term 'toxaemias of pregnancy' is an inaccurate, but useful, term for three distinct disease entities, which have a similar constellation of signs and symptoms, namely hypertension, proteinuria and marked oedema. The three disease entities are: (1) the specific hypertensive disease of pregnancy, or pre-eclampsia; (2) essential hypertension complicating pregnancy and (3) chronic renal disease. Both essential hypertension and chronic renal disease tend to deteriorate during pregnancy in about 30 per cent of cases, although this deterioration is related to the height of the diastolic blood pressure in early pregnancy in the case of essential hypertension, and to the degree of renal impairment in the case of chronic renal disease. In the former condition proteinuria appears; in the latter the degree of hypertension increases, so that the two conditions become indistinguishable from pre-eclampsia, except by knowing the previous history. Since many patients do not obtain pre-natal care until after the 20th week of pregnancy, the diagnostic differentiation may be impossible. All three conditions, with increasing deterioration, can lead to epileptiform fits—the condition of eclampsia, which has a very high mortality.

The toxaemias of pregnancy complicate between 5 and 12 per cent of all pregnancies, being more common amongst primiparae (10 to 15 per cent) and older grande multiparae (6 to 12 per cent) than other groups. Pre-eclampsia is predominantly a disease of young nulliparae, although all parities are affected. Essential hypertension and chronic renal disease tend to be found more often amongst older multiparae. About 75 per cent of all cases of 'toxaemia of pregnancy' are due to pre-eclampsia, about 20 per cent to essential hypertension and less than 5 per cent to chronic renal disease.

The danger of toxaemia of pregnancy to the mother is the danger of delay in receiving skilled treatment. Despite a considerable research programme, the cause of pre-eclampsia remains unknown, and the disease cannot be prevented. However, if the condition is detected in its mildest and earliest stages, deterioration to potentially lethal severity can be prevented. Similarly, knowledge in the first ten weeks of pregnancy that a pregnant woman has essential hypertension, or chronic renal disease, enables the medical attendants to plot a strategic plan to deal with the problem and to ensure a live mother and child.

The crux of reducing the maternal mortality from the toxaemias of pregnancy is pre-natal care from the first quarter of pregnancy. The essential investigation is to determine the level of the woman's blood pressure and to examine her urine for the presence of protein. If a diastolic blood pressure of 90 mm mercury or more is found, which persists after half an hour's rest, or if protein is detected in a specimen of urine, the patient must be referred without delay for the opinion of a doctor who has received postgraduate obstetric training. As is well known, the frequency with which the toxaemias of pregnancy appear is related to the duration of pregnancy. This implies that the patient must be examined at increasingly shorter intervals as term approaches, and if a patient fails to attend, a visit to the house must be made, or some other arrangement instituted to ensure that she is examined. The technology for detecting the toxaemias of pregnancy is simple and inexpensive. It is the proper use of the sphygmomanometer by a trained person.

Since patients who are diagnosed as having mild toxaemia of pregnancy require admission to hospital, sufficient pre-natal beds must be available in strategically sited hospitals or health centres, and appropriate medical care must be given.

Mild pre-eclampsia, mild essential hypertension and mild renal disease have a very low mortality; however, with increasing severity the maternal mortality rises, whilst if eclampsia develops it reaches 3 to 20 per cent—a death rate fifty times that of pre-eclampsia. Deaths are due to cardiorespiratory failure in 50 per cent of cases; to a cerebrovascular accident in 25 per cent; to renal failure in 10 per cent; to hepatic failure in 5 per cent; to infection in 5 per cent, and to miscellaneous causes in the remaining 5 per cent.

With good pre-natal care the incidence of eclampsia falls from more than 1 case in 500 pregnancies to less than 1 case in 5,000 pregnancies, and severe pre-eclampsia, which is about ten times as common, shows an even greater fall.

TRAUMA AND DIFFICULT LABOUR

In the developed nations deaths from trauma and difficult labour are tending to decline as obstetric services cover a greater proportion of the population, and as fewer women neglect to obtain pre-natal care. This has reduced very considerably the importance of trauma and difficult labour as a cause of maternal death, but constant assessment of training procedures and standards of practice are necessary if the decline is to continue. In the developing nations, neglected obstructed labour, ruptured uterus, and haemorrhage from improperly conducted emergency obstetrics, are significant causes of maternal death. Most of these deaths can be prevented if good obstetrics is practised.

THROMBO-EMBOLISM

With the reduction of other factors in the developed nations, deaths from pulmonary embolism have acquired a much greater significance. For example, 15 per cent of the 512 deaths reported in Australia between 1964 and 1969 were due to pulmonary embolism. In Britain pulmonary embolism in the first four Confidential Enquiry reports (1955–66) accounted for 13 per cent of all maternal deaths. Women aged 30, or more, had a higher than average risk and the risk increased with increasing age. Pulmonary embolism is a sequel of deep venous thrombosis, usually in the iliofemoral or pelvic segments of the venous network, but clinical evidence of preceding venous thrombosis is found in fewer than 25 per cent of cases. The diagnostic accuracy could be raised by the use of sophisticated techniques using radioactive fibrinogen, but such investigatory measures are only available in special centres and are of doubtful cost-benefit. There is an increased association with increasing age, increasing parity, increasing obesity and with operative delivery, particularly delivery by Caesarean section. There is also some suggestion that in this group of patients, the use of oestrogens to inhibit or suppress lactation is a factor, although this is denied by Drill (see Chapter 12).

Currently, there seems no way in which these deaths can be reduced significantly, although family limitation would have some effect by eliminating the older women of higher parity from child-bearing. This factor may account for the decrease in the numbers of deaths from pulmonary embolism in the puerperium reported from Britain in each of the triennial reports since 1955 (Table **19/7**).

Table 19/7

Maternal deaths due to pulmonary embolism, England and Wales, since 1952

Year	*In pregnancy (excluding abortion)*	*In the puerperium*	*Total*
1952–54	4	134	138
1955–57	17	140	157
1958–60	30	102	132
1961–63	36	93	129
1964–66	23	68	91

INFECTION

From the time maternal mortality statistics were recorded until the 1940s, infection constituted the most important cause of maternal death. Childbed fever was an ever-present hazard to pregnant women. Following Colebrook's work in London on droplet cross-infection, and especially since the introduction of potent chemotherapeutic and antibiotic agents, the dangers of infection have been reduced. The level will only remain low if meticulous care is taken to avoid the introduction of infection during childbirth, and if women receive adequate nutrition, especially of protein, during pregnancy so that their resistance to infection is increased. In developed nations, fever in the puerperium now occurs in less than one per cent of all deliveries, and infection has ceased to be a major danger. However, infection remains a constant threat after illegally induced abortion, and these cases continue to pose problems.

In the developing nations, where the standard of obstetric care still leaves much to be desired, infection in pregnancy and childbirth, and especially that following illegally induced abortion, is still a major threat to the life of mothers.

ANAESTHETIC DEATHS

In developed nations anaesthetic deaths as a proportion of all maternal deaths are increasing, but are rare, the rate being less than 0·2 per 10,000 live births. In over 60 per cent of cases the death is due to inhalation of vomited gastric contents and is therefore avoidable. Many of the deaths follow an anaesthetic given by a relatively inexperienced anaesthetist, particularly if he fails to intubate the patient's larynx.

CARDIAC DISEASE

The Confidential Enquiries into Maternal Deaths reported from Britain have shown that whilst anaesthetic deaths have been rising slightly, deaths due to cardiac disease have dropped in each 3-year period. Cardiac disease has consequently ceased to be a major problem. This has occurred because the importance of constant attention to the cardiac state in pregnancy has been appreciated, as has the need for rest in pregnancy and, even more importantly, in the puerperium. However, 8 per cent of all maternal deaths in Britain were due to cardiac or respiratory conditions in the years 1955–66, and in Australia the proportion was 12 per cent of all deaths between 1964 and 1969.

ANAEMIA IN PREGNANCY

The adverse effect of maternal anaemia on the death rate, particularly in nations where anaemia is widespread, is well known. Not only does severe anaemia (defined as a haemoglobin level of 6·5 g or less) carry a mortality of its own because of anaemic heart failure, but the anaemic woman is much less able to withstand blood loss in pregnancy or the puerperium. There is also evidence that anaemic patients are less well able to resist infection. Deaths in which anaemia plays a significant, but contributory part, form a large proportion of maternal deaths in the developing nations, and anaemia is one of the factors for the five- to ten-fold maternal mortality in these nations as compared with the developed nations.

Anaemia in pregnancy is completely preventible. When facilities exist, haemoglobin estimations should be made on all patients at the first pre-natal visit, at the 30th week and again at the 36th week. In addition, all pregnant women in developing nations should be given iron salt supplements, together with small doses of folic acid. As a routine, ferrous sulphate tablets providing 200 mg thrice daily, and folic acid 0·5 to 1 mg daily, is sufficient to treat the majority of cases. Such medication should also be given routinely when facilities do not exist for estimating, accurately, the haemoglobin level of the pregnant woman.

The Reduction of Maternal Mortality

Since the death rate is so much higher in the under-developed countries, and amongst the submerged 20 per cent of the people in the affluent societies, the following suggestions for reducing maternal deaths apply, in the main, to these two groups.

1. Conveniently-sited antenatal clinics should be built and a continuing educational campaign should be initiated to induce all pregnant women to use the facilities provided. Whilst the State and the family doctor can provide antenatal clinics, it is up to the community leaders, the press and all educated people to show the poorer and less-educated sections of the population that care during the 40 weeks of pregnancy is as important as care during the 14 hours of labour.

   Unfortunately, evidence from several nations, and most recently that of Klein and Karten in New York, shows that inability to induce high risk mothers to seek pre-natal care is a most significant factor in maternal death. They report that 'Forty per cent of the current deaths, or 3·8 deaths per 10,000 live births, occurred in women who either failed to obtain medical care prior to their hospitalization or death, or received inadequate care. This group included self-inflicted complications and criminal abortions. This is unbelievable in view of the availability of pre-natal and family planning clinics in municipal and voluntary hospitals, as well as neighbourhood satellite clinics that are open evenings in order to accommodate those women who cannot attend the usual clinics. Evidently, availability of medical care is not the only factor contributing to patient welfare. Socio-economic status appears to be a more potent force, affecting patient attitude as well as outcome. Seventy-two per cent of the patients who died in the various institutions were in the "low socio-economic" category. Thus, poverty with all its complications contributed disproportionately to our current mortality rate. The decline in maternal death rate has been significantly greater among the higher income groups than among the poorer class.' In another survey of deaths occurring over a 14-year period in Chicago, Webster concluded that poverty, rather than race, is the major factor in the maternal mortality rate. Poverty is associated with poor education; with fear of institutions, particularly if the staff are distant, dictatorial and condescending; and with a lack of motivation to seek medical care. Such help is only sought when the disability or discomfort becomes sufficiently severe to constitute a crisis, which is invariably late in the disease process. The remedy lies in a multidisciplinary health education programme which starts at primary school and continues after school in community educational enterprises, involving local key persons, and for which the full impact of radio and television is utilized. Even this will fail unless the health staff of clinics are trained to deal with problems without condescension. As a first step the pejorative terms 'public' (i.e. charity) patient and 'indigent' patient must be replaced. The ability to pay for medical care should not produce a higher standard for the affluent, and a lower standard 'charity' medicine for the poor.

2. Properly designed, adequately equipped district obstetric hospitals must be provided, which will receive from the peripheral hospitals, the health centres, the maternity homes, and family doctors, all patients who would more suitably be delivered in units where specialist care is available. Where this is economically possible, these would include all women pregnant for the fourth or subsequent time; all primigravidae over the age of 30; all patients with a multiple pregnancy; all patients who have had an abnormality in a previous pregnancy or labour, or who develop an abnormality in

the present pregnancy; and all women whose labour has lasted more than 24 hours, for whatever cause. The hospitals should have sufficient antenatal beds to admit all patients requiring treatment; in the developed countries an antenatal: postnatal bed ratio of 1 to 8, and in the developing countries a ratio of 1 to 4 is required. The hospitals should also be designed to ensure that the operating theatre is adjacent to the delivery suite, and that the blood bank and pathological laboratory are accessible to both.

3. The provision of a central obstetric hospital with medical staff in sufficient numbers to permit teaching and research to be conducted as well as routine clinical care of patients. The specialist obstetricians and gynaecologists in the hospital should have undergone a course of training of not less than three years in their speciality. The director of the hospital, who might well also be the Professor of Obstetrics, would organize the obstetric services of the area, in conjunction with the health authorities. He would ensure that good person-to-person communication existed and that visits were made to the peripheral units, and to midwives working in the field to assess the quality of obstetric care (including family planning) and to encourage the obstetric health workers at all levels in their endeavours. He would ensure that ready, easy, transfer of problem patients could be effected from the periphery to the centre should this be required, and that skilled expert attention from the centre could be brought to the seriously ill patient at the periphery without delay. This presupposes the development of a mobile obstetric 'flying squad'. The idea behind the flying squad is that in cases of emergency, particularly severe pre-eclampsia, eclampsia, and postpartum haemorrhage, skilled medical attention is better given in the patient's home before transferring her to hospital. The team consists of a trained obstetrician and a nurse who has been trained to give anaesthetics (or in developed nations, additionally, an anaesthetist). The team travels by ambulance Land-Rover as far as is possible, and then by foot, and takes with them previously packed equipment, and supplies of Group O blood, which in areas where rhesus iso-immunization is a problem is also rhesus negative. Experience has shown that resuscitation by

blood transfusion and the removal of a retained placenta are the most common procedures required. In certain nations, notably Malaysia, this service has been supplemented by the use of a helicopter air ambulance to bring in help and to evacuate the ill patient. The central hospital would be 'linked' to the district hospitals, and both would be linked to a web-network of pre-natal clinics held in health centres, or in sub-centres. The smaller clinics would be conducted by midwives, under supervision; the clinic in health centres by midwives or doctors; those in hospitals by doctors and midwives. In this way the patient is 'screened' and can be transferred rapidly and safely to the next link in the chain should an abnormality arise in pregnancy or labour. At all levels of the chain, health education, nutritional information, child health care and motivation to family planning is undertaken by the appropriate person.

To be effective, the organization of the obstetric service demands that at all levels there is an awareness of the social problems of obstetrics, and the staff function as a co-ordinated team, specialist obstetricians, family doctors, and midwives working in a close relationship with frequent contacts, so that each knows his strengths and his limitations.

4. The provision of permanent senior trained nursing staff in the larger obstetric hospitals and, in the developing countries, the intensive training of sufficient midwives to work in the hospitals, the towns, the villages and the rural areas, so that one midwife is available to every 1000 of the population.
5. The provision of facilities for all family doctors, who intend to care for pregnant women, to spend six months to one year after graduation in a selected, properly equipped and adequately staffed obstetric hospital, where continued education is possible. It is also recommended that all family doctors practising obstetrics return every three to five years for two- to four-week organized courses of instruction in the subject.
6. Facilities for family planning and population control should be provided in convenient locations so that the hazard of frequent, repeated childbearing is minimized. Such family planning information, advice and supplies are best introduced in the puerperium, when patients are more motivated to accept birth control, or in conjunction with maternal and

child health services. The death of a mother in pregnancy or childbirth is the greatest tragedy which can befall a family, and the reduction of the maternal mortality is one of the most important indications of the efficiency of the medical care provided in any country. It is a challenge which can be met, and is being met increasingly in all nations.

The example of the Republic of Singapore is a model in this respect. Singapore is a tropical island of 226 sq. miles and a population in 1972 of 2 million. It is highly urbanized and has a predominantly Chinese population, most of whom are urban dwellers. In contrast, the 10 per cent Malay population is largely rural. In 1955, the maternal mortality (excluding abortion) was

Table 19/8

Maternal death rate (excluding abortion) per 10,000 births in Singapore related to the ethnic group of the mother

Year	*Ethnic Group*		
	Chinese	*Malay*	*Indian*
1957	4·9	41·0	5·9
1960	3·7	10·0	1·9
1962	2·1	10·6	2·1
1964	2·7	13·5	13·1
1965	4·3	6·3	6·8

7·7 per 10,000 births. By 1967 it had dropped to 3·1 per 10,000 births, a rate comparable with that of many developed nations. Even more significantly there had been a very much greater reduction in the maternal mortality of the Malay community (Table **19/8**). This decline can be attributed to several factors. Firstly, there has been an active campaign in the Republic to bring maternity and child care to the people. To effect this, 36 MCH clinics have been established in key areas 'with the objective of carrying health services to the very door of the house of the people'. Secondly, because of the good communications in the island, and the free maternity services, increasing numbers of women have sought hospital confinement, and are prepared to be admitted to hospital when complications arise. Thirdly, the

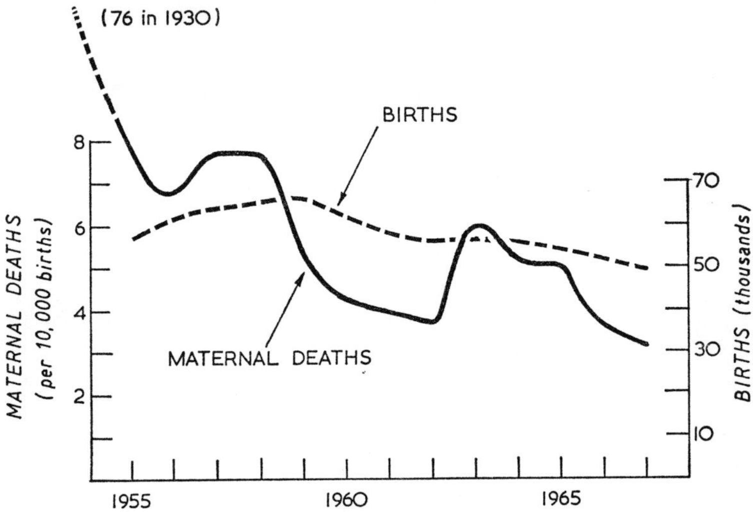

Figure **19/6** Maternal deaths in the Republic of Singapore 1955–67. Source: Lean, T. H., in *Trans. 4th Asian Cong. of Obstetrics and Gynaecology.*

main hospital has increased the quality of the services offered over the 12 years surveyed. Fourthly, a campaign for increased motivation for, and usage of, contraceptives has been successful. Singapore is a model of what can be done to reduce maternal mortality in a developing nation (Figure **19/6**).

Bibliography

Chapter 1 The Problem of Population Growth

BORRIE, W. D., 'Malthusian Reflections on the South Pacific'. *Trans. Roy. Soc., N.Z.*, **2**, 19 (1967).

CALDWELL, J. C., 'Family Planning Sub-Saharan Africa'. Mimeographed *A.N.U.* (1972).

CALDWELL, J. D., and IGUN, A., 'The spread of anti-natal knowledge and practice in Nigeria'. *Pop. Studies*, **24**, 21 (1970).

HAYTER, T., *Aid as Imperialism*. Penguin, London (1971).

MEADOWS, D., et alia, *The Limits to Growth*. Potomac, Washington (1972).

TITMUSS, R., ABEL-SMITH, B. and LYNES, T., *Social Policies and Population Growth in Mauritius*. Allen and Unwin, London (1968).

United Nations, *The World Population Situation in* 1970. U.N., New York (1971).

U.S. Commission on Population Growth, *Population and the American Future*. Signet, New York (1972).

Chapter 2 The Development of Demography

CARR-SAUNDERS, A. M., *The Population Problem*. Clarendon Press, Oxford (1922).

DE CASTRO, J., *The Geography of Hunger*. Little Brown and Co., Boston (1952).

DOUBLEDAY, T., *The True Law of Population*. 2nd Edition, G. Pierce, London (1847).

DUMONT, A., *La Morale basée sur la Demographie*.

GLASS, D. V. (ed.), *Introduction to Malthus*, Watts and Co., London (1953).

HO PING, T., *Studies on the population of China*. Cambridge Mass. (1959).

LORIMER, F., The Development of Demography in *The Study of Population*. Eds. Hauser, Philip M., and Duncan, Otis D., Univ. Chicago Press, Chicago, p. 124 (1951).

MALTHUS, T. M., *An Essay on Population*, 2 Volumes (Everyman's Library) J. M. Dent and Sons. *A Summary View of Population* 1830, reprinted in Glass, D. V., *Introduction to Malthus*. q.v.

RUSSELL, BERTRAND, *A History of Western Philosophy*. Allen and Unwin, London (1947).

SADLER, M. T., *The Law of Population*, 2 Volumes. J. Murray Ltd., London (1830).

SILBERMAN, L., 'Hung Liang Chi: a Chinese Malthus'. *Population Studies*, **13,** 257 (1960).

SMITH, K., *The Malthusian Controversy*. Routledge and Kegan Paul, London (1951).

SPENCER, H. S., *The Principles of Biology*, Vol. 2.

Chapter 3 The Collection of Demographic Data

HAWLEY, A. H., Population Composition in *The Study of Population*. Eds. Hauser, Philip M., and Duncan, Otis D., Univ. Chicago Press, Chicago, p. 361 (1959).

KAPLAN, D. L., 'Plans for the 1970 Census of Population and Housing'. *Demography*, **7,** 1 (1970).

MAUDLIN, W. P., 'Estimating Rates of Population Growth' in *Family Planning and Population Programs*. Ed. Berelson, B., p. 635. Univ. Chicago Press (1966).

United Nations, *Principles and Recommendations for National Censuses*, U.N., New York (1958).

United Nations, *Handbook of Vital Statistics Methods*, Series F, No. 7, New York (1955).

United Nations, *Handbook of Population Census Methods*, Vol. 1, 'General Aspects of a Population Census', Series F., No. 5, New York (1958).

United Nations, *Population Bulletin*, **7,** 12 (1965).

United Nations, *Principles and Recommendations for the* 1971 *Population Censuses*. U.N., New York (1967).

Chapter 4 The Methodology of Population Dynamics

BARCLAY, G. W., *Techniques of Population Analysis*. Chapman and Hall, London (1958).

SHYROCK, H. S., and SIEGAL, J. S. (editors), *The Methods and Materials of Demography*. U.S. Dep. Commerce, Washington (1971). In two volumes.

Chapter 5 The Composition of Population

HAJNAL, J., 'The Marriage Boom'. *Population Index*, **19,** 80 (1963).

HAJNAL, J., 'Differential changes in marriage patterns', *Amer. Sociol. Review*, **19,** 148 (1954).

Chapter 6 Natality

JAIN, A. K., et alia, 'Demographic aspects of lactation and post-partum amenorrhoea'. *Demography* **7,** 255 (1970).
NOTESTEIN, F. W., 'Decrease in Size of Families 1890 to 1910.' *Milbank Mem. Fund Quarterly,* **9,** 181.
POTTER, R. G., NEW, M. L., WYON, J. D., and GORDON, J. E., 'Lactation and its effects on birth intervals' in *Public Health and Population Change.* Eds. Sheps, M. L., and Ridley, J. C. Univ. Pennsylvania Press, Pittsburgh (1965).
RYDER, N. B., and WESTOFF, C. F., 'Oral Contraception and American Birth Rates' in Liu, W. P. (editor), *Family and Fertility.* Univ. Notre Dame Press (1967).
WHELPTON, P. K., and KISER, C. V., *Milbank Mem. Fund Quarterly,* **26,** 224 (1948).
United Nations, 'The Mysore Population Study'. *Population Studies,* No. **34,** New York (1961).

Chapter 7 Mortality

GLASS, D. V., 'Some indicators of differences between urban and rural mortality'. *Population Studies,* **17,** 273 (1964).
LOGAN, W. P. D., 'Social Class Variations in Mortality'. *Public Health Reports,* **59,** 1217 (1954).
Registrar General, *Occupational Mortality,* Part 1, H.M. Stationery Office, London (1954).
RICHARDS, G., 'Infant Mortality in Scotland'. *Scottish Health Service Studies,* No. **16,** Scottish Home and Health Dept. Edinburgh (1971).
RUTSTEIN, S., 'Relation of child mortality to fertility in Taiwan'. Univ. Mich. *Pop. Studies Centre Reprint,* **87** (1971).
RUZICKA, L. T., 'Infant and Childhood Mortality in the Countries of South East Asia'. *Trans. Second Asian Population Conference,* Tokyo, 1–13 November 1972.
United Nations, 'The Situation and Recent Trends of Mortality in the World'. *Population Bulletin* No. **6,** New York (1963).
World Health Organisation, 'Congenital Malformations'. *Bulletin Supp.* Vol. **34,** Geneve (1966).

Chapter 8 Migration

ARDREY, R., *The Social Contract,* Collins, London (1970).
BORRIE, W. D., 'The Great Migrations' in *The Growth and Control of Population.* Weidenfeld and Nicholson, London (1970).

HANDLIN, O. (editor), *Immigration as a factor in American history.* Prentice Hall, New Jersey (1959).

LEE, E. S., 'A Theory of Migration'. *Demography*, **3**, 47 (1966).

SHARP, P., 'Why Continue Migration'. Unpublished (1971).

THOMAS, B., *Migration and Economic Growth.* Cambridge Univ. Press (1954).

United Nations, *The World Population Situation in* 1970. U.N., New York (1971).

Chapter 9 The Growth of the World's Population

BOGUE, D. J., *Principles of Demography*. J. Wiley, New York, pp. 879–83 (1969).

COLE, G. D. K., *The Intelligent Man's Guide to the Post War World.* Gollancz, London (1947).

COMMONER, B., *The Closing Circle*. Cape, London (1972).

DAVIS, K., 'Will Population Policies Succeed'. *Science*, **158,** 730 (1967).

EHRLICH, P. R., and EHRLICH, A. H., *Population, Resources and Environment*. Freeman and Co., San Francisco (1970).

HARLAN, J. R., 'Agricultural Origins: Centres and Noncentres'. *Science*, **174,** 468 (1971).

KEYFITZ, N., 'On the momentum of population growth'. *Demography*, **8,** 71 (1971).

MCKEOWN, T., *Medicine in Modern Society*. Allen and Unwin, London (1965).

MCKEOWN, T., BROWN, R. G. and RECORD, R. G., 'An Interpretation of the Modern Rise of Population in Europe'. *Demography*, **26,** 345 (1972).

NOTESTEIN, F. W., 'Population—the long view' in Schultz, T. W. (editor), *Food for the World.* Univ. Chicago Press, Chicago (1945).

PLUMB, J. H., *England in the Eighteenth Century*. Penguin Books, London (1950).

REDDAWAY, W. B., *The Economics of a Declining Population*. Allen and Unwin, London (1939).

RYTHER, J. H., 'Photosynthesis and Fish Production in the Sea'. *Science*, **166,** 72 (1969).

THOMPSON, W. S., *Plenty of People*. Jacques-Cattel Press, Lancaster, Pa. (1944).

United Nations, 'The Past and Future Growth of World Population —A Long View'. *Population Bulletin* 1, New York (1952).

United Nations, *The Future Growth of World Population.* U.N., New York (1956).

United Nations, 'World population prospects as assessed in 1963'. *Population Studies*, No. **41,** New York (1966).

United States Bureau of the Census, 'Projections of the Population of the United States Current Population Reports'. *Population Estimates*, Series P-25, No. **359,** Washington (1967).

U.S. Dept. of Commerce/Bureau of the Census, *The two-child family and population growth: an international view.* Washington, U.S.A., Sept. (1971).

WHELPTON, P. K., 'Population'. *Amer. J. Sociol.* **38,** 825 (1933).

WOODHAM-SMITH, C., *The Great Hunger—Ireland* 1845–9. Hamish Hamilton, London (1962).

YOUNG, A., *Tour of Ireland*, quoted by Woodham-Smith.

Chapter 10 History of Contraception

AQUINAS, T., *Summa Theologica*; quoted by Hines, p. 167.

Contraceptives in NHS from 1974. See *Brit. Med. J.*, **2,** 4 (1973).

DAVIS, K. B., *Factors in the Sex Life of Twenty-two Hundred Women.* Harper, New York, (1929).

HINES, N. E., *A Medical History of Contraception*, 2nd Edition. Gamut Press, New York (1963).

JORDAN, J. A., and STUDD, J. W. W., '900 unmarried young women seeking contraceptive advice'. *Psychosomatic Medicine in Obstetrics and Gynaecology.* Ed. Morris, N. Karger, London (1972).

KOPP, M. E., *Birth Control in Practice.* MacBride, New York (1934).

LLEWELLYN-JONES, D., 'Conception Control' in *Fundamentals of Obstetrics and Gynaecology*, Vol. 2 Gynaecology. Faber, London (1970).

NEWTON, J., et alia, 'Contraceptives for unmarried people'. *Brit. Med. J.*, **2,** 642 (1972).

PINCUS, E., *Proc. 5th Int. Conf. Planned Parenthood.* Tokyo, Japan (1955).

Chapter 11 The Technology of Contraception: I

BILLINGS, J. J., *The Ovulation Method.* Advocate Press, Melbourne, Australia (1969).

BILLINGS, E. L., BILLINGS, J. J., BROWN, J. B., and BURGER, H. G., 'Symptoms and Hormonal Changes Accompanying Ovulation'. *Lancet*, **1,** 282 (1972).

BOUTSELIS, J. G., DICKEY, R. P., and JORYS, N., 'Control of ovulation time'. *Amer. J. Obst. Gynec.*, **112,** 171 (1972).

BRAYER, F. T., CHIAZZE, L., and DUFFY, B. J., 'Birth Control by the Calendar Method'. *Fert. and Steril.*, **20,** 279 (1969).

GORER, G., *Sex and Marriage in England and Wales*. Nelson, London (1972).

HANLEY, H. G., 'Vasectomy for Voluntary Male Sterilization'. *Lancet*, **2,** 207 (1968).

International Planned Parenthood Federation, *Medical Handbook (of contraceptive practice)*, 3rd Edition, London (1969).

KOTHARI, L. K., and MISHRA, P., 'Vasectomy and endocrine function of the testes'. *Lancet*, **1,** 438 (1972).

LASAGNA, L., *Public Health and Population Change*. Eds., Sheps, M. C., and Ridley, J. C., Univ. Pittsburgh Press (1965).

MARSHALL, J., 'Basal Body Temperature Method of Regulating Births'. *Lancet*, **2,** 8 (1968).

PEARL, R., 'Contraception and Fertility in 2000 Women'. *Human Biol*, **4,** 363 (1932).

PEEL, J., and POTTS, M., *Textbook of Contraceptive Practice*. Cambridge Univ. Press (1969).

PHADKE, G. M., and PHADKE, A. G., 'Reanastomosis of the vas deferens'. *J. Urol.*, **97,** 888 (1967).

POTTER, R. G., 'Additional Measures of Use-effectiveness of Contraception'. *Millbank Memorial Quarterly Fund*, **41,** 400 (1963).

PRESSER, H. B., 'Voluntary Sterilisation'. *Reports on Population/Family Planning*, **5,** 1 (1970).

STYCOS, J. M., *Exploding Humanity*. Eds. Regier, H., and Falls, J. B., Anansi, Toronto, Canada (1969).

TEITZE, C., 'Advances in Family Planning'. *Excerpta Medica*, Vol. VI, 117 (1971).

TEITZE, C., and LEWIT, S., 'Comparison of diaphragm with jelly or cream, vaginal foam and jelly/cream alone'. *J. Sex Research*, **3,** 295 (1967).

WEISSMANN, M. C., et alia. 'A Trial of the Ovulation Method in Tonga', *Lancet* **2,** 813 (1972) (and letters from Marshall, J., *Lancet* **2,** 1027 (1972); Rochat, R. W., *Lancet* **2,** 1027 (1972); Moseley, W. H., *Lancet* **2,** 1028 (1972).)

Chapter 12 The Technology of Contraception: II

Hormonal contraceptives

ANDREWS, W. E., 'Oral contraceptives—a review of physiological and pathological effects'. *Obst. Gynec. Surv.*, **26,** 477 (1971).

BICK, R. L., and THOMPSON, W. B., 'Fibrinolytic activity'. *Obst. Gynec.*, **39,** 213 (1972).

CHIDELL, M. P., 'Oral contraceptives and blood pressure'. *Practitioner*, **205,** 58 (1970).

CLAMAN, A. D., 'One dose a month oral contraceptive'. *Amer. J. Obst. Gynec.*, **107,** 461 (1970).

DIDDLE, A. W., et alia, 'Oral contraceptives headaches'. *Amer. J. Obst. Gynec.*, **105,** 507 (1969).

DRILL, V. A., 'Oral contraceptives and thromboembolic disease'. *J. Amer. Med. Ass.*, **219,** 583 (1972).

DRILL, V. A., and CALHOUN, D. W., 'Oral contraceptives and thromboembolic disease II: oestrogen content of oral contraceptives'. *J. Amer. Med. Ass.*, **219,** 593 (1972).

FECHNER, R. F., 'Oral contraceptives and breast cancer'. *Cancer*, **26,** 1204 (1970).

GOLDZIEHER, J. W., et alia, 'A placebo-controlled double-blind crossover investigation of the side effects attributed to oral contraceptives'. *Fert. and Steril.*, **22,** 609 (1971).

HEFNAWI, F., 'Attempts to select a suitable hormonal contraceptive during lactation'. *Int. J. Gyn. & Obst.*, **8,** 115 (1970).

HERZBERG, B., et alia, 'Oral contraceptives, depression and libido'. *Brit. Med. J.*, **3,** 495, (1971).

I.P.P.F., 'Comments on steroidal contraception', IPPF Central Office, London (1970).

KUCHERA, L. K., 'Post-coital contraception with diethylstilboestrol'. *J. Amer. Med. Ass.*, **218,** 562 (1971).

KUTNER, S. J., 'Oral contraceptives, depression, sexual adjustments and fear of pregnancy' (letter), *Lancet*, **1,** 1180 (1972).

Lancet, Editorial, 'Hypertension and oral contraceptives'. *Lancet* **1,** 485 (1971).

LARAGH, T. H., et alia, 'Oral contraceptives and high blood pressure.' *J. Amer. Med. Ass.*, **201,** 918 (1967).

MARTINEZ-MANAUTOU, J., 'Low level progestogens', in *Control of Human Fertility*. Ed. Diczfalusy, E., and Borrell, V., Almqvist, Stockholm (1971).

MELAMED, M. R., et alia, 'Prevalence Rates of Uterine Cervical Carcinoma in situ for Women Using the Diaphragm or Contraceptive Oral Steroids'. *Brit. Med. J.*, **3,** 195 (1969).

ORR, A. H., and ELSTEIN, M., 'Luteinizing hormone levels in plasma'. *J. Endocrin.*, **43,** 617 (1969).

PINCUS, G., *The Control of Fertility*. Academic Press, London (1965).

POLLER, L., 'Coagulation changes in oral contraceptive users'. *Advances in Fertility Control*, **4,** 31 (1969).

PUGOT-AMAT, P., et alia, 'Ovarian response to gonadotrophins. *J. Obst. Gynaec. Brit. Cwlth*, **78,** 261 (1971).

ROMAN, W., and HECKER, R., 'Oral contraceptives and liver function—a review'. *Med. J. Aust.*, **2,** 682 (1968).

Royal College of General Practitioners, 'Oral contraception and thromboembolic disease'. *J. Coll. Gen. Practit.*, **13,** 267 (1967).

RUDEL, H. W., and KINEL, F. A., 'Long acting steroid injectables', in *Control of Human Fertility*. Eds. Diczfalusy, E., and Borrell, V., Almqvist, Stockholm (1971).

SALMON, M. L., et alia, 'Migraine and oral contraceptives'. *J. Amer. Med. Ass.* **206,** 85 (1968).

SARTWELL, P. E., et alia, 'Thrombo-embolism and oral contraceptives'. *Amer. J. Epidemol.*, **90,** 365 (1969).

SHEARMAN, R. P., 'Prolonged secondary amenorrhoea after oral contraceptive therapy'. *Lancet*, **2,** 64 (1971).

SPELLACY, W. N., 'Carbohydrate metabolism and oral contraceptives'. *Amer. J. Obst. Gynec.*, **104,** 448 (1969).

STERN, E., et alia, 'Contraceptives and dysplasia'. *Science*, **169,** 407 (1970).

VESSEY, M. P., and DOLL, R., 'Relation between use of oral contraceptives and thromboembolic disease'. *Brit. Med. J.*, **2,** 651 (1969).

VESSEY, M. P., et alia, 'Randomized double-blind trial of four oral progestagen-only contraceptives'. *Lancet*, **1,** 915 (1972).

WINIKOFF, D., 'Oral contraceptives and thyroid function'. *Med. J. Aust.*, **2,** 13 (1968).

The intra-uterine contraceptive device

BERNARD, R., 'IUD performance patterns'. *Int. J. Obst. Gynec.*, **8,** 926 (1970).

CHAN, K. C., 'The Hong Kong IUD reassurance project'. *Studies in Family Planning*, **2,** 225 (1971).

GOLDSMITH, A., et alia, 'Immediate post-partum IUD insertion'. *Amer. J. Obst. Gynec.*, **112,** 957 (1972).

GUTTMACHER, A. F., Intra-uterine contraceptive devices'. *J. Reprod. Fert.*, **10,** 115 (1965).

ISHIHAMA, 'Clinical experience with intra-uterine rings'. *Yokohama Med. J.*, **10,** 89 (1959).

MAKHLOUF, A. M., and ABDEL-SALAM, A. F., 'Kymographic studies of fallopian tubes'. *Amer. J. Obst. Gynec.*, **106,** 759 (1970).

MARCUS, S. L., 'Effect of Induced Leukopenia on the Contraceptive Action of a Intra-uterine Device in the Rat'. *Obst. & Gynec.*, **38,** 55 (1971).

MORRIS, N. F., and EDELSTEIN, M., 'Gonorrhoea and the IUCD'. *Brit. Med. J.*, **4,** 828 (1968).

OPPENHEIMER, W., 'Prevention of pregnancy by the Grafenberg ring method'. *Amer. J. Obst. Gynec.*, **78,** 446 (1959).

ROSENFELD, A. G., and VARAKAMIN, S., 'The post-partum approach to family planning'. *Amer. J. Obst. Gynec.*, **113,** 1 (1972).

SAGIROGLU, N., and SAGIROGLU, E., 'Biologic mode of action of Lippes loop'. *Amer. J. Obst. Gynec.*, **106,** 506 (1970).

SIVIN, I., 'Fertility decline and contraceptive use'. *Studies in Family Planning*, **2,** 241 (1971).

TATUM, H. J., 'Intra-uterine contraception'. *Amer. J. Obst. Gynec.*, **112,** 1000 (1972).

TEITZE, C., 'Complications with IUDs'. *Brit. Med. J.*, **2,** 444 (1969).

WOLFERS, D. 'Pharmacologically active IUDs'. *Brit. Med. J.*, **1,** 112 (1972).

World Health Organization, 'Intra-uterine devices: physiological and clinical aspects'. *Tech. Rep. Series* **397,** Geneve (1968).

ZIPPER, J., et alia, 'Intra-uterine contraception'. *Amer. J. Obst. Gynec.*, **105,** 1224 (1969).

Tubal ligation

JORDON, J. A., et alia, 'Laparoscopic sterilization'. *J. Obstet. Gynaec. Brit. Cwlth.*, **78,** 460 (1971).

PRESSER, H. B., 'Voluntary sterilisation'. *Rep. Population/Family Planning* **5,** 1 (1970).

STEPTOE, P., *Laparoscopy in Gynaecology*. Livingstone, Edinburgh (1967).

Chapter 13 Abortion

BEAZLEY, J. M., and HAERI, A. D., 'Termination of pregnancy refused'. *Lancet*, **1,** 1059 (1971).

BELLER, F. K., et alia, 'Consumption coagulopathy associated with intra-amniotic infusion of hypertonic salt'. *Amer. J. Obst. Gynec.*, **112,** 534 (1972).

BENGTSSON, L. P., in *Trans. 5th World Cong. Obstet. Gynaec.*, p. 774, Butterworth, Sydney (1967).

British Medical Association, 'Memorandum for Inquiry into the Working of the Abortion Act'. *Brit. Med. J. Suppl.*, **33** (1972).

CLAMAN, D., et alia, 'Impact on hospital practise of liberalising abortions'. *Canad. Med. Assn., J.*, **105,** 35 (1971).

CORNER, G., *Ourselves Unborn!* Yale Univ. Press (1944).

DEVEREUX, G., *A Study of Abortion in Primitive Societies*. Julian Press, New York (1955).

Family Planning Association, *Abortion in Britain*. Pitman Medical Books, London (1966).

FORSSMAN, H., and THUWE, I., *Act. Psychiatric Scand.*, **42,** 71 (1966).

FUCHS, F., 'Termination of Pregnancy by Intra-amniotic Saline', in *Advances in Obstetrics and Gynaecology*. Ed. Marcus S. Williams and Wilkins, Baltimore (1967).

GEIJERSTAM, G. K., *An Annotated Bibliography of Induced Abortion*. Univ. Michigan Press, Ann Arbor (1969).

GOLDSMITH, A., et alia, 'IUD insertion immediately after incomplete abortion'. *IPPF Med. Bull.*, **6,** 1 (1972).

GUSTAVII, B., 'Mode of action of hypertonic saline in abortion'. *Acta Obstet. et Gynec. Scand.* Supp. 25 (1973).

HALL, R. E. (editor), *Abortion in a Changing World* (2 volumes), Columbia Univ. Press, New York (1970).

I.P.P.F., Seminar, Induced Abortion—a Hazard to Public Health (1971).

KARIM, S. M. M., and FILSHIE, G. M., 'The use of prostaglandin E_2 for therapeutic abortion'. *J. Obst. Gynaec. Brit. Cwlth.*, **79,** 1 (1972).

KARMAN, H., and POTTS, M., 'Syringe vacuum curettage'. *Lancet*, **1,** 1051 (1972).

KOTASEK, A., *Int. J. Gynaecology and Obstetrics*, **9,** 118 (1971).

KUMMER, J. M., in *Abortion in a Changing World*, p. 96.

LAMBERT, J., 'Survey of 3,000 Unwanted Pregnancies'. *Brit. Med. J.*, **4,** 156 (1971).

LEWIS, S. C., LAI, S., BRANCH, B., BEARD, R. W., 'Outpatient termination of pregnancy'. *Brit. Med. J.*, **4,** 606 (1971).

MEANS, C. C., 'The Ethical Aspects of Abortion—an Historian's View' in *Abortion in a Changing World*, Ed. Hall, p. 16.

MEHLAN, K., 'Abortion on a Global Scale', *Trans. 5th World Cong. Gynaec. Obst.*, Butterworth, Sydney (1967).

NOONAN, J. T., 'Abortion and the Catholic Church', *The Dublin Review*, **241,** 300 (1967).

OTTOSSON, J. O., 'Legal Abortion in Sweden', *J. Biosol. Sci.*, **3,** 173 (1971).

ROVINSKY, J. J. 'Abortion in New York City—Preliminary Experience with a Permissive Abortion Statute'. *Obst. & Gynec.*, **38,** 333 (1971).

SCHULMAN, H., KAISER, I. H. and RANDOLPH, G., 'Outpatient Saline Abortion.' *Obst. Gynaec.*, **37,** 521 (1971).

Select Committee on Science and Technology, 'Population in the United Kingdom'. H.M.S.O., London (1971).

SHAPIRO, H. L., in *Abortion in a Changing World*, Ed. Hall.

SHAPIRO, S., LEVINE, H. S., and ABRAMOWICZ, M., in 'Factors Associated with Early and Late Fetal Loss', in *Advances in Planned Parenthood*, Vol. 6, Excerpta Medica, Amsterdam (1971).

SHEARMAN, R. P., et alia, 'Abortifacient action of prostaglandins.' *Trans. IPPF Med. Cong.* Sydney (1972).

SIMMS, M., in *Nova*, p. 83 (October 1971).

SLOME, J., 'Abortion and the unmarried mother', *Psychosomatic medicine in obstetrics and gynaecology.* Ed. Morris, N., p. 540, Kager, London (1972).

STEVENSON, A. C., 'Causes of Spontaneous Abortion', in *Trans. 5th World Cong. Gynec. and Obst.*, Butterworth, Sydney (1967).

TEITZE, C. and LEWIT, S., 'Early Complications of Legal Abortion'. *Studies in Family Planning*, **3,** 97 (1972).

TOPPAZADA, M., et alia, 'Induction of abortion by intra-amniotic prostaglandin $F_{2\alpha}$'. *Contraception*, **4,** 293 (1971).

VIEL, B., *Abortion in a Changing World*, Ed. Hall, p. 226.

WIQVIST, N., personal communication.

World Health Organization, 'Spontaneous and Induced Abortion'. *Tech. Rep. Series* **461,** (1970), Geneve.

WRIGHT, C. S. W., et alia, 'Second-trimester abortion after vaginal termination of pregnancy'. *Lancet*, **1,** 1278 (1972).

Chapter 14 The Campaign for Fertility Control and Family Welfare

ARDREY, R., *The Social Contract.* Collins, London (1970).

BERELSON, B., 'K.A.P. Studies in Fertility' in *Family Planning and Population Programs*, Ed. Berelson, University of Chicago Press (1966).

BOGUE, D. J., and HERSKANEN, F. S., 'How to Improve Written Communication for Birth Control'. National Committee on Maternal Health Inc., New York (1963).

LAPHAM, R. J., and MAUDLIN, W. P., 'National Family Planning Programs Review and Evaluation'. *Stud. in Family Planning*, **3,** 30 (1972).

NORTMAN, D., 'Family Planning Programs in Relation to Demographic Targets'. *Pop. Studies*, **26,** 1 (1972).

Royal College of Obstetricians and Gynaecologists, *Unplanned Pregnancy.* London (1972).

STYCOS, J. M., *Exploding Humanity*, Eds. Regier, H., and Falls, J. B., Aransi, Toronto, Canada (1969).

U.S. Population Commission, *Population Trends in the U.S.A.* Washington (1972).

WAYLAND, SLOAN, R., 'Family Planning and the School Curriculum' in *Family Planning and Population Programs.* Ed. Berelson, B., Univ. Chicago Press, p. 353, (1966).

World Health Organization, 'Health Aspects of Family Planning'. *WHO Tech. Rep.* **442,** Geneve (1970).

Chapter 15 Social Factors in Reproductive Efficiency—I

Teenage pregnancy

CLARK, J. F. J., WONG, J. A., and NILES, J. H., *Ann. NY Acad. Sciences*, **142,** 813 (1967).

GABRIELSON, I. W., KLERMAN, L. V., CURRIE, J. B., TYLER, N. C., and JEKEL, J. F., *Amer. J. Publ. Health and Nation's Health*, **60,** 2289 (1970).

HARRIS, J., *Bull. Johns Hopkins Hosp.*, **33,** 12 (1922).

ISRAEL, S. L., and WOUTERSZ, T. B., 'Teenage Obstetrics'. *Amer. J. Obst. Gynec.* **85,** 659 (1963).

MARCHETTI, A. A., and MENAKER, J. S., 'Pregnancy and the Adolescent'. *Amer. J. Obst. Gynec.*, **59,** 1013 (1950).

National Council for the Unmarried Mother, 'Pregnancy in Adolescence'. Conference Report. NCUMC, London (1967).

RUSSELL, J. K., 'Pregnancy in the Young Teenager'. *Practitioner*, **204,** 401 (1970).

SEMMENS, J. P., and LAMERS, W. M., *Teenage Pregnancy*. Thomas, Springfield, Illinois (1968).

TANNER, J. M. (editor), *Human Growth*. Pergamon Press (1960).

UTIAN, W. H., *Brit. Med. J.*, **2,** 734, 1967. (Contains references to other papers.)

WALLACE, H. M., 'Teenaged Pregnancy'. *Amer. J. Obst. Gynec.*, **92,** 1125 (1965).

WEIR, S., *Study of Unmarried Mothers in Scotland.* Scottish Home and Health Dept., Edinburgh (1971).

Pregnancy in the Unmarried

BOWLBY, J., *Maternal Care and Mental Health*, W.H.O. Geneva (1952.)

CHOLMONDELEY, C., et alia, 'Psychosocial characteristics of illegitimate pregnancy in England'. *Psychosomatic Medicine in Obstetrics and Gynaecology, 3rd Cong.* Ed. Morris, N. Karger, Basel (1972).

COBLINER, W. G., 'Teenage out of wedlock pregnancy'. *Bull. NY Acad. Med.*, **46,** 438 (1970).

CRELLIN, E., PRINGLE, M. L. K., and WEST, *Born Illegitimate—Social and Educational Implications*. Nat. Found. for Educational Research, London (1971).

PAAVOLA, A., 'The illegitimacy rate and other factors influencing the pregnancy and delivery of unmarried mothers'. *Acta Obst. Gynec. Scand.* **47,** Supp. 3 (1968).

WEARING, M. P., KINCH, R. A. H., LOVE, E. J., and MCMAHON, D., *Obst. Gynec.*, **29,** 792 (1967).

WEIR, S., *Study of Unmarried Mothers in Scotland.* Scottish Home and Health Dept. Edinburgh (1971).

WIMPERIS, V., *The Unmarried Mother and her Child.* Allen and Unwin, London (1960).

World Health Organization, Conference on 'Mental Health of Adolescents and Young Persons', Stockholm (1969).

YOUNG, L., *Out of Wedlock.* McGraw-Hill, New York (1954).

Older Primigravida

BAIRD, D., HYTTEN, F. E., and THOMSON, A. M., *J. Obst. Gynaec. Brit. Emp.*, **65,** 865 (1958).

BUTLER, N. R., and ALBERMAN, E. D., *Perinatal Problems.* E. and S. Livingstone, Edinburgh (1969).

BUTLER, N. R., and BONHAM, D., *Perinatal Mortality.* E. and S. Livingstone, Edinburgh (1963).

NELSON, T. R., *J. Obst. Gynaec. Brit. Emp.*, **62,** 48 (1954).

STEWART, D. B., and BERNARD, R. M., *J. Obst. Gynaec. Brit. Emp.*, **61,** 319 (1954).

Chapter 16 Social Factors in Reproductive Efficiency—II

Parity and Obstetric Efficiency

BUTLER, N. R., and BONHAM, D. G., *Perinatal Mortality*, E. and S. Livingstone, Edinburgh (1963).

LAW, R. G., *Standards of Obstetric Care.* E. and S. Livingstone, Edinburgh (1967).

Royal Commission on Population, *Report of the Family Census*, 1946, H.M.S.O., London (1954).

U.S. Bureau of the Census, *Women by Number of Children Ever Born.* Report PC (2) 3A (1960).

Socio-economic Status

ILLSLEY, R., 'Social Class Selection'. *Brit. Med. J.*, **2,** 1520 (1955).

TANNER, J. M., *Growth at Adolescence.* 2nd Ed. Blackwell, Oxford (1962).

TANNER, J. M., 'The Secular Trend to Earlier Maturation'. *J. Soc. Geneesk*, **44,** 524 (1966).

TANNER, J. M., 'The Study of Growth'. *Eugen. Rev.*, **58,** 122 (1964).

VENTATACHALAM, P. S., and GOPALAN, C., *Indian J. Medical Research*, **48,** 507 (1960).

Chapter 17 Low Birth Weight

BAIRD, D., 'Epidemiology of Prematurity'. *J. Paediat.*, **65,** 909 (1964).

Bishop, E. H., 'Prematurity: Etiology and Management'. *Post Grad. Med.*, **35,** 185 (1964).

Butler, N. R. et alia, 'Cigarette Smoking in Pregnancy'. *Brit. Med. J.*, **2,** 127 (1972).

Cavanagh, D., and Talisman, M. R., *Prematurity and the Obstetrician*. Appleton-Century Crofts, New York (1969).

Day, R. L., 'Factors Influencing Offspring'. *Amer. J. Dist. Child.*, **113,** 179 (1967).

Douglas, J. W. B., 'Factors Associated with Prematurity'. *J. Obst. Gynaec. Brit. Cwlth.*, **57,** 143 (1950).

Drillien, C. M., 'Social and Economic Factors in Prematurity'. *J. Obst. Gynaec. Brit. Emp.*, **64,** 161 (1967).

Gruenwald, P., 'Growth and Maturation of the Fetus', in *Perinatal Problems*. Eds. Butler, N. R., and Alberman, E. D. E. and S. Livingstone, Edinburgh (1969).

Jansen, A. A., 'Birthweight and Neonatal Mortality in New Guinea.' *Trop. and Geog. Med.* **14,** 341 (1962).

Kloosterman, G. J., 'Intra-uterine Growth.' *Int. J. Gynec. Obst.*, **8,** 895 (1970).

Lichty, J. A., Ting, J. Y., Bruns, P. D. and Dyar, E., 'Babies born at high altitude'. *Amer. J. Dis. Child.*, **93,** 666 (1957).

Mitchell, R. G. (editor), *Child Life and Health*, Fifth Edition. J. & A. Churchill, London (1970).

Thomson, A. M., Billewicz and Hytten, F. E., 'Assessment of Fetal Growth'. *J. Obst. Gynec. Brit. Cwlth.*, **75,** 903 (1968).

Verhoestrate, L. J. and Puffer, R. R., 'The Challenge of Fetal Loss—A World View'. *J.A.M.A.*, **167,** 950 (1958).

World Health Organization, 'Expert Group on Prematurity', *WHO Tech. Rep. Ser.* **27,** Geneva (1950).

World Health Organization, 'Public Health Aspects of Low Birth Weight'. *WHO Tech. Rep. Ser.* **217,** Geneva (1961).

Yerushalmy, J., 'Longitudinal Studies in Pregnancy'. *Amer. J. Obst. Gynec.*, **71,** 80 (1956).

Yerushalmy, J., 'Birth Weight and Intra-uterine Growth'. *Clin. Obst. Gynec.*, **13,** 107 (1970).

Yerushalmy, J., 'Birth Weight, Gestational Age and Intra-uterine Growth'. *Clin. Obst. Gynec.*, **13,** 107 (1970).

Chapter 18 Perinatal Mortality

Baird, D., 'Perinatal Mortality'. *Lancet*, **1,** 511 (1969).

Butler, N. R., and Alberman, E. D., *Perinatal Problems*. E. and S. Livingstone, Edinburgh (1969).

BUTLER, N. R. and BONHAM, D. G., *Perinatal Mortality*. Livingstone, Edinburgh (1963).

CHASE, H. C., 'International Comparison of Perinatal and Infant Mortality'. *US Dept. of Health, Education and Welfare, Vital and Health Stat.*, Ser. 3, No. 6 (1967).

DALY, C., HEADY, J. A., and MORRIS, J. N., *Lancet*, **1,** 445 (1955).

GILES, P. F. H., Reactions of Women to Perinatal Death'. *Aust. N.Z. J. Obst. Gynaec.*, **10,** 207 (1970).

HUNT, E. P., and HUYUK, E. E., *Health Education and Welfare Indicators*, Washington (1966).

KOHL, S. G., *Community Obstetrical Study*, Brooklyn New York Progress Report (1960).

Leading Article, *British Medical Journal*, **4,** 2 (1967).

LLEWELLYN-JONES, D., 'Severe Anaemia in Pregnancy'. *Aust. N.Z. J. Obst. Gynaec.*, **5,** 191 (1965).

LLEWELLYN-JONES, D., 'Accidental Haemorrhage'. *Aust. N.Z. J. Obst. Gynaec.*, **3,** 197 (1963).

NISWANDER, K. R., and GORDON, M., *The women and their pregnancy*. Saunders, Philadelphia (1972).

THOMPSON, J. F., Perinatal deaths in Indiana'. *Am. J. Obst. Gynec.*, **101,** 43 (1968).

USHER, R., MCLEAN, F., and MAUGHAN, G., 'Respiratory distress syndrome in infants delivered by caesarean section'. *Am. J. Obst. Gynec*', **88,** 806 (1964).

World Health Organization, 'The Prevention of Perinatal Mortality and Morbidity'. *WHO Tech. Rep. Series* **457,** Geneva (1970).

Chapter 19 Maternal Mortality

American Medical Association, *A Guide to Maternal Death Studies* (1957).

Australia: National Health and Medical Research Council: *Maternal Deaths in the Commonwealth of Australia.* First Report published in 1969, second Report published in 1972. Government Printing Office, Canberra.

BRONTE, J. T. P., and VERBRUGGE, H. P., 'Maternal Mortality' (in the Netherlands), *Acta. Obst. et Gynec. Scand.*, **46,** 445 (1967).

KLEIN, M. D., and KARTEN, I., 'Maternal deaths: A Health and Socio-economic Challenge'. *Amer. J. Obst. Gynec.*, **110,** 299 (1971).

LEAN, T. H., 'Maternal Deaths in Singapore'. *Trans. 4th Asian Congress of Obstetrics and Gynaecology* (1969).

MARMOL, J. G., VOLLMAN, R. E., GORDON, M., PETTERSON, S. P., and REID, W.A., 'Maternal Death and High Risk Pregnancy', *Obstet. Gynec.*, **30**, 816 (1967).

Marmol, J., Scriggins, A. C., and Vollman, R. F., 'History of Maternal Mortality Study Committees in the United States'. *Obst. and Gynec.*, **34,** 123 (1969).

Ministry of Health, England and Wales. *Confidential Reports into Maternal Deaths:* No. 97 (1957); No. 103 (1960); No. 108 (1963); No. 115 (1966); No. 119 (1969). H.M.S.O., London.

Ohio State Medical Association. 'Maternal Mortality Report for Ohio, 1955–1964.' *Ohio Med. J.*, **63,** 323 (1967).

New York Department of Health. *Criteria for High Risk Patients* (Jan., 1965.)

Stallworthy, J. S., and Bourne, G., *Recent Advances in Obstetrics and Gynaecology*, 11th Edition. Churchill, London (1966).

Webster, A., 'Maternal Deaths in Cook County Hospital'. *Amer. J. Obst. Gynec.*, **101,** 244 (1968).

Index